Directed Drug Delivery

Experimental Biology and Medicine

Directed Drug Delivery

A Multidisciplinary Problem

Edited by

Ronald T. Borchardt, Arnold J. Repta, and Valentino J. Stella

University of Kansas, Lawrence, Kansas

Humana Press · Clifton, New Jersey

Library of Congress Cataloging in Publication Data

Main entry under title:
Directed drug delivery.
(Experimental Biology and Medicine)

   Based on the proceedings of a symposium held in
Lawrence, Kan., on Oct. 17-19, 1984, and sponsored by
the Dept. of Pharmaceutical Chemistry, School of
Pharmacy, University of Kansas.
   Includes index.
   1. Drugs—Dosage forms—Congresses. 2. Pharmaco-
kinetics—Congresses. 3. Chemistry, Pharmaceutical—
Congresses. I. Borchardt, Ronald T. II. Repta, Arnold.
III. Stella, Valentino, 1946- . IV. University of
Kansas. Dept. of Pharmaceutical Chemistry. [DNLM:
1. Chemistry, Pharmaceutical—congresses. 2. Delayed-
Action Pharmaceuticals—congresses. 3. Drugs—adminis-
tration & dosage—congresses. QV 785 D598 1984]
RS200.D57 1985   615'.7   85-2291
ISBN 0-89603-089-X

©1985 The Humana Press Inc.
Crescent Manor
PO Box 2148
Clifton, NJ 07015

Printed in the United States of America

PREFACE

This book is based on the proceedings of the symposium entitled "Directed Drug Delivery: A Multidisciplinary Problem," which was held in Lawrence, Kansas on October 17–19, 1984. The purpose of the symposium and this book is to focus on the multidisciplinary nature of drug delivery. Development of a successful drug delivery system requires contributions from various scientific disciplines, including pharmaceutical chemistry, analytical chemistry, medicinal chemistry, biochemistry, pharmacology, toxicology, and clinical medicine. The contents of this volume illustrate the importance of the various disciplines in identifying the problems and approaches for the development of a rational and effective drug delivery system. Thus the information provided herein will be of value not only to the pharmaceutical chemists who are responsible for dosage form design, but also to the pharmacokineticists, pharmacologists, and clinicians involved in biological evaluation of drug delivery systems. The volume should also be of interest to the analytical chemists who must provide technology to quantitatively evaluate drug delivery. Additionally, this work will also interest the biochemists and medicinal chemists involved in drug discovery, since the drug delivery system often plays a major role in determining the success or failure of a new drug entity.

Each speaker at the symposium was requested to contribute a chapter reviewing the contribution of their major discipline to the development of a successful drug delivery system. Topics covered in this volume include pharmacokinetics and pharmacodynamic factors (Section A) and physiological and biochemical factors (Section B) that influence directed drug delivery, various approaches to controlled and targeted drug delivery, including physical (SectionC) and biological (Section D) systems, as well as appropriate and important analytical chemistry topics (Section E).

The individual chapters in this volume represent comprehensive, up-to-date reviews of the subject material. However, to gain maximum appreciation for the multidisciplinary nature of drug delivery, the editors suggest a thorough reading of the entire volume.

Ronald Borchardt
Arnold Repta
Valentino Stella

v

A Tribute to

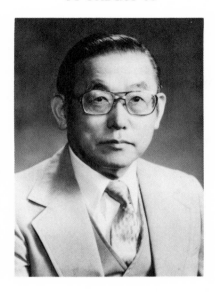

Takeru Higuchi

Teacher, Researcher, Innovator, Entrepreneur, Colleague, and Friend

It is only appropriate that this symposium and these proceedings be dedicated to Professor Higuchi, who for nearly forty years has contributed so immensely to those aspects of the pharmaceutical sciences addressed in these proceedings. His leadership and contributions in pharmaceutical analysis, prodrug research, and controlled release have, by all measures, had a major impact on the emergence of drug delivery as an important aspect in improving drug utilization and therapy.

Additionally, his enthusiasm and guidance as mentor to over 250 graduate students and postdoctoral fellows has had tremendous impact around the world, since those former students have continued to make research contributions in the many and diverse areas they first encountered while studying with Professor T. Higuchi, a truly unique individual.

ACKNOWLEDGMENTS

The symposium entitled "Directed Drug Delivery: A Multi-disciplinary Problem," which served as a basis for this book, was organized and sponsored by the Department of Pharmaceutical Chemistry, School of Pharmacy, The University of Kansas. We acknowledge with pleasure the assistance of Nancy Helm in organization of the symposium.

The symposium was made possible by the financial support provided by the following companies:

Abbott Laboratories
Alcon Laboratories, Inc.
ALZA Corporation
American Critical Care, Division of American Hospital Supply
    Corporation
Berlex Laboratories, Inc., Subsidiary of Schering AG
Boehringer-Ingelheim Ltd.
Bristol-Myers Company
Burroughs Wellcome Company
Ciba-Geigy Corporation
Dorsey Laboratories, Division of Sandoz, Inc.
E. I. DuPont de Nemours & Company
Hoffmann-LaRoche, Inc.
Key Pharmaceuticals, Inc.
Lederle Laboratories, American Cyanamid Company
Luitpold-Werk GmbH & Co. KG
Marion Laboratories, Inc.
McNeil Pharmaceutical
Menley & James Laboratories, Ltd.
Merck & Co.
Monsanto Company
Nyegaard & Co. A/S
Ortho Pharmaceutical Corporation
Pennwalt Corporation
Pfizer Central Research, Pfizer, Inc.
Revlon Health Care
Riker Laboratories, Inc.
A. H. Robins Company
R. P. Scherer Corporation
Schering Corporation

G. D. Searle & Co.
Smith Kline & French Laboratories
E. R. Squibb & Sons, Inc.
Syntex Research, Division of Syntex (USA)
Travenol Laboratories, Inc.
The Upjohn Company
Vicks Research Center, Richardson-Vicks, Inc.
Winthrop-Breon Labs, Division of Sterling Drug, Inc.
Wyeth Laboratories, Inc.

Contents

A. PHARMACODYNAMIC AND PHARMACOKINETIC FACTORS INFLUENCING DIRECTED DRUG DELIVERY

B. PHYSIOLOGICAL AND BIOCHEMICAL FACTORS INFLUENCING DIRECTED DRUG DELIVERY

E. ANALYTICAL ASPECTS OF DRUG DELIVERY

CONTRIBUTORS

*RALPH N. ADAMS • Department of Chemistry, University of Kansas, Lawrence, Kansas

B. D. ANDERSON • College of Pharmacy, University of Utah, Salt Lake City, Utah

*LESLIE Z. BENET • Department of Pharmacy, University of California-San Francisco, San Francisco, California

*S. S. DAVIS • The University of Nottingham, University Park, Nottingham, England

BOBBE L. FERRAIOLO • Department of Pharmacy, University of California-San Francisco, San Francisco, California

G. L. FLYNN • College of Pharmacy, University of Utah, Salt Lake City, Utah

J. L. FOX • College of Pharmacy, University of Utah, Salt Lake City, Utah

*COLIN R. GARDNER • INTERx Research Corporation, Lawrence, Kansas

MITSURU HASHIDA • Faculty of Pharmaceutical Sciences, Kyoto University, Kyoto, Japan

*JORGE HELLER • Polymer Sciences Department, SRI International, Menlo Park, California

*WILLIAM HIGUCHI • College of Pharmacy, University of Utah, Salt Lake City, Utah

K. J. HIMMELSTEIN • INTERx Research Corporation, Lawrence, Kansas

*RUDY JULIANO • Department of Pharmacology, The University of Texas Medical School, Houston, Texas

K. KNUTSON • College of Pharmacy, University of Utah, Salt Lake City, Utah

THOMAS MALEFYT • Smith Kline & French Laboratories, Philadelphia, Pennsylvania

*DAVID NEVILLE, JR. • Laboratory of Molecular Biology, National Institutes of Health, Bethesda, Maryland

*WILLIAM PARDRIDGE • Department of Medicine, UCLA School of Medicine, University of California-Los Angeles, Los Angeles, California

*IAN H. PITMAN • *Victorian College of Pharmacy, Ltd., Parkville, Victoria, Australia*

*JOSEPH R. ROBINSON • *School of Pharmacy, University of Wisconsin-Madison, Madison, Wisconsin*

*WOLFGANG SADÉE • *School of Pharmacy, The University of California-San Francisco, San Francisco, California*

*GÖRAN SCHILL • *Department of Analytical Pharmaceutical Chemistry, Uppsala University, Uppsala, Sweden*

*HITOSHI SEZAKI • *Faculty of Pharmaceutical Sciences, Kyoto University, Kyoto, Japan*

*T. Y. SHEN • *Merck Sharp & Dohme Research Laboratories, Rahway, New Jersey*

*V. J. STELLA • *Department of Pharmaceutical Chemistry, University of Kansas, Lawrence, Kansas*

*LARRY A. STERNSON • *Smith Kline & French Laboratories, Philadelphia, Pennsylvania*

*FELIX THEEUWES • *ALZA Research Corporation, Palo Alto, California*

*JOHN URQUHART • *ALZA Research Corporation, Palo Alto, California*

*Presenter and principal author.

A. PHARMACODYNAMIC AND PHARMACOKINETIC FACTORS INFLUENCING DIRECTED DRUG DELIVERY

PHARMACEUTICS AND THE EVOLVING TECHNOLOGY OF DRUG DELIVERY-A PERSPECTIVE

Joseph R. Robinson

University of Wisconsin

School of Pharmacy Madison, Wisconsin

To be the lead speaker at a symposium to honor Professor Takeru Higuchi is of special significance to me. Aside from the enormous impact Dr. Higuchi has had on the pharmaceutical sciences, by virtue of his own research activities, and that of students he has trained, he is also my academic godfather and has had a significant impact on my career. It is also fitting that the topic of drug delivery has been selected to honor Professor Higuchi since his entire career reflects an interest in and impact on the broad issue of drug delivery.

My task is to explore the discipline of pharmaceutics and the evolving technology of drug delivery. The historical perspective and forecasting of both pharmaceutics and drug delivery to be described subsequently is based on my own perspective and is therefore personal opinion. Others may have a different historic view and may see the growth of drug delivery in a different light. These differences will encourage further discussion to help shape the course of academic and industrial programs.

As a starting point it is helpful to begin with some definitions of both pharmaceutics and drug delivery. From these definitions we will proceed to an examination of Pharmaceutics, its past and projected future and, finally, make comment on the evolving nature of drug delivery and the role of pharmaceutics in drug delivery.

3

DEFINITIONS

The term <u>drug</u> <u>delivery</u> is fashionable at present and
is intended to emphasize the complex nature of delivering
drug in an optimal fashion. Indeed, we now employ the term
drug-delivery system rather than dosage form, presumably to
indicate the complex nature of the drug-carrier system,
especially as they evolve in the future. The important mes-
sage of this change of emphasis in terminology is that <u>drug</u>
<u>delivery carries with it the implication that drug therapy</u>
<u>will be optimized.</u>

Some individuals have made drug delivery synonymous
with pharmaceutics. This is acceptable provided a clear
understanding of this implication is made. It is difficult
to provide a precise definition of pharmaceutics given
that the discipline(s) appear to be in a fluid state. Indeed it is undesirable to try to be specific with a definition at this time. Listed below are two general definitions
of pharmaceutics:

> <u>Pharmaceutics</u> - A discipline that is interested in the
> formulation, manufacture, quality control and biologi-
> cal application of drug delivery systems.

> <u>Pharmaceutics</u> - A heterogenous discipline tied together
> by an interest in drugs and drug delivery systems.

The first definition emphasizes several discrete activities
that are traditional to pharmaceutics. I find this definition restrictive and therefore prefer the second which permits considerable room for interpretation and growth. The
definition of a discipline is on the basis of activities of
scientists in that discipline. In the coming years the
activities of pharmaceutical scientists will be broadened
considerably, thus blurring the traditional definition of a
pharmaceutical scientist. One already sees an increasingly
heterogenous faculty in pharmaceutics departments of Schools
of Pharmacy and the composition of industrial Pharmacy R & D
groups is much more interdisciplinary than ever before. As
these "new" Pharmaceutical scientists contribute to the
literature the definition of Pharmaceutics will crystallize.
In my view, pharmaceutics is in a transition state and a
broad definition is therefore required.

HISTORICAL PERSPECTIVE ON PHARMACEUTICS

In order to appreciate the present state of pharmaceutics and its projected role(s) in the area of drug delivery, it is helpful to review some of the major developments in pharmaceutics over the past few decades. As with most disciplines, developments are generally of an evolutionary nature but for discussion purposes they will be described as discrete activities.

The modern era of pharmacy can be considered to date from World War II. It is approximately 40-50 years ago that major pharmaceutical firms developed with a primary mission of consistency in the preparation of drug-delivery systems. In the late 1940's and early 1950's the application of physical-chemical principles to pharmaceutical systems was made. Professor Higuchi made major contributions in this regard. These quantitative applications were intended to insure that the dosage form containing drug was stable, with an accurate dose of drug. Note that the fate of drug in the body was not a serious consideration or research discipline. As an outgrowth of so-called "physical pharmacy", pharmacokinetics evolved and it was an attempt to provide a mass-balance accounting of drug in the body in terms of rates and equilibria. Interestingly, Teorell had provided the framework for pharmacokinetics in two classic papers in the late 1920's but it was not until some 20 years later in North America that concern over the fate of drugs in-vivo became a serious issue. In Europe, and Germany in particular, the concern over drug disposition in the body seemed to appear somewhat earlier, as judged by the 1949 publication of "Der Blutspiegel" by Dost and the pioneering work of Kruger-Thiemer. In these early days of pharmacokinetics, and lingering today in many respects, the body was considered as a black box, or series of compartments and much of the work was based on the rise and fall of drug levels in the blood. A cellular or subcellular approach was limited by analytical capabilities.

Thus from the mid to late 1950's pharmacokinetics became an important part of pharmaceutics. A natural consequence of pharmacokinetics was to consider the impact of the dosage form on the biological disposition of the drug and thus in the 1960's the area of Biopharmaceutics was ushered in. In my view the level of understanding of routes of ad-

ministration was so primitive in most cases that the area
of biopharmaceutics was treated with long extrapolations,
usually from pharmacokinetic data.

Coincidental with these developments attempts were
made to improve the efficiency of manufacturing processes
and to understand the underlying mechanisms of dosage form
fabrication, i.e., tablet compression and suspension
flocculation. In addition, synthetic, or at least improved
dosage form constituents, were introduced to replace many
of the natural materials used in the preparation of dosage
forms.

It is of interest that pharmaceutical analysis was not
a part of pharmaceutics and, indeed, in Schools of Pharmacy,
analysts were placed in medicinal chemistry groups. The
more modern approach is to recognize the importance of analysis in the area of drug delivery research and to have
within Pharmaceutics groups, analysts with an interest in
drug delivery questions.

Controlled Drug Delivery

An important subset of the historical development of
Pharmaceutics is the area of sustained/controlled drug release systems. In the early 1950's, Smith Kline & French,
introduced the Spansule dosage form. Whether the reasons
for this work were marketing or for therapeutic advancement
is not clear to me, but what is clear is that the potential
therapeutic benefits of correct spatial and temporal drug
delivery was not picked up as a general theme by the biomedical community. Admittedly, from the early 1950's through
the mid 1960's a sizeable number of relatively primitive
sustained release dosage forms appeared on the market. Interestingly, these systems did not capture a significant portion of the market in most cases, nor did they capture the
imagination of the medical community. The modern era of
controlled drug delivery probably began in the late 1960's
with formation of the ALZA Corporation

Great credit is due, in my view, to Alex Zaffaroni, the
founder of ALZA, and his advisors, one of which was Professor T. Higuchi. Interestingly, the thrust of the ALZA program was to make drug-delivery systems where the release
rate of drug could be controlled with precision and the
systems would, hopefully, be independent of the environment.

The marriage of these technological advances to biology has evolved subsequently but is still primitive.

There appeared to be two major disease classes that had an important bearing on the evolving nature of controlled drug delivery. The finding that long term vascular effects could be minimized in diabetes, if fluctuations in insulin/glucose levels could be minimized, spoke to the need of better control over the rate of drug delivery (temporal control). On the other hand in cancer therapy there was and is a need to target drugs to a specific subset of abnormal cells without involvement of normal cells. This then spoke to the need of spatial placement of the drug in the body. Both spatial placement and temporal release are actually inseparable in a drug-delivery system.

I would be remiss if I did not mention the economic and regulatory impact on the present drug-delivery research emphasis. Quite clearly the present 10-12 years from drug discovery to market with an estimated price tag of $75-100 million for new drug entities suggests that a modest investment in drug-delivery research may prove profitable. The economic impact of transdermal nitroglycerin, sustained release theophylline, phenylpropanolamine and potassium chloride products, drug entities that are rather old, captured the imagination of management in the various pharmaceutical firms.

It is of interest to note the divergent approaches to controlled drug delivery over the past two decades. In the case of targetted drug delivery, the principal scientists involved in this research are mostly all biologists, e.g., tumor biologists or polymer/engineering scientists. For controlled drug delivery, where precision of release rate is an issue, the key players appear to be pharmaceutical/polymer/engineering scientists. A happy marriage of these disciplines has yet to be made.

PRESENT AND PROJECTED AREAS OF RESEARCH IN PHARMACEUTICS

Aside from the changing nature of Pharmaceutics research there are a number of research areas that have a bearing on drug delivery development and which will receive increasing attention in the future. The list is not exhaustive but representative of some areas of inquiry. Actually,

the list reflects my personal bias of the need for better
integration of several disciplines with a focus on drug
delivery. Indeed, the last entry in the Table summarizes
this view. Others may draw up a different menu than I have
created but I believe there would be general agreement on
the framework of producing a better scientist-technologist
and specifically a physico-chemical-biological scientist-
technologist.

The above discussion is of a general nature and simply
attempts to identify broad areas of inquiry. Essential to
each of these is the level of support both in industry and
academia and the level of support will undoubtedly be tied
to perceived need. Unfortunately, some of these areas have
suffered from benign neglect in the past and this will probably continue in the future. Thus, for example, the area
of material science for pharmaceutical application has not
been well funded in the past. However, it is likely that
materials properties will be of increasing importance in
the future. Thus, for example, it has been stated by some
that penetration enhancement of skin is a problem only at
present and that in the near future the barrier function of
skin will have been eliminated with penetrant enhancers. At
this point the interaction of dosage form constituents with
the skin will be an important issue and the physico-chemical
properties of the materials in question will dominate.

THE ROLE OF PHARMACEUTICS IN DRUG DELIVERY

RESEARCH AND DEVELOPMENT

There are some who believe that Drug Delivery is an
alternate definition of pharmaceutics. While it is true
that pharmaceutics has always been closely associated with
drug delivery, and probably will continue in the future,
there are now other players in the game and it is likely
that the nature of Pharmaceutics research will change to
accommodate these new players. Minimally, the role of Pharmaceutics research in an industrial setting can be as an
effective interface between discovery groups and development
groups. However, this interface is not the usual development activity and in Scheme 1 I have purposefully moved the
pharmaceutics group midway between discovery and development
to emphasize the dual roles to be played by the scientist-
technologist in the Pharmacy R & D group.

TABLE 1. SOME PRESENT AND PROJECTED AREAS

OF PHARMACEUTICS RESEARCH

-Continued work in Material sciences
-Expanded Activities in Polymers
    a. Better biocompatibility
    b. More predictable behavior in-vivo, e.g., dissolu-
       tion rate, drug diffusion, interaction with bio-
       polymers or biological surfaces
-Expanded work in routes of drug delivery
    a. Understand anatomy/physiology/biochemistry
    b. Modify or control physiology/anatomy/biochemistry
-Improvements in control and efficiency of processes
-Expanded work on Analogs/Prodrugs
-Expanded work on drug disposition on/in cells
-Expanded work on solute interaction with the cell sur-
    face
-Pharmacodynamics
-Stabilization and delivery of peptides and proteins
-Improved and expanded interface between the physical-
    chemical-technology areas and the biological sci-
    ences at a good level of inquiry.

Pharmaceutical scientists, by virtue of their exposure
to biology-physical-chemical science and technology in the
undergraduate, and to a lesser extent, graduate program,
in some sense, therefore, are   generalists. However,
we are aware that depth in an area is required for a fundamental contribution. Thus, the generalist background is
needed to communicate at a research level with other dis-
covery/development groups, recognizing that the specific
areas of research will be more focused.

One expected fallout of an improved understanding of
drug delivery is perhaps to salvage more drug candidates in
the discovery phase. Presumably, the development of better
screens, for drug delivery purposes, as well as a more fundamental understanding of factors influencing transit, will
not only suggest new and better approaches to drug delivery
but also to aid the synthetic chemist and pharmacologist
who will screen these compounds. Hopefully, these screens
will permit optimization of the discovery process.

I find it amusing to receive phone calls inquiring

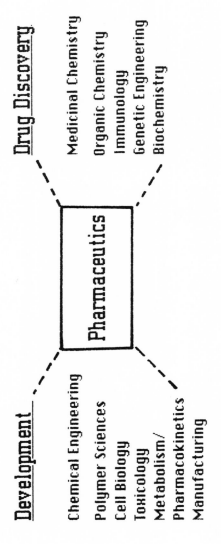

Scheme 1

about individuals with education/training in drug delivery. Drug delivery is a concept not a discipline. I say this, despite the fact that some schools have unfortunately begun describing their programs as drug delivery programs. In my view all graduate programs in the pharmaceutical sciences produce budding scientists that will work in the general area of drug delivery. To describe the graduate program as a drug delivery program is unfortunate at best and dishonest at worst.

PROJECTED DRUG DELIVERY DEVELOPMENTS

It is difficult to predict with accuracy, developments that will occur in drug delivery in the future. However, there are some low risk statements that can be made.

1. Within the next five years we will actually see a novel drug delivery system which will then allow re-examination of all the earlier novel-drug delivery systems.

2. It is unlikely that antacids will be given trans-dermably.

3. It is unlikely that hominy grits will be recognized by the reticuloendothelial system and not be endocytosed.

4. In the future, all arguments as to which manufacturer has a release rate closest to zero order will be settled by a cross-over study in freshly cloned 75 kg subjects identically diseased.

5. The nanoparticle enthusiasts will merge with the liposome workers to produce the universally applicable nanosome which will be dispensed in a loaded red blood cell for recognition purposes.

Now that I have these low risk pet peeves out of the way we can move on to the higher risk area. Others during this symposium will give a more accurate reflection of the state of their respective areas and where the area is heading. On this basis I can afford to be more global in my comments. Listed below are some general statements reflecting a few trends that I anticipate and these are general thoughts borrowed from others with which I agree.

1. Drug delivery programs in industrial settings will need to be incorporated, on a research and a development level, to be maximally effective.

2. Pharmaceutics will play a pivotal role in drug delivery system development but the pharmaceutical scientists participating will be a heterogeneous collection: The "classical" pharmaceutical scientist, however you define that, will have a more fundamental biological background.

3. There will be a continuing merger of the fluid liposome and solid particulate carrier programs to some central position where the physical properties of the carrier are constant. At this point surface chemical properties will dictate host compatibility and recognition factors.

4. Prodrug and Analog research will focus on optimizing transit, all uptake and internalization as well as receptor characteristics.

5. Skin penetrant enhancement will be overcome in the near future and at that point formulation biocompatibility will be the dominant theme.

6. There must be a greater reliance on pharmacodynamics and subsequent calculation of release rate kinetics that are dictated by need of the condition. The continued use of zero-order drug delivery systems is artificial and primitive.

7. There needs to be a serious examination of routes of drug administration by several disciplines to fully characterize these routes at the best level possible. Useful strategies for drug delivery will emerge from such inquiries.

This wish list could be expanded considerably. The major point to be made that at its best a focused effort on drug delivery will not only aid the drug discovery process but will truly begin to optimize drug utilization. However, to accomplish such a goal requires a commitment to the process, an integration of research and development efforts and a challenge for pharmaceutics to participate in this process.

PHARMACODYNAMIC CONSIDERATIONS IN THE DEVELOPMENT OF

NEW DRUG DELIVERY CONCEPTS

Bobbe L. Ferraiolo and Leslie Z. Benet

Department of Pharmacy
University of California, San Francisco
San Francisco, California

RELATIONSHIP BETWEEN PHARMACOKINETICS AND PHARMACODYNAMICS: EQUILIBRATION HALF-TIME

The ultimate therapeutic value of a drug depends upon its pharmacodynamic effects and the temporal expression of these effects. A dosing regimen that is appropriate for the treatment of a disease state in a specific patient population is best instituted when one knows the plasma concentration which will maximize the efficacy of the drug and the level below which drug concentrations or amounts in the body must be maintained to avoid toxicity (Benet, 1984). Effective and toxic concentration values for a number of drugs have been reported (Benet and Sheiner, 1980) and these may be useful in defining drug dosage regimens, however, there is no general agreement about the best way to describe the relationship between the concentration of drug in plasma and its effect. For many drugs the form of this relationship between effect and plasma concentration is unknown. For those concentration-effect correlations that have been defined, it is important to realize that the relationships are only meaningful at steady state or at a time when the ratio of the drug concentrations at the site of action and in plasma can be expected to remain constant over time; that is, during the terminal log-linear phase of the concentration versus time

13

curve. Thus, when one attempts to correlate pharmacokinetics with pharmacodynamics, the time of distribution of
drug to the site of action must be taken into account.

Sheiner et al. (1979) have proposed a model of drug
pharmacodynamic response that integrates the pharmacokinetic model and allows the temporal aspects of pharmacodynamics as well as the time-independent sensitivity
component to be characterized. Holford and Sheiner (1981)
list the equilibration half-times for five drugs which
have been modelled by the simultaneous assessment of pharmacokinetics and pharmacodynamics (Table I). This
parameter indicates at what time following drug dosage one
may expect to see a relationship between the measured
plasma concentration and the effect that is similar to the
concentration-effect relationship expected when the system
is at equilibrium. For example, this equilibration occurs
quite rapidly following doses of disopyramide (Table I).
Considering that after 3 to 4 half-lives 90% of the equilibration will have occurred, a correlation between the QT
interval prolongation caused by disopyramide and the
drug's plasma levels may be assumed after 6-8 minutes. In
contrast, the equilibration half-time for digoxin is 200
min. Therefore, one should not expect to see a reasonable

Table I. Half-times of equilibration between plasma
concentrations and pharmacodynamic effect*.

Drug	Equilibration half-time (min)	Effect
Disopyramide	2	QT interval prolongation
d-Tubocurarine	4	Muscle paralysis
Quinidine	8	QT interval prolongation
Cimetidine	30	Inhibit gastric acid secretion
Digoxin	200	Left ventricular ejection time shortening

*After Holford and Sheiner (1981).

direct correlation between digoxin plasma levels and a shortening of the left ventricular ejection time until 10-12 h following drug dosage. It is probable that patient population or disease state characteristics may affect a drug's equilibration half-time. It has already been shown that drug-drug interactions can alter the time it takes to achieve this equilibration. Stanski et al. (1979) have shown that halothane anesthesia enhances the steady-state effects for a particular plasma concentration of curare, apparently without changing its pharmacokinetics, and that this type of anesthesia lengthens the time required for equilibration between a particular curare concentration and its effect. A factor yet to be considered is that the equilibration time between plasma concentration and the desired therapeutic effect may not be the same as the equilibration time between plasma concentrations and toxic (or merely undesirable) effects.

DEFINITION OF A RELEVANT HALF-LIFE

Although half-life suffers the limitation of being a composite parameter that reflects changes in both clearance and volume of distribution, it determines the maximum and minimum blood concentrations obtained for a particular dosage regimen, important quantities in defining the pharmacodynamic response to a drug. Therefore, the relevance of a particular half-life for a drug must be interpreted in terms of its correlation with either effective or toxic concentrations. Most drugs appear to follow multicompartment pharmacokinetics. That is, the equation describing the time course of the plasma concentration requires more than one exponential term:

$$C_p = A_1 e^{-\lambda_1 t} + A_2 e^{-\lambda_2 t} + \ldots + A_n e^{-\lambda n t} \qquad \text{(Eq. 1)}$$

For example, digoxin pharmacokinetics following intravenous dosing is best described by a three exponential equation (Kramer et al., 1974), yet digoxin kinetics are usually discussed in terms of only one half-life, that which corresponds to the smallest disposition rate constant, where the half-life is approximately 1.6-2 days in healthy volunteers with normal renal function. Ethambutol has also been shown to follow three compartment kinetics following intravenous dosing (Lee et al., 1980). However, in this case the shortest and longest half-lives are generally ignored; the reported half-life value corresponds to the second disposition constant (3.1 h).

A number of factors must be considered in defining whether a particular half-life has relevance in terms of drug therapy. This determination, however, can only be made when the investigator has some knowledge as to the concentration (or amount)-effect (or toxicity) relationship as well as the equilibration time between the measured concentration and the pharmacodynamic response. If it is known that the pharmacodynamic effect is related to plasma concentrations following multiple dosing or at steady state, then a decision can be made concerning the relevance of a particular half-life in terms of the fractional clearance related to that half-life. If instead, the pharmacodynamic effect, usually a toxic effect, is more closely related to the total amount of drug in the body (or in a particular organ), then the relevance of a particular half-life may be defined in terms of the fraction of the steady-state volume of distribution related to that half-life. Whether toxicity will occur also depends upon the dosing interval as well as the total time over which the patient receives the drug. These concepts will be discussed in terms of gentamicin, ethambutol, digoxin and lidocaine pharmacokinetics (Table II).

Nomograms that relate gentamicin dosing to renal function assume a half-life of 2-4 h in young subjects with normal renal function, which then increases to 13 h or greater in patients with creatinine clearances less than 25 mL/min (Benet and Sheiner, 1980). Schentag et al. (1977), using very sensitive analytical methods, have indicated that gentamicin exhibits a significantly longer terminal half-life. They have described the gentamicin plasma concentration-time relationship in terms of two exponential terms. The following equation describes the average plasma concentration (µg/mL) following an 80 mg i.v. dose in 16 patients whose renal function was considered to be normal:

$$C_p = 5.38 \ e^{-0.195t} + 0.060 \ e^{-0.013t} \qquad \text{(Eq. 2)}$$

The disposition constants in the exponents correspond to half-lives of 3.56 and 53.3 h. In most cases, we can ignore the longer half-life. The area under the plasma concentration-time curve (AUC) can be calculated as the ratio of the coefficients and exponents based on the following relationship:

$$AUC = \frac{A_1}{\lambda_1} + \frac{A_2}{\lambda_2} + \cdots + \frac{A_n}{\lambda_n} \qquad \text{(Eq. 3)}$$

Applying this relationship to gentamicin:

$$AUC \ (\mu g \cdot h/mL) = \underset{(86\%)}{27.6} + \underset{(14\%)}{4.6} \qquad \text{(Eq. 4)}$$

Note that 86% of the AUC relates to the coefficient and exponent for the 3.56 h half-life (Table II). Rearrangement of the following equation:

$$\text{Dosing rate} = CL \cdot C_{ss} \qquad \text{(Eq. 5)}$$

Table II. Fractional areas under the curve in normal volunteers.

Drug	$(t_{\frac{1}{2}})1$	%AUC	$(t_{\frac{1}{2}})2$	%AUC	$(t_{\frac{1}{2}})3$	%AUC
Gentamicin	3.56 h	86	53.3 h	14	--	--
Digoxin	9 min	3	1.2 h	20	45 h	77
Ethambutol	5 min	26	3.1 h	47	10.2 h	27
Lidocaine	9 min	2	92 min	98	--	--

and substitution for clearance in terms of a single i.v. dose as described by the relationship:

$$CL = Dose_{iv}/AUC = F \; Dose/AUC \qquad \text{(Eq. 6)}$$

reveals that the predicted steady-state level (C_{ss}) is directly correlated to AUC:

$$
\begin{aligned}
C_{ss} &= Dosing \; rate/CL \\
       &= Dosing \; rate \cdot AUC/Dose_{iv} \qquad \text{(Eq. 7)}
\end{aligned}
$$

If we ignore the 53.3 h half-life in this normal population, the value for AUC and therefore the steady-state plasma concentration will be underestimated by only 14%, since this long half-life represents a small fraction of the total gentamicin clearance. This error in plasma levels can be ignored with confidence since this difference may often by within analytical error as well as within the day-to-day variability in a particular patient.

The above calculations assume that plasma levels are important in defining the efficacy of gentamicin. If this is true, the clinician can safely ignore this longer half-life in patients with normal renal function since little change in steady-state plasma levels will be observed. However, it may be that the response (particularly toxicity) is related to the amount of drug in the body rather than the plasma concentration. The amount in the body at steady state (A_{ss}) is the product of the plasma concentration and the steady-state volume of distribution:

$$A_{ss} = C_{ss} \cdot V_{ss} \qquad \text{(Eq. 8)}$$

V_{ss} may be calculated from the area under the moment curve (AUMC) and AUC as defined by Benet and Galeazzi (1979):

$$V_{ss} = \frac{(Dose_{iv}) \; AUMC}{AUC^{2}} \qquad \text{(Eq. 9)}$$

where AUMC can be calculated from the coefficients and

exponents of the polyexponential plasma concentration versus time relationship:

$$AUMC = \frac{A_1}{\lambda_1^2} + \frac{A_2}{\lambda_2^2} + \ldots + \frac{A_n}{\lambda_n^2} \qquad (Eq. 10)$$

If the second exponential term for gentamicin is ignored, the volume of distribution is 14.9 L; including the second exponential, V_{ss} is 38.3 L. When the amount at steady state is calculated including and excluding the second exponential term the values differ significantly; the ratio of these amounts equals 2.9 while the plasma concentrations differ only slightly.

Schentag et al. (1977) also described gentamicin kinetics following an 80 mg dose in 7 subjects with renal failure. In this patient population mean plasma concentrations were defined by the following equation:

$$C_p = 4.03 \; e^{-0.053t} + 0.46 \; e^{-0.004t} \qquad (Eq. 11)$$

The disposition constants represent half-lives of 13.1 h and 173 h (7.2 days). Calculating AUC from the ratio of coefficients and exponents:

$$AUC = 76.0 + 115.0 \qquad (Eq. 12)$$
$$\quad (40\%) \quad (60\%)$$

The ratio of amounts in the body at steady state when the second exponential is either included or excluded is 8.4. In these patients with renal insufficiency, steady-state plasma levels would be underestimated by 60% if the 7.2 day half-life were ignored. In addition, significant differences in the amount of drug in the body at steady state would be predicted depending upon whether the long terminal half-life was included or excluded.

In patients with both normal and decreased renal function the extent of gentamicin accumulation both in terms of plasma concentration and amount in the body will depend upon the dosing interval <u>and</u> the total time that the drug is administered to the patient. Since gentamicin is generally dosed as a function of the shorter half-life, accumulation might be expected to occur. Recall though that half-life is a measure of the time required to attain and decay from steady-state conditions. For patients with renal insufficiency the longer half-life is approximately 1 week. Therefore, only 50% of the accumulation predicted at steady state will occur after 1 week. Thus, in these patients, major accumulation will not occur unless the drug is dosed over a long period.

From the above discussion it is apparent why clinical investigators have found it difficult to validate nomograms which supposedly can predict and prevent toxicity with gentamicin. These nomograms are generally based on plasma concentration measurements which are relatively insensitive to the long terminal half-life. Ignoring the long half-life for patients with normal renal function results in a 14% error in the predicted plasma concentrations, but a 290% error in the predicted <u>amount</u> of drug in the body. If toxicity is related to the amount of amino-glycoside accumulated either in the kidney or in the ear endolymph it can readily be understood why plasma concentration changes may not predict this toxicity. It has been shown (Schentag et al., 1977) that up to 40% of the amount of drug in the body accumulates in the kidneys, which is the major site of gentamicin toxicity. Since the kidney accounts for less than 1% of the total body mass, the "concentration" of gentamicin in the kidney is extremely large. Therapeutic plasma level monitoring will never succeed for this drug because plasma level changes are too insensitive to reflect this change of "concentration" in the kidneys.

The relationship between dosing interval, accumulation and the importance of a terminal half-life may be illustrated using ethambutol kinetics. Lee et al. (1980) reported a terminal half-life for ethambutol of 10.2 h which accounted for 27% of the AUC (Table II). The accumulation ratio was 2.1 for the amount at steady state when this half-life was included or excluded. However, ethambutol is usually dosed only once daily. Since this drug is dosed at an interval greater than 2 times the terminal half-life the accumulation that could result from this longer half-life will not be very significant. The maximum accumulation will be only 25% of the predicted steady-state increase in plasma concentration and amount of drug in the body.

Digoxin pharmacokinetics following i.v. dosage in normal volunteers may be described by a three-exponential equation (Table II and Kramer et al., 1974). Obviously, the longest half-life (45 h) is most important in defining digoxin steady-state plasma concentrations (77% AUC). However, since digoxin is a drug with a narrow therapeutic index, one might be concerned that initial plasma concentrations, which fall off rapidly, may reach levels which correspond to toxic effects. However, as mentioned previously, the equilibration time between measured plasma concentrations and pharmacodynamic effect must be taken into consideration. The half-time of this equilibration is 200 min for digoxin (see Table I), a value longer than the two distribution half-lives following intravenous dosage of the drug. Because of this prolonged equilibration half-time, high initial plasma concentrations are not important in predicting toxic effects. Therefore, for digoxin we may safely ignore the 9 min and 1.2 h half-lives, both with respect to the predicted steady-state concentrations as well as with respect to initial concentrations which may lead to acute toxicity.

The situation is quite different for the antiarrhythmic lidocaine. Rowland et al. (1971) described lidocaine pharmacokinetics with two exponential terms relating to two half-lives (Table II). Obviously, the 9 min half-life (2% AUC) would be insignificant in predicting steady-state plasma concentrations. In addition, initial half-lives always represent a small fraction of the volume of distribution, so estimates of accumulated amounts of drug in the body would be little affected if this half-life were ignored. However, the equilibration half-time for

lidocaine is quite short, probably 2 min or less. Therefore, initial plasma concentrations following an
intravenous dose cannot be ignored if they are in the
toxic concentration range for this drug (Benet and
Sheiner, 1980).

The above examples illustrate when a particular half-
life is clinically relevant. The factors which must be
considered in defining the relevance of a half-life are
thus: 1) the concentration (or amount)-effect (or toxicity) relationship; 2) the half-time for equilibration
between a measured plasma concentration and the pharmacodynamic effect; 3) the fractional clearance related to a
particular half-life as defined in terms of AUC; 4) the
increase in the amount of drug in the body at steady state
which may be related to a prolonged terminal half-life; 5)
the dosing interval with respect to the terminal half-
life; and 6) the total period of drug dosage with respect
to the terminal half-life.

The concepts described above may be important in
controlled drug delivery systems where zero-order drug
delivery over long periods of time is the goal, approxi-
mating an i.v. infusion of drug. Under these conditions,
maximum drug accumulation may be expected to occur.
Whereas the possibility for maintenance of constant therapeutic plasma drug levels may be realized with these
systems, the accumulation factor, especially with regard
to the amount of a drug or metabolites in the body and
their relationship to toxicity, must be taken into account.

FACTORS INFLUENCING PHARMACODYNAMICS

Therapeutic agents are usually characterized in
healthy, often young adult male volunteers under carefully
controlled conditions, but these conditions may not be
applicable to the clinical situation (Table III). In
reality, the patient under consideration may be pediatric,
geriatric or female, and the drug is likely to be administered with numerous other drugs and in the presence of

various disease states. All of these factors may affect the drug's pharmacodynamics as well as its pharmacokinetics. Whereas it is relatively easy to extrapolate from the kinetics in healthy volunteers to the kinetics in specific disease states or specific patient populations based on known pathophysiological changes such as altered blood flow or protein binding, little work has been done on the relationship between specific disease states or patient populations and the pharmacodynamic response.

Since in disease states or specific patient populations the pharmacokinetics and/or the pharmacodynamics of a drug may be modified, it is impossible to separate the effects of these factors on pharmacokinetics or pharmacodynamics without investigating the clinical response of the patient as well as the time course of the drug in biological fluids. This is a serious limitation of many of the studies where a change in response in a particular patient population or disease state has been reported. This requirement for investigation of both the dynamics and kinetics may also account for the relatively small number of reports that are available. Another complication to be considered in the presence of disease states is that the disease may not present an unvarying clinical picture or result in stable alterations in func-

Table III.   Factors that may influence the pharmacodynamic response to a drug.

Patient population factors
        pediatric (developmental)
        geriatric (chronological vs. biological age)
        gender
Disease states
        heterogeneity of pathophysiology
        changing course of disease
Concomitant drug administration (and/or drug metabolites)
Drug dosage regimen

---

tion or response; the patient's condition may improve or deteriorate with therapy (or spontaneously) and, as a result, the response may also change. Another consideration is the heterogeneity of the severity of disease states. Models of human disease in animals may not be of general relevance to human disease because these models may provide a much narrower spectrum of severity (Vessel, 1981). Further complications may arise depending upon a drug's dosage form, route of administration or the drug dosage regimen.

EFFECT OF DISEASE STATES ON PHARMACODYNAMICS

There is some evidence in the literature suggesting that hepatic dysfunction may alter a patient's sensitivity to drugs (Williams, 1984). A study of the disappearance of chlorpromazine from plasma and its effect on EEG activity in patients with cirrhosis versus normal controls (Maxwell et al., 1972) reported that while there were only minor differences in plasma concentrations and elimination constants between the two groups, the patients with cirrhosis exhibited an increased sensitivity to the CNS depressant effects of the drug, especially in those patients with a history of encephalopathy. Marcantonio et al. (1983) found that although bumetanide serum concentrations in patients with hepatic disease were higher than in normal subjects, these patients demonstrated an impaired diuretic response to the drug. The authors suggested that this drug resistance may be related to the secondary hyperaldosteronism present in liver disease. A study of tranylcypromine (an MAO inhibitor) in patients with liver cirrhosis versus normal volunteers (Morgan and Read, 1972) indicated that the cirrhotic patients were more sensitive to the EEG slowing effects of the drug compared with the control subjects, again especially if there was a history of encephalopathy. No kinetic data were provided in this study.

There are also indications that changes in renal function may alter a patient's response to certain drugs.

In a study of acute renal failure patients and age-matched normal controls, Levitan et al. (1982) found that norepinephrine infusion produced smaller increments in mean blood pressure in the renal failure group than in the controls. It has been suggested that this dysfunction may be partly due to a reduced ability to respond to norepinephrine (Campese et al., 1981). The blood pH disturbances associated with renal disease may be a factor contributing to the decreased pressor response to catecholamines and other vasopressor drugs. Nash and Heath (1961) reported that low blood pH resulted in a reduced peripheral vascular response to epinephrine and norepinephrine in dogs. In a study of the cardiac effects of pindolol in renal failure patients versus normal volunteers (Galeazzi et al., 1979), similar total body clearance of the drug was demonstrated for the two groups but for each plasma drug concentration the uremic patients exhibited an increased sensitivity to the beta-blocking effects of the drug. Lowenthal et al. (1983) studied the pharmacodynamic effects of clonidine in endstage renal disease. Although it has been suggested that plasma concentrations of more than 2 ng/ml are associated with decreased antihypertensive effect through peripheral α-receptor stimulation, very high clonidine plasma concentrations (30 ng/ml) in these patients were associated with a maintenance of blood pressure control. The authors suggest that one explanation for this effect may be decreased peripheral α-receptor sensitivity in this patient population. It has also been postulated that electrolyte abnormalities such as magnesium, potassium or sodium depletion, or increased calcium, potassium or magnesium may affect a patient's sensitivity to cardiovascular (digitalis glycosides) and other drugs (Brater and Chennavasin, 1984; Smith, 1975).

SPECIAL PATIENT POPULATIONS AND PHARMACODYNAMICS

Biological maturation may affect the relationship between pharmacokinetics and pharmacodynamics (Green and Mirkin, 1984). Few combined pharmacokinetic/pharmacodynamic studies have been done in children, partly due to ethical and legal problems in conducting controlled clinical trials in these patients.   There are some reports, however, that suggest that the pediatric population possesses altered pharmacodynamic responses to certain drugs. Newborns may exhibit an increased sensitivity to nondepolarizing blockers such as d-tubocurarine used as muscle relaxants in pediatric operative procedures (Bush and Stead, 1962).   A second study (Bennett et al., 1975) confirmed the finding that the newborn has an increased sensitivity to nondepolarizing muscle relaxants (pancuronium),   and reported that this hypersensitivity decreases with age.   Neither of these studies, however, provided pharmacokinetic data in these populations.   Tricyclic antidepressant drugs, which may be used in pediatrics to treat enuresis, hyperactivity and psychiatric disorders, elicit a hypertensive response in these patients (Lake et al., 1979).   This contrasts with the systolic hypotension that usually occurs in adult populations.   Recently, Morselli et al. (1983) have reported that children seem to be more sensitive to the effects of haloperidol; therapeutic and toxic effects of the drug occur at lower plasma concentrations than in adults.   Lower therapeutic and toxic thresholds in children may also apply with chlorpromazine (Rivera-Calimlim et al., 1979).

The geriatric population is another special group that may exhibit altered pharmacodynamic responses to certain drugs. A factor complicating drug therapy in this population is the heterogeneity inherent in the "geriatric" classification.   Age-induced dynamic changes probably occur at different rates in different subjects; chronological age may not correspond to biological age. As yet there is no overall measure of functional age. The rate of aging of a given system in a patient cannot be used to predict the rate of aging of a second organ system.

Some clinical observations in the literature suggest that there are changes in drug effects in the elderly that are independent of pharmacokinetic changes.   There seems to be an increase in adverse behavioral reactions in elderly patients treated with hypnotic drugs. In addition, the elderly may exhibit drug reactions that are qualitatively different than those described in younger populations (Stevenson, 1984). Castleden et al. (1977) studied the CNS depressant effects of nitrazepam in healthy young and elderly patients. Plasma concentrations and the elimination half-life of the drug were similar in the two groups, but the elderly subjects appeared to be more sensitive to the drug's effects on cognitive functions. Other studies suggest that increased receptor site sensitivity may account for the increased depression of clotting factor synthesis in response to warfarin administration in elderly subjects (Husted and Andreasen, 1977; Shepherd et al., 1977). Kinetic studies revealed that the plasma clearance and protein binding of warfarin were identical in elderly and young subjects (Shepherd et al., 1979). Conversely, the elderly population may be more resistant to the effects of certain pharmacologic agents such as isoproterenol and propranolol (Vestal et al., 1979).

REGIMEN-DEPENDENT PHARMACODYNAMIC EFFECTS

It has recently been pointed out that the regimen employed for drug administration may influence the pharmacodynamic (efficacy/toxicity) response for certain drugs [see Urquhart et al. (1984) for review]. The importance of the timing and route of drug administration is well-known for drug therapy with antibiotics and in cancer chemotherapy. With antibiotics one tries to strike a delicate balance between killing the bacteria without selecting for resistant strains. Cancer chemotherapy is characterized by complicated schedules of drug administration and combinations. Sikic et al. (1978) and Peng et al. (1980) found that bleomycin administered by constant-rate infusion to tumor-bearing mice was more efficacious in tumor size reduction and less toxic than injections of similar doses of the drug. Lower pulmonary toxicity with continuous i.v. infusion of bleomycin has also been found in human studies (Cooper and Hong, 1981). This phenomenon of regimen-dependence of pharmacodynamic effects has also been observed for other drugs. Nau (1983) describes a study comparing the embryotoxicity of similar doses of valproic acid administered to pregnant mice by a once-daily subcutaneous injection regimen or constant-rate administration with an osmotic minipump. The impact on the developing fetus was greater after s.c. injection of the drug than after controlled-rate delivery with respect to resorptions and teratogenicity. The author concluded that the transient high drug concentrations that are inevitable with an injection regimen were responsible for the higher terato-genicity. In contrast, intermittent injections were shown to be superior to infusions in rats (Tam et al., 1982) and dogs (Podbesek et al., 1983) treated with parathyroid hormone. The injection regimen was more effective than the continuous infusion in promoting increased bone deposition.

It is apparent that the spectrum of pharmacodynamic effects for a drug may depend, in part, on the delivery regimen and/or the rate of its delivery. This provides an opportunity to optimize therapy for those drugs with regimen-dependent pharmacodynamics. The goal of controlled drug delivery has been to achieve constant therapeutic plasma levels, but there must be constraints upon such devices applied to approved drugs to show that the new regimen is safe (safer) or (more) efficacious. The importance of this issue may be illustrated by the example of deaths among insulin-dependent diabetics using pumps for the administration of their insulin (Urquhart, 1983). In these patients the application of controlled drug delivery was over the short term more convenient, but over the long term too inflexible to be safe or practical. The development and incorporation of physiological feedback mechanisms into controlled delivery devices may aid in the treatment of specific disease states with these systems.

SUMMARY

Pharmacodynamic responses may be affected by numerous patient variables including age and the presence of disease states. The actual method and timing of drug administration may also change the spectrum of pharmacodynamic effects. The rational use of drug delivery systems will require further pharmacodynamic research to identify the appropriate combinations of patients, drugs and delivery systems.

ACKNOWLEDGEMENTS

Preparation of this manuscript was supported in part by NIH Center Grant GM 26691. Dr. Ferraiolo was supported by National Research Service Award GM 09027. The authors thank Ms. Susana Atwood and Mrs. Martha Barba for excellent technical assistance in the preparation of this manuscript.

REFERENCES

Benet, L.Z. and Galeazzi, R.L., Noncompartmental determination of steady-state volume of distribution. J. Pharm. Sci., 68 (1979) 1071–1074.

Benet, L.Z. and Sheiner, L.B., Design and optimization of dosage regimens; pharmacokinetic data. In Gilman, A.G., Goodman, L.S. and Gilman, A. (Eds) The Pharmacological Basis of Therapeutics, Macmillan Publishing, New York, 1980, pp. 1675–1737.

Benet, L.Z., Pharmacokinetic parameters: which are necessary to define a drug substance? Eur. J. Resp. Dis. (Suppl. 134), 65 (1984) 45–61.

Bennett, E.J., Ramamurthy, S., Dalal, F.Y. and Salem, M.R., Pancuronium and the neonate. Br. J. Anaesth., 47 (1975) 75–78.

Brater, D.C. and Chennavasin, P., Effects of renal disease: pharmacokinetic considerations. In Benet, L.Z., Massoud, N. and Gambertoglio, J.G. (Eds) Pharma-

cokinetic Basis for Drug Treatment, Raven Press, New
York, 1984, pp. 119-147.

Bush, G.H. and Stead, A.L., The use of d-tubocurarine in
neonatal anesthesia.   Brit. J. Anaesth., 34 (1962)
721-728.

Campese, V.M., Romoff, M.S., Levitan, D., Lane, K. and
Massry, S.G., Mechanisms of autonomic system dysfunction in uremia. Kidney Int., 20 (1981) 246-253.

Castleden, C.M., George, C.F., Marcer, D. and Hallett, C.,
Increased sensitivity to nitrazepam in old age.   Br.
Med. J., 1 (1977) 10-12.

Cooper, K.R. and Hong, W.K., Prospective study of the
pulmonary   toxicity   of   continuously   infused
bleomycin. Cancer Treat. Rep., 65 (1981) 419-425.

Galeazzi, R.L., Gugger, M. and Weidmann, P., Beta blockade
with pindolol: differential cardiac and renal effects
despite similar plasma kinetics in normal and uremic
man. Kidney Int., 15 (1979) 661-668.

Green, T.P. and Mirkin, B.L., Clinical pharmacokinetics:
pediatric considerations.   In Benet, L.Z., Massoud, N.
and Gambertoglio, J.G. (Eds) Pharmacokinetic Basis for
Drug Treatment, Raven Press, New York, 1984, pp. 269-
282.

Holford, N.H.G. and Sheiner, L.B., Understanding the dose-
effect relationship: clinical application of pharmacokinetic-pharmacodynamic   models.   Clin.   Pharmacokinet., 6 (1981) 429-453.

Husted, S. and Andreasen, F., The influence of age on the
response to anticoagulants.   Br. J. Clin. Pharmacol.,
4 (1977) 559-565.

Kramer, W.G., Lewis, R.P., Cobb, T.C., Forester, W.F. Jr.,
Visconti,   J.,   Wanke,   L.A.,   Boxenbaum,   H.G.   and
Reuning, R.H., Pharmacokinetics of digoxin: comparison
of a two- and a three-compartment model in man.   J.
Pharmacokinet. Biopharm., 2 (1974) 299-312.

Lake, C.R., Mikkelsen, E.J., Rapoport, J.L., Zavadil III,
A.P. and Kopin, I.J., Effect of imipramine on norepi-
nephrine and blood pressure in enuretic boys.   Clin.
Pharmacol. Ther., 26 (1979) 647-653.

Lee, C.S., Brater, D.C., Gambertoglio, J.G. and Benet, L.Z., Disposition kinetics of ethambutol in man. J. Pharmacokinet. Biopharm., 8 (1980) 335–346.

Levitan, D., Massry, S.G., Romoff, M.S. and Campese, V.M., Autonomic nervous system dysfunction in patients with acute renal failure. Am. J. Nephrol., 2 (1982) 213–220.

Lowenthal, D.T., Affrime, M.B., Meyer, A., Kim, K.E., Falkner, B. and Sharif, K., Pharmacokinetics and pharmacodynamics of clonidine in varying stages of renal function. Chest (Suppl. 2), 83 (1983) 386–390.

Marcantonio, L.A., Auld, W.H.R., Murdoch, W.R., Purohit, R., Skellern, G.G. and Howes, C.A., The pharmacokinetics and pharmacodynamics of the diuretic bumetanide in hepatic and renal disease. Br. J. Clin. Pharmacol., 15 (1983) 245–252.

Maxwell, J.D., Carrella, M., Parkes, J.D., Williams, R., Mould, G.P. and Curry, S.H., Plasma disappearance and cerebral effects of chlorpromazine in cirrhosis. Clin. Sci., 43 (1972) 143–151.

Morgan, M.H. and Read, A.E., Antidepressants and liver disease. Gut, 13 (1972) 697–701.

Morselli, P.L., Bianchetti, G. and Dugas, M., Therapeutic drug monitoring of psychotropic drugs in children. Pediatr. Pharmacol., 3 (1983) 149–156.

Nash, C.W. and Heath, C., Vascular responses to catecholamines during respiratory changes in pH. Am. J. Physiol., 200 (1961) 755–758.

Nau, H., The role of delivery systems for the toxicological evaluation of drugs: potential for new drug discovery and development. In McCloskey, J. (Ed) Drug Delivery Systems, Aster Publishing, Springfield, Oregon, 1983, pp. 15–18.

Peng, Y.M., Alberts, D.S., Chen, H.S.G., Mason, N. and Moon, T.E., Antitumor activity and plasma kinetics of bleomycin by continuous and intermittent administration. Br. J. Cancer, 41 (1980) 644–647.

Podbesek, R., Edouard, C., Meunier, P.J., Parsons, J.A., Reeve, J., Stevenson, R.W. and Zanelli, J.M., Effects of two treatment regimens with synthetic human parathyroid hormone fragment on bone formation and the tissue balance of trabecular bone in greyhounds. Endocrinology, 112 (1983) 1000–1006.

Rivera-Calimlim, L., Griesbach, P.H. and Perlmutter, R., Plasma chlorpromazine concentrations in children with behavioral disorders and mental illness. Clin. Pharmacol. Ther., 26 (1979) 114–121.

Rowland, M., Thomson, P.D., Guichard, A. and Melmon, K.L., Disposition kinetics of lidocaine in normal subjects. Ann. N.Y. Acad. Sci., 179 (1971) 383–398.

Schentag, J.J., Jusko, W.J., Vance, J.W., Cumbo, T.J., Abrutyn, E., DeLattre, M. and Gerbracht, L.M., Gentamicin disposition and tissue accumulation on multiple dosing. J. Pharmacokinet. Biopharm., 5 (1977) 559–577.

Sheiner, L.B., Stanski, D.R., Vozeh, S., Miller, R.D. and Ham, J., Simultaneous modeling of pharmacokinetics and pharmacodynamics: application to d-tubocurarine. Clin. Pharmacol. Ther., 25 (1979) 358–371.

Shepherd, A.M.M., Hewick, D.S., Moreland, T.A. and Stevenson, I.H., Age as a determinant of sensitivity to warfarin. Br. J. Clin. Pharmacol., 4 (1977) 315–320.

Shepherd, A.M.M., Wilson, N. and Stevenson, I.H., Warfarin sensitivity in the elderly. In Crooks, J. and Stevenson, I.H. (Eds) Drugs and the Elderly, University Park Press, Baltimore, 1979, pp. 199–209.

Sikic, B.I., Collins, J.M., Mimnaugh, E.G. and Gram, T.E., Improved therapeutic index of bleomycin when administered by continuous infusion in mice. Cancer Treat. Rep., 62 (1978) 2011–2017.

Smith, T.W., Digitalis toxicity: epidemiology and clinical use of serum concentration measurements. Am. J. Med., 58 (1975) 470–476.

Stanski, D.R., Ham, J., Miller, R.D. and Sheiner, L.B., Pharmacokinetics and pharmacodynamics of d-tubocurarine during nitrous oxide-narcotic and halothane anesthesia in man. Anesthesiology, 51 (1979) 235–241.

Stevenson, I. H., Drugs in the elderly. In Lemberger, L. and Reidenberg, M.M. (Eds) Proceedings of the Second World Conference on Clinical Pharmacology and

Therapeutics, American Society for Pharmacology and Experimental Therapeutics, Bethesda, Maryland, 1984, pp. 64–73.

Tam, C.S., Heersche, J.N.M., Murray, T.M. and Parsons, J.A., Parathyroid hormone stimulates the bone apposition rate independently of its resorptive action: differential effects of intermittent and continuous administration. Endocrinology, 110 (1982) 506–512.

Urquhart, J., Implantable pumps in drug delivery. In McCloskey, J. (Ed) Drug Delivery Systems, Aster Publishing, Springfield, Oregon, 1983, pp. 53–54.

Urquhart J., Fara, J.W. and Willis, K.L., Rate-controlled delivery systems in drug and hormone research. Ann. Rev. Pharmacol. Toxicol., 24 (1984) 199–236.

Vesell, E.S., The influence of host factors on drug response. V. Endocrinological, gastrointestinal and pulmonary diseases. Ration. Drug Ther., 15 (1981) 1–6.

Vestal, R.E., Wood, A.J.J. and Shand, D.G., Reduced β-adrenoceptor sensitivity in the elderly. Clin. Pharmacol. Ther., 26 (1979) 181–186.

Williams, R.L., Drugs and the liver: clinical applications. In Benet, L.Z., Massoud, N. and Gambertoglio, J.G. (Eds) Pharmacokinetic Basis for Drug Treatment, Raven Press, New York, 1984, pp. 63–75.

MOLECULAR MECHANISMS OF DRUG ACTION AND PHARMACOKINETIC-PHARMACODYNAMIC MODELS

Wolfgang Sadée

School of Pharmacy, University of California

San Francisco, CA 94143

ABSTRACT

Drug response triggered by receptor activation arises from a chain of events that are regulated by many factors. Molecular changes associated with drug sensitization or tolerance are currently being elucidated on the molecular level, e.g. for adenylate cyclase coupled systems. Despite the complexity of the drug-response mechanism, simple empirical pharmaco-dynamic models on the basis of the law of mass action are widely applicable to describe drug-effect relationships. In combination with a pharmacokinetic model and suitable delay functions, such models are capable of simulating the complete time course of drug action in vivo. The predictive potential of the pharmacokinetic-pharmacodynamic models should prove useful in evaluating pharmaceutical formulations with controlled drug delivery.

INTRODUCTION

Significant insights have recently been gained into the molecular events during and after ligand-receptor binding. The number of neurotransmitter systems identified has proliferated to 50 and more, mostly neuropeptides that are processed from larger precursor molecules (Krieger, 1983; Snyder and Goodman, 1980). With such complexity, drug action is not readily understood on the basis of interaction with one single receptor system,

35

even though some drugs are thought to be specific. First,
each transmitter system does not operate in isolation, but
it can cause changes throughout several pathways, and
second, many drugs are already known to interact with
multiple receptor systems. For example, antidepressants
bind to dopaminergic, α-adrenergic, muscarinic
cholinergic, serotonergic and histaminergic receptors to
varying degrees (Hall and Ögren, 1981). Similarly, many
opioid drugs cross-react with each of the μ, δ, and κ
opioid types of the opioid receptor (Snyder and Goodman,
1980). Such receptor promiscuity of drugs must be
considered with their mechanism of action.

In case of coupling of the neurotransmitter receptor
to a catalytic unit, e.g. adenylate cyclase, many factors
are known to change the responsiveness of the signal
transduction (Table I). Of pharmacological importance are
changes caused by continuous exposure to agonist drugs,
that frequently lead to desensitization, tolerance or
tachophylaxis by various mechanisms. Involvement of
several receptor systems and the complex regulation of
each individual system, taken together,

Table I. Changes in responsiveness to drug effects
(sensitization, up-regulation; tolerance, tachophylaxis,
down-regulation). Examples are limited to molecular
changes of signal transducing systems across membranes of
the receptor-adenylate cyclase type system and related
coupled systems (e.g. Rodbell, 1980). Such systems are
thought to consist of at least three components, the
receptor (R), a coupling protein (G) and a catalytic unit
(C; e.g. adenylate cyclase). Coupling proteins can either
stimulate (G_s) or inhibit (G_i) the catalytic activity;
they consist of at least two subunits ($G_{s\alpha}$ or $G_{i\alpha}$ and G_β,
where G_β apparently is common to G_s and G_i) (Gilman,
1984). Physiological changes of several interacting
receptor systems are not included.

Biochemical-molecular change	Selected references
1. Increase or decrease in the number of receptors; up- and down-regulation.	Tempel et al., 1984; Law et al., 1983 and 1984, etc.
2. Changes in the receptor reserve i.e., the ratio of receptors to regulatory-	Chavkin and Goldstein, 1982

catalytic units.

3. Covalent modification (e.g. phosphorylation) of the receptor with altered coupling efficiency.	Strulovici et al., 1984
4. Covalent modification of the coupling protein G (e.g. ADP-ribosylation of G_s by cholera toxin and of G_i by bordetella toxin.	Katada and Ui, 1982
5. Genetic deficiency of the coupling protein (postulated in certain types of hyperparathyroidism.	Farfel et al., 1980
6. Genetic alteration of various components of the transducing system resulting in impaired coupling.	Various mechanisms
7. Possible exchange of the G_β subunit among G_s and G_i, changing their integrating regulatory capacity.	Gilman, 1984
8. Changes of the response cascade, e.g. altered cycl. AMP response, changes of phospho-diesterase and proteo-phosphatases.	Various mechanisms
9. Interaction of stimulatory receptors with the inhibitory coupling unit.	Asano et al., 1984
10. Enhancement of guanine nucleotide stimulation of adenylate cyclase.	Menkes et al., 1983
11. Coupling changes during the cell cycle.	Scheideler et al., 1983

should caution one with the interpretation of pharmacodynamic models that greatly simplify the relationship between dose and effect. In many instances, pharmacodynamic models may serve to simply describe and possibly predict a pharmacological outcome, while their use as mechanistic tools may be rather limited when applied to whole organisms.

RECEPTOR OCCUPANCY – EFFECT RELATIONSHIP

Most pharmacodynamic models are based on a linear

relationship between occupied receptors and effect, i.e. the fractional occupancy hypothesis where effect is proportional to the fractional receptor occupancy (see Ariens and Simonis, 1964a,b). Hence, drug concentration-effect models can be written in terms of the law of mass action, assuming that drug receptor-binding follows the law of mass action. Moreover, half-maximal effect should be achieved at 50% receptor occupancy. However, the effect is usually not directly linked to the activated receptor, but rather an intermediate second messenger (e.g., cyclic AMP), and an amplification cascade (e.g. protein kinases) precedes cellular response (Fig. 1). It can be argued on theoretical grounds that receptor occupancy by an agonist in indirect receptor-effect systems is necessarily lower than expected from the fractional occupancy hypothesis (Holford, 1984; Strickland and Loeb, 1981). Furthermore, low fractional occupancy by agonists might be expected from saturation of the amplification cascade and the presence of spare receptors among other factors (Perry et al., 1982). In particular, the presence of spare receptors, i.e., more receptors than available effector units, may be a widespread phenomenon that varies from one tissue to another and can profoundly affect the actions of partial agonists (Ariens and van Rossum, 1960).

Whether pharmacodynamic models based on the law of mass action remain valid or useful under these conditions remains to be investigated. We have recently shown that the antinociceptive action of etorphine and sufentanil indeed occurs at an exceedingly low fractional occupancy at the μ opioid receptor (Rosenbaum et al., 1984a,b). In contrast, the fractional μ receptor occupancy of the competitive antagonists naloxone and diprenorphine paralleled the inhibition of the agonist's action, which suggests that the fractional receptor occupancy hypothesis applies here, but only in the case of the antagonist action.

DRUG CONCENTRATION-EFFECT RELATIONSHIP

In the simplest case we may assume a linear relationship, $E = S \cdot C + I$ (E = effect, S = proportionality factor; C = drug concentration, I = initial baseline measurement). The log-linear model, $E = S \cdot \log C + I$, often provides a reasonable approximation

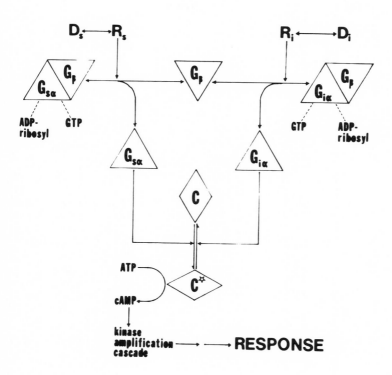

Fig. 1 Schematic representation (adopted from Gilman, 1984) of the proposed interactions among the various components of the receptor–adenylate cyclase coupled system, consisting of the receptor units R, the coupling proteins G and the cata-lytic units C. The subunits of G_s (stimulatory) and G_i (inhibitory) are further discussed in the legend of Table I. Note the competition of G_s and G_i for the proposed common G_β subunit. G_β may inhibit G_s stimulation of adenylate cyclase (Gilman, 1984). Any drug intervention sets all of these reactions into motion. ADP-ribosylation of the G_s or G_i subunits by bacterial toxins can lead to permanent activation of the coupling units. Many receptor–adenylate cyclase systems demonstrate receptor reserve, i.e., a larger number of R than G–C units.

in the range of 20 to 80% of maximum effect (Levy, 1966), but it fails to describe drug effects at very high or low

doses. This can be accomplished with the help of the Emax
model that is

$$E = \frac{E_{max} \cdot C}{EC_{50} + C} \ ,$$

where EC_{50} is the concentration causing half maximum
effect. If dose and drug concentration in the body are
proportional to each other, C can also be expressed in
drug dosage units. However, this model fails to fit many
dose-response curves, and more flexibility is gained with
the sigmoidal Emax model:

$$E \ \frac{E_{max} \cdot C^n}{EC_{50}^{\ n} + C^n} \ .$$

This model was originally proposed by Hill (1910) to
describe oxygen-hemoglobin association with the exponent n
representing the number of ligands combining with a
receptor. The Hill equation was later suggested by Wagner
(1968) to be applied to drug concentration-effect
relationships in vivo. In this case, n does not assume
any relevance regarding molecular stoichiometry, but it is
simply used to reflect the steepness of the dose-effect
curve.

The sigmoidal Emax system can be extended to the
interaction of agonists and antagonists, on the basis of
receptor theory (Ariens and Simonis, 1984a,b).

$$E = \frac{E_{max} \cdot A^n}{A^n + [ED_{50}(1 + \frac{B}{ID_{50}})]^n} \ ,$$

where A = dose of agonist, B = dose of antagonist, and
ID_{50} = antagonist dose which doubles the agonists dose
required to produce 50% effect. We have employed this
equation to fit the dose-response curve of etorphine in
the presence of increasing doses of the antagonist
naloxone (Fig. 2) (Rosenbaum et al., 1984). The fit
provides good estimates of ED_{50}, ID_{50} and n, which was 3.6
in this case. The n value for sufentanil in a similar
experiment was found to be n=16, essentially indicating an
all-or-none response. These values can then be compared
to in vivo receptor occupancy (Rosenbaum et al., 1984b) to
determine fractional occupancy at the ED_{50} and ID_{50} as
discussed above.

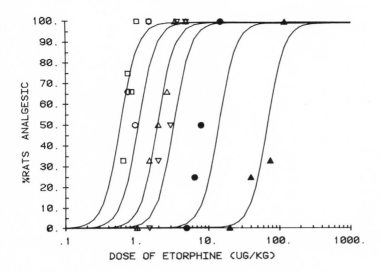

Fig. 2. Dose-response curves for etorphine (rat tail-flick test) in the presence of increasing naloxone doses. □ , etorphine alone; ○ , + 5 µg/kg naloxone; △ , + 15)g/kg naloxone, ▽ , + 30 µg/kg naloxone; ● , + 150 µg naloxone; ▲ , + 750 µg/kg naloxone. Each point represents the percentage of the rats at that dose which did not flick their tails by cutoff (3-5 rats/dose). The curves represent the computer-generated predictions for the competitive equation of the sigmoidal Emax model where the ED_{50} of etorphine = 0.59 µg/kg, the ID_{50} of naloxone = 6.5 µg/kg and n = 3.6. The dose-response curves were constructed in 3 sets of experiments with different batches of rats from the same lot (i.e. different days) which may account for the relatively poor fit for some of the response data. (Reproduced from Brain Research; Rosenbaum, et al., 1984a).

Such studies represent one example of the application of pharmacodynamic models to identify receptor function with the use of agonists and, more importantly, antagonist. However, the empirical nature of the pharmacodynamic model must be clearly recognized. Nevertheless, the ability to directly connect receptor binding events with a pharmacological response of great complexity, i.e., analgesia, supports the validity of the use of pharmacodynamic models on the basis of the law of mass action.

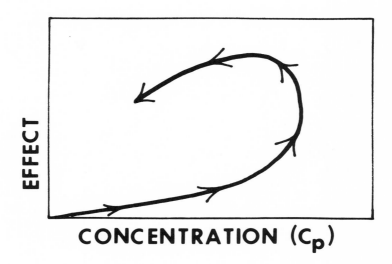

EFFECT

CONCENTRATION (C_p)

Fig. 3. Relationship between Drug Concentration (Cp) and
Effect when there is a delay in equilibrium between C and
the effect compartment.   A counter-clockwise hysteresis loop
is obtained by joining the observation points in time
sequence. (The arrow indicates the sequence of observations.) An inverse hysteresis loop may bo obtained when
drug tolerance occurs over the observation period.

THE PHARMACOKINETIC-PHARMACODYNAMIC LINK

     To assess the time course of drug effects in the body
requires the simultaneous modeling of drug concentration
and pharmacological effect. Since drug plasma levels are
most readily accessible, they usually serve as a basis for
the pharmacokinetic-pharmacodynamic link. In the simplest
case one might assume that the drug levels in plasma, i.e.
in the central compartment, are in immediate equilibrium
with the target site and that the effect ensues without
delay. Hence, drug plasma levels could be fitted into the
sigmoidal Emax model without further manipulations.
However, in most cases a significant delay occurs until
the effect is established (for reviews see Holford and
Sheiner, 1982; Colburn, 1981; Sheiner et al., 1979;
Holford, 1984). The hysteresis loop shown in Fig. 3

exemplifies the relationship between plasma level and effect when a significant delay occurs. The effect delay can result from slow equilibration of drug access and binding to its receptor or from slow expression of the effect after receptor activation. The delayed action of warfarin as a function of prothrombin turn-over rates represents an example of the latter case. The two pharmacodynamic models are quite different, as the delay time is independent of the drug dosage only in the latter case.

To solve the delay during access to the target site, it was first suggested to employ a "deep" or tissue compartment rather than the central compartment as the effect site (e.g. Wagner et al., 1968). However, Sheiner and coworkers pointed out that the effect site may not contain a sizeable fraction of the drug in the body, and therefore, may prove to be kinetically different from a peripheral compartment. Indeed, Dahlström et al. (1978) found that morphine brain levels correlated poorly with analgesia in rats. Sheiner proposed a model with a hypothetical (infinitesimal volume) entity that is linked to Cp by a first order rate process (Fig. 4), but whose exponential does not enter into the pharmacokinetic solution for the mass of the drug in the body (Sheiner et al., 1979). Changes of drug in the effect compartment (C_e) are thus given by

$$dC_e/dt = k_{eo} \ (C_p - C_e),$$

where k_{eo} represents the first order rate constant out of the effect compartment. In this model the first order rate constant k_{eo} determines the rate of equilibration with the effect compartment and hence the delay. Typical equilibration half-lives for the effect compartment are (Holford and Sheiner, 1982):

disopyramide	2 min
d-tubocurarine	4 min
quinidine	8 min
cimetidine	~ 1 hr
digoxin	~ 3 hrs

The hypothetical amount of drug in the effect compartment is then related to the observed effect by the Hill equation (sigmoidal Emax model). The elegance of this linking model stems from the introduction of only three new parameters (in addition to the pharmacokinetic

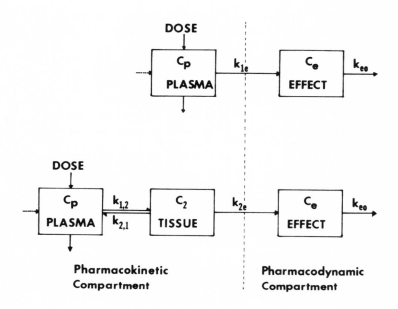

Fig. 4. Pharmacokinetic-pharmacodynamic models connecting the central or a peripheral compartment with the effect compartment. Because of the hypothetical infinitesimal size of the effect compartment, drug amount in the body is not affected and k_{eo}, the rate that regulates equilibration with the effect compartment, does not feed back into the body compartments (Holford and Sheiner, 1982; Colburn, 1981).

parameters) that must be estimated to completely characterize the time course of drug action:

   n, the exponent of the Hill equation which
   determines the steepness of the dose-response curve.
   k_{eo}, the equilibration rate constant (rate out) of
   the effect compartment.
   $C_{pss}(50)$, drug concentration at steady state under
   constant infusion that causes 50% effect.

Modifications of the linking model by Sheiner and coworkers have been proposed by Colburn (1981), where the hypothetical effect compartment is connected to a peripheral compartment rather than the central compartment. These pharmacodynamic models have proven quite useful in describing the relationships among drug dosage, plasma level and effect. However, it is imperative to keep in mind the empirical nature of this descriptive tool.

RECEPTOR MICRO-COMPARTMENT

While the simple effect compartment model of Sheiner et al. is sufficient to describe and predict the time course of action for many drugs, it cannot accommodate more complex dose-response relationships. For example, the biphasic effect curve of clonidine which lowers blood pressure at low drug concentrations but raises it at high concentrations, requires a more flexible model, for example on the basis of the interaction of the drug with two different receptors with opposite effects (Paalzow and Edlund, 1979). Furthermore, Sheiner suggested that certain drugs (e.g., neostigmine) do not equilibrate rapidly with the receptor in the effect compartment, such that after stopping the drug infusion the effect declines rather slowly while the C_p falls rapidly. To solve this problem it is necessary to explicitly model the drug receptor interaction in vivo.

We have noticed previously that certain potent neurotransmitter antagonists bind tenaciously to their receptor sites in vivo. Thus, ^{3}H labeled tracers of quinuclidinyl benzilate, spiroperidol and diprenorphine are retained in the brain over many hours, while the tracers are rapidly eliminated from other tissues that lack specific receptors (Perry et al., 1980; and references therein). This retention phenomenon suggested to us the possible existence of a micro-compartment with restricted drug diffusion next to the receptor sites. Such a model is depicted in Fig. 5. Within the micro-compartment the drug molecule can either diffuse away or associate with the receptor. If the rate of diffusion out of the micro-compartment is slower than the rate onto the receptor, a ligand molecule reassociates several times before diffusing away. Diprenorphine served as the model drug to test this model, since ~ 70% of the ^{3}H activity in the brain is receptor bound after tracer doses. Both tracer dilution and pulse-chase experiments with ^{3}H-diprenorphine conformed well with the micro-compartment model (Fig. 5), while certain other models were ruled out. We found that if the model is valid diprenorphine

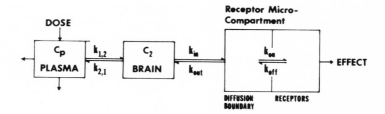

Fig. 5. The receptor micro-compartment model (Perry et al., 1980). A diffusion boundary compartment (e.g. the synaptic cleft or a similar physiological correlate) is introduced to account for an additional delay in drug-receptor interaction. If $k_{out} < k_{on}$, significant accumulation of drug in the receptor micro-compartment may occur, and tracers are retained for prolonged time periods (given sufficiently high receptor affinity or a small k_{off}). This model was capable of fitting the time course of diprenorphine disposition in the brain, 70% of which is bound to the receptor at tracer doses (Perry et al., 1980). Given a proportionality of fractional receptor occupancy and response for diprenorphine (Rosenbaum et al., 1984a), this receptor micro-compartmental model can readily be converted into a pharmacodynamic model that may be more suitable for diprenorphine's pharmacological effects than the models show in Figure 3.

reassociates ~ 7 times with the receptor before diffusing away. Taken together with its rather slow in vivo receptor dissociation rate (~ 10 min half-life), (Kurowski et al., 1982), the overall half-life of tracer elimination from the brain was ~ 2 hrs, while it was much more rapid from plasma.

The receptor binding kinetics of diprenorphine represent a clear example where rapid equilibrium does not occur and receptor equilibration should be part of a pharmacodynamic model. A physical representation of the receptor micro-compartment could be the synaptic cleft and a receptor cluster embedded in the cell membrane; hence, the model might apply more generally to potent neurotransmitter drugs. Moreover, the diprenorphine example shows that pharmacokinetic-pharmacodynamic models need to be fine-tuned to extend their general utility and to better account for the physiological and biochemical events during the expression of drug action. Significant advances in our understanding of drug action in the intact body could thus arise from the joint application of pharmacokinetic-pharmacodynamic models and controlled drug delivery.

REFERENCES

Ariens, E.J. and Simonis, A.M., A molecular basis of drug action. J. Pharm. Pharmacol., 16 (1964a) 137–157.

Ariens, E.J. and Simonis, A.M., A molecular basis for drug action. The interaction of one or more drugs with different receptors. J. Pharm. Pharmacol., 16 (1964b), 289–312.

Ariens, E.J., van Rossum, J.M. and Koopman, P.C., Receptor reserve and threshold phenomena. I. Theory and experiments with autonomic drugs tested on isolated organs. Arch. Int. Pharmacodyn. 127 (1960) 459–478.

Asano, T., Katada, T., Gilman, A.G. and Ross, E.M., Activation of the inhibitory GTP-binding protein of adenylate cyclase, G_i, by β-adrenergic receptors in reconstituted phospholipid vesicles. J. Biol. Chem., 259 (1984) 9351–9354.

Chavkin, C. and Goldstein, A., Reduction in opiate receptor reserve in morphine tolerant guinea pig ilea. Life Sci., 31 (1982) 1687–1690.

Colburn, W.A., Simultaneous pharmacokinetic and pharmacodynamic modeling. J. Pharmacokin. Biopharm., 9 (1981) 367–388.

Dahlström, B.E., Paalzow, L.K., Segre, G. and Ågren, A.J., Relation between morphine pharmacokinetics and analgesia. J. Pharmacokin. Biopharm., 6 (1978) 41–53.

Farfel, Z.A., Brickman, A.S., Kaslow, H.R., Brothers, V.M. and Bourne, H.R., N. Engl. J. Med., 303 (1980) 237–242.

Gilman, A.G., Proteins and dual control of adenylate cyclase. Cell, 36 (1984) 577–579.

Hall, H. and Ögren, S.-O., Effects of antidepressant drugs on different receptors in the brain. Europ. J. Pharmacol., 70 (1981) 393–407.

Hill, A.V., The possible effects of the aggregation of the molecules of haemoglobin on its dissociation curves. J. Physiol. (Lond.), 40 (1910) iv–vii.

Holford, N.H.G., Drug concentration, binding and effect in vivo. Pharm. Res., (1984) 102–105.

Holford, N.H.G. and Sheiner, L.B., Kinetics of
    pharmacological response. Pharmac. Ther., 16
    (1982) 143–166.
Katada, T. and Ui, M., ADP ribosylation of the specific
    membrane protein of CG cells by islet activating
    protein associated with modification of adenylate
    cyclase activity. J. Biol. Chem., 257 (1982) 7210–
    7216.
Kurowski, M_3, Rosenbaum, J.S_3, Perry, D.C. and Sadée,
    W., ^{3}H–Etorphine and ^{3}H–diprenorphine receptor
    binding in vitro and in vivo. Differential effects
    of Na^+ and GPP(NH)P. Brain Res. 249 (1982) 345–
    352.
Krieger, D.T. Brain peptides. What, where, why?
    Science, 222 (1983) 975–985.
Law, P.Y., Hom, D.S. and Loh, H.H., Opiate receptor
    down–regulation and desensitization in
    neuroblastoma x glioma NG–108–15 hybrid cells are
    two separate cellular adaptation processes. Molec.
    Pharmacol., 24 (1983) 413–424.
Law, P.-Y., Hom, D.S. and Loh, H.H., Down–regulation of
    opiate receptor in neuroblastoma x glioma NG 108–15
    hybrid cells. J. Biol. Chem., 259 (1984) 4096–
    4104.
Levy, G., Kinetics of pharmacological effect. Clin.
    Pharmacol. Ther., 7 (1966) 362–372.
Menkes, D.B., Rasenick, M.M., Wheeler, M.A. and Bitensky,
    M.W., Guanosine triphosphate activation of brain
    adenylate cyclase: Enhancement by long–term
    antidepressant treatment. Science, 219 (1983) 65–
    67.
Paalzow, L.K. and Edlund, P.O., Multiple receptor
    responses: A new concept to describe the
    relationship between pharmacological effects and
    pharmacokinetics of a drug: Studies on clonidine
    in the rat and cat. J. Pharmacokin. Biopharm., 7
    (1979) 495–510.
Perry, D.C., Mullis, K.B., Oie, S. and Sadée, W.,
    Opiate antagonist receptor binding in vivo:
    Evidence for a new receptor binding model. Brain
    Res., 199 (1980) 46–61.
Perry, D.C., Rosenbaum, J.S., Kurowski, M. and Sadée
    W., [^{3}H]Etorphine receptor binding in vivo: Small
    fractional occupancy elicits analgesia. Molec.
    Pharmacol., 21 (1982) 272–279.
Rodbell, M., The role of hormone receptors and GTP–

     regulatory proteins in membrane transduction.
     Nature, 284 (1980) 17–22.

Rosenbaum, J.S., Holford, N.H.G. and Sadée, W.,
     Opiate receptor binding-effect relationship:
     Sufentanil and etorphine produce analgesia at the
     μ-site with low fractional occupancy. Brain Res.,
     291 (1984a) 317–324.

Rosenbaum, J.S., Holford, N.H.G., Richards, M.L., Aman,
     R.A. and Sadée, W., Discrimination of three types
     of opiate binding sites in rat brain in vivo.
     Molec. Pharmacol., 25 (1984b) 242–248.

Scheideler, M.A., Lockney, M.W. and Dawson, G., Cell
     cycle-dependent expression of specific opiate
     binding with variable coupling to adenylate cyclase
     in a neurotumor hybrid cell line NG 108–15. J.
     Neurochem., 41 (1983) 1261–1268.

Scheiner, L.B., Stanski, D.R., Vozeh, S., Miller, R.D.
     and Ham, J., Simultaneous modeling of
     pharmacokinetics and pharmacodynamics: Application
     to d-tubocurarine. Clin. Pharmacol. Ther. 25
     (1979) 358–371.

Snyder, S.H. and Goodman, R.R., Multiple neurotrans-
     mitter receptors. J. Neurochem., 35 (1980) 5–15.

Strickland, S. and Loeb, J.N. Obligatory separation of
     hormone binding and biological response curves in
     systems dependent upon secondary mediators of
     hormone action. Proc. Natl. Acad. Sci. USA, 78
     (1981) 1366–1370.

Strulovici, B., Cerione, R.A., Kilpatrick, B.F., Caron,
     M.G. and Lefkowitz, R.J. Direct demonstration of
     impaired functionality of a purified desensitized
     β-adrenergic receptor in a reconstituted system.
     Science, 225 (1984) 837–840.

Tempel, A., Gardner, E.L. and Zukin, R.S., Visualization
     of opiate receptor upregulation by light microscopy
     autoradiography. Proc. Natl. Acad. Sci. USA, 81
     (1984) 3893–3897.

Wagner, J.G., Kinetics of pharmacological response.
     I. Proposed relationship between response and drug
     concentration in the intact animal and man. J.
     Theoret. Biol., 20 (1968) 173–201.

Wagner, J.G., Aghajanian, G.K. and Bing, O.H.L.,
     Correlation of performance test scores with "tissue
     concentration" of lysergic acid diethylamide in
     human subjects. Clin. Pharmacol. Ther., 9 (1968)
     635–638.

THE THERAPEUTIC SYSTEM: THERAPEUTIC IMPLICATIONS OF RATE-
CONTROLLED DRUG DELIVERY

John Urquhart, M.D.
ALZA Corporation
950 Page Mill Road
Palo Alto, California 94304 USA

The concept of the therapeutic system (Anonymous, 1970, 1971; Heilmann, 1982) brought Tak Higuchi and Alex Zaffaroni together in a day-to-day working collaboration that continued for over 4 years between 1969 and 1972. Higuchi's laboratory played a major role in developing the first two therapeutic system products, which have embodied a number of pharmaceutical "firsts". These are the pilo-carpine ocular therapeutic system and the progesterone uterine therapeutic system.

The ocular therapeutic system pilocarpine, for example, is the first pharmaceutical to carry strength labelling by rate and duration of drug delivery, rather than simply by drug content. It was also the first gamma-sterilized ophthalmic and only the 2nd gamma-sterilized pharmaceutical to enter the U.S. market (Urquhart, 1980). This product gave the first clear demonstration of how constant-rate drug delivery could make important changes in the side-effects profile of a drug. These results stimu-lated the pharmacodynamic thinking that led to the concept of "steady-state" or "zero-order" pharmacology (Urquhart, 1979, 1981, 1985).

The uterine therapeutic system progesterone was the first hormonal contraceptive based upon a physiological steroid, rather than a pharmacological one. It is the first intra-uterine contraceptive with registered therapeutic claims (reduced menstrual blood loss and cramps) in most

51

major markets, in addition to a contraceptive claim
(Pizarro et al., 1979; Bergqvist and Rybo, 1983). Moreover, recent European work (Volpe et al., 1982) shows the
product's ability to reverse endometrial hyperplasia; if
and when this claim is registered, it will be another first
in the intra-uterine contraceptive field.

Another facet of Higuchi's contribution to the therapeutic systems field was the miniaturization of the osmotic
pump. Miniaturization made possible the development of the
osmotic pump implants (Theeuwes and Yum, 1976) that are now
internationally used for multiday or multiweek programmed
drug delivery in laboratory animals. These osmotic pump
implants bring the functional capability of the therapeutic
system down to the animal research level, allowing drugs to
be assessed with rate-controlled, constant or programmed
delivery. By the fall of 1984 there were about one thou-
sand publications based upon use of these delivery systems,
which have opened up a wide variety of new investigative
techniques in drug and hormone research (Urquhart et al.,
1984).

Other papers in this symposium will consider the
physicochemical, pharmaceutical, mass transport, and membrane aspects of these and other delivery systems. My aim
is to discuss how osmotic pump implants in preclinical
studies, and therapeutic systems in clinical studies are
influencing therapeutics, pharmacology, and pharmacodynamics.

With registration and introduction of the transdermal
scopolamine product for motion sickness, the therapeutic
system concept was extended from localized to systemic
action. This product is supported by extensive data in
both the pharmacodynamic and the biopharmaceutical areas
(Shaw and Urquhart, 1980; ALZA Corporation NDA 17-784). It
is the first systemically-acting pharmaceutical to have its
label strength rated by in vivo rate/duration of delivery,
and is also the first rate-controlled pharmaceutical to
execute a specified time-varying pattern of drug delivery
rate: a loading dose, followed by a constant rate for three
days. On the pharmacodynamic side, the development of this
product wrote a new chapter on the steady-state pharmacology of scopolamine, with an unprecedented separation
between the drug's beneficial vestibular effects and its
other undesirable effects (Shaw and Urquhart, 1980; ALZA

Corporation, NDA 17-784). This product did not arise out of
work here in Lawrence, but it is an important step in the
history of therapeutic systems.

When you consider jointly the steady-state pharma-
cologies of pilocarpine and of scopolamine, quite a strong
and encouraging picture emerges of the prospects of using
rate-control to enhance the selectivity of drug action. To
be sure, both agents act within the parasympathetic nervous
system, and fortunately have therapeutic actions that are
elicited at the lowest rates of drug delivery. With other
agents, acting upon other physiological systems, it does
not necessarily follow that the therapeutically useful
action will be elicited by the lowest rate of drug administration. It remains for future work to know which drugs
have a steady-state pharmacology that shows their most
useful actions to be elicited by the lowest rates of administration.

In animal pharmacology, a very important new concept
in pharmacodynamic testing has emerged from work stimulated
by the availability of the miniature osmotic pumps
(Theeuwes and Yum, 1976). The first prototypes of these
pumps were designed and made here in Lawrence by Felix
Theeuwes, working under Tak's direction (Higuchi et al.,
1976). Felix was recruited by Tak Higuchi into pharmaceutical research from his original field of low temperature
physics.

Pharmacological research done with the miniature
osmotic pump implants has led to the concept of comparing
dose-response relations when drug is given by a sequence of
injections vs by a constant infusion.

A landmark study and, to the best of my knowledge, the
one that both defined and first systematically exploited
the injection-infusion comparison (IIC) principle, was done
by Sikic et al. (1978) on both the anti-tumor and the
toxicity dose-response relations of bleomycin. This work
showed that the constant-rate infusion mode of administration shifts the anti-tumor dose-response curve to the left,
but concomitantly shifts the toxicity dose-response curve
to the right, relative to the injection mode of administration. These results thus demonstrate that the therapeutic
index of bleomycin in the mouse tumor model is regimen- or
delivery-mode dependent to a striking degree. It suggests

that the drug might be more beneficially administered
clinically by constant infusion than by a series of injections (Carlson and Sikic, 1983), although that conclusion
is still the subject of some controversy (Osieka, 1984).

Another landmark IIC study was done by Nau et al.
(1981, 1984) on the embryotoxic effects of sodium valproate. They showed that the dose-response curves for the
drug's various embryotoxic effects in the mouse are shifted
markedly to the right when the drug is infused continuously
versus when it is injected once daily. This result is all
the more striking because the plasma half-life of injected
drug is less than an hour in the mouse; consequently, the
once-daily injection produces a high early peak of drug
concentration in plasma, followed by a rapid decline, with
undetectable concentrations from hours 4-5 until the next
injection at hour 24.

Nau's work suggests several important conclusions.
First, most drugs have much longer plasma half-lives in
humans than in the small animals that are widely used in
embryotoxicity testing; hence, the typical 1-3X/day regimens of human therapeutics may give very different plasma
concentration-time curves in the test animals than in man.
Second, one of the major pharmacokinetic differences to be
expected with the injection regimen is a period of some
hours prior to the next dose when the drug concentrations
in plasma and tissues are undetectably low; this is a basis
for under-estimating toxicity. Third, another major pharmacokinetic difference to be expected with the injection
regimen is a higher peak concentration in the test animals
than in humans; this is a basis for over-estimating toxicity. Thus, the IIC protocol might be thought of as a
pharmacodynamic probe that will identify drugs whose
regimen-dependent actions may give rise to errors of either
kind in embryotoxicity and other toxicologic evaluations.

One should not over-interpret these initial studies
with the IIC protocol. They involve two very differently
acting drugs for which the constant-rate regimen emerges as
preferable to the injection regimen. However, there are
bound to be other drugs that will show superiority of the
injection regimen. It seems reasonable to conclude that
the IIC protocol provides a practical means of identifying
regiment-dependent pharmacodynamics. Studies using this
protocol will can be expected to yield one of three dif-

ferent results: (1) the constant-rate delivery pattern is advantageous; (2) the intermittent pulse (injection) pattern is advantageous; (3) neither regimen has a pharmacodynamic advantage over the other (Fara and Urquhart, 1984).

John Fara and I have also pointed out that it may sometimes be advantageous to examine the dose-response characteristics of a "combined" regimen of intermittent injections superimposed upon a constant-rate infusion, in order to see how peak concentrations of the drug may interact with unremitting drug presence (Fara and Urquhart, 1984).

At the September 1984 European Teratology Society meetings in The Netherlands, further work with the IIC protocol was reported from Nau's group in Berlin on sodium valproate, and from the group of Gabrielson, Larsson, and Paalzow in Uppsala on salicylates. Nau led a workshop on the use of the IIC protocol in embryotoxicity testing, which was well-attended and evoked much interest. It appears that the IIC protocol is an important, practical advance in embryotoxicity testing. The IIC protocol seems not only applicable but also important in general pharmacology and toxicology, adding the usually missing pharmacodynamic element to dose-response relations.

Here one should note that many people abuse the term "pharmacodynamics" by using it to describe practically any kind of study in which a drug is given and some of its effects are observed, which is just garden-variety pharmacology with an extra syllable. The term "pharmacodynamics" should be reserved for some kind of systematic study of the comparative effects of different temporal patterns of administration of a particular drug. That is certainly consistent with how the term "dynamics" is used in physiology, the engineering sciences, and systems theory (cf. Urquhart, 1970). The IIC protocol appears to be a logical starting point for systematic pharmacodynamic studies.

The past decade has focussed almost exclusively on delivery systems and regimens that provide constant-rate ("zero-order") drug delivery. Current research is beginning to turn toward temporal patterning of drug administration, prompted in no small measure by Ernst Knobil's stunning discovery of how GnRH is normally secreted in a pulsatile pattern (cf. Knobil, 1980). As a consequence of its novel pharmacodynamics, GnRH (and its various synthetic analogs) is either an agonist or an antagonist for gonadotropin secretion, depending on the temporal pattern of its secretion or exogenous administration. Temporal patterning challenges pharmaceutical technologists to make the necessary hardware for therapeutic applications, but good tools for research in this area are already available. Thus, the much larger challenge confronts the pharmacologists to devise the protocols, i.e. the software, that can reveal therapeutically and toxicologically important pattern-dependencies. The past emphasis on constant-rate drug delivery notwithstanding, Alejandro Zaffaroni's original conception of the therapeutic system (Anonymous, 1970, 1971) anticipated that some drugs would need temporally patterned delivery for optimum action.

CONCLUSION

Both the concept of rate-control and the dimension of time in drug deployment in the body are opened up by the advent of practical embodiments of the therapeutic system concept: constant-rate and programmed-rate drug delivery systems. In new drug development, it is now practical to consider experimentally defining the optimum pattern of drug administration. The injection-infusion comparison (IIC) protocol can provide basic data from dose-response models in animals that can give direction to the always difficult task of defining the best regimen for a drug's use in humans. Delivery system technology now makes such considerations practical, in contrast to the situation fifteen years ago when the first work on therapeutic systems began here in Lawrence. Tak Higuchi and his colleagues made the first therapeutic systems hardware, and its accessibility has in turn stimulated very important advances in the software that is known as pharmacodynamics.

ACKNOWLEDGMENT

Many people at ALZA worked on the development of the various therapeutic systems. Two who merit special acknowledgment are Dr. John W. Shell, who led the development of the ocular therapeutic systems, and Dr. Virgil A. Place, whose innovative medical, regulatory, and other judgments have had a strong and beneficial influence on the development of all of ALZA's products.

REFERENCES

Anonymous, Towards a new concept of precision in drug administration. Pharm. J., 205 (1970) 400–402.

Anonymous, ALZA's approach to controlled medication. Pharm. J., 207 (1971) 414–415.

Bergqvist, A. and Rybo, G., Treatment of menorrhagia with intrauterine release of progesterone. Br. J. Obstet. Gynaecol., 90 (1983) 255–258.

Carlson, R. W. and Sikic, B. I., Continuous infusion or bolus injection in cancer chemotherapy. Ann. Intern. Med., 99 (1983) 823–833.

Fara, J. and Urquhart, J., The value of infusion and injection regimens in assessing efficacy and toxicity of drugs. Trends Pharmacol. Sci., 5 (1984) 21–25.

Heilmann, K., Therapeutische Systeme—Konzept und Realisation programmierter Arzneiverabreichung. 2. uberarbeitete und erweiterte Auflage, Ferdinand Enke Verlag, Stuttgart, 1982.

Higuchi, T., Leeper, H. M., and Theeuwes, F., U.S. Patent 3,995,631, Osmotic dispenser with means for dispensing active agent responsive to osmotic gradient, issued 7 December 1976.

Knobil, E., The neuroendocrine control of the menstrual cycle. Rec. Prog. Horm. Res., 36 (1980) 53–88.

Nau, H., Merker, H. J., Brendel, K., Gansau, C., Häuser, I., and Wittfoht, W., Disposition, embryotoxicity, and teratogenicity of valproic acid in the mouse as related to man. In Levy, R. H., Ritlick, W. H., Eichelbaum, M., and Meijer, J. (Eds) Metabolism of Antiepileptic Drugs, Raven Press, New York, 1984, pp. 85–96.

Nau, H., Zierer, R., Spielmann, H., Neubert, D., and Gansau, C., A new model for embryotoxicity testing: teratogenicity and pharmacokinetics of valproic acid following constant-rate administration in the mouse using human therapeutic drug and metabolite concentrations. Life Sci., 29 (1981) 2803–2813.

Osieka, V. R., Continuous infusion vs. bolus injection of bleomycin in a human testicular cancer xenograft system. Arzneim. Forsch., 34 (1984) 460–464.

Pizarro, E., Gomez-Rogers, C., and Rowe, P. J., A comparative study of the effect of the PROGESTASERT and GRAVIGARD IUDs on dysmenorrhoea. Contraception, 20 (1979) 455–466.

Shaw, J. and Urquhart, J., Programmed systemic drug delivery by the transdermal route. Trend Pharmacol. Sci., 1

(1980) 208-211.

Sikic, B. I., Collins, J. M., Mimnaugh, E. G., and Gram, T.
E., Improved therapeutic index of bleomycin when admin-
istered by continuous infusion in mice. Cancer Treat.
Rep., 62 (1978) 2011-2017.

Theeuwes, F. and Yum, S. I., Principles of the design and
operation of generic osmotic pumps for the delivery of
semisolid or liquid drug formulations. Ann. Biomed.
Eng., 4 (1976) 343-353.

Urquhart, J., Endocrinology and the systems paradigm.
Behav. Sci., 15 (1970) 57-71.

Urquhart, J., Opportunities for research: methods of drug
administration. In Proceedings of the Institute of
Medicine Conference on Pharmaceuticals for Developing
Countries, National Academy of Sciences, Washington,
D. C., 1979, pp. 329-348.

Urquhart, J., Development of the OCUSERT pilocarpine ocular
therapeutic systems--a case history in ophthalmic product development. In Robinson, J. (Ed) Ophthalmic Drug
Delivery Systems, American Pharmaceutical Association,
Academy of Pharmaceutical Sciences, Washington, D. C.,
1980, pp. 105-118.

Urquhart, J., Performance requirements for controlled-
release dosage forms: therapeutic and pharmacological
perspectives. In Urquhart, J. (Ed) Controlled-Release
Pharmaceuticals, American Pharmaceutical Association,
Academy of Pharmaceutical Sciences, Washington, D. C.,
1981, pp. 1-48.

Urquhart, J., Drug development and preclinical research
applications of steady-state pharmacology. In Prescott,
L. F. and Nimmo, W. S. (Eds) Rate Control in Drug
Therapy, Churchill Livingstone, Edinburgh, 1985, pp.
19-29.

Urquhart, J., Fara, J., and Willis, K. L., Rate-controlled
delivery systems in drug and hormone research. Ann.
Rev. Pharmacol. Toxicol., 24 (1984) 199-236.

Volpe, A., Botticelli, A., Abrate, M., Vecchia, E. D.,
Mantovani, M., Carani, C., Grasso, A., Mazza, V., and
Di Renzo, G. C., An intrauterine progesterone contraceptive system (52 mg) used in pre- and peri-menopausal
patients with endometrial hyperplasia. Maturitas, 4
(1982) 73-79.

. PHYSIOLOGICAL AND BIOCHEMICAL FACTORS INFLUENCING DIRECTED DRUG DELIVERY

GASTROINTESTINAL BARRIER TO ORAL DRUG DELIVERY

Colin R. Gardner

INTERx-Merck Sharp & Dohme Research Laboratories

Lawrence, Kansas USA

INTRODUCTION

During the last ten to twenty years there have been major changes in the drug discovery process. As a result of a greater understanding of the pathology and biochemical defects responsible for disease processes the drug industry has moved from large scale screening operations to much more rational approaches to drug design in which active molecules are synthesized and tested on the basis of in vitro measurements of interactions with specific receptors or enzymes. While this process is very efficient in defining and refining structures active at the desired target site, it leaves problems of drug delivery largely unexplored until active lead compounds are tested in whole animal models. Questions of rate and extent of absorption, degree of pre-systemic metabolism and optimal delivery pattern are critical to the success of a therapeutic agent and deserve important attention in the development of new drug entities.

Despite growing interest in and use of other routes of delivery, oral drug administration predominates and will probably continue to do so for the foreseeable future. Therefore, optimizing the pattern of drug delivery to the patient involves controlling accurately and predictably the oral bioavailability of the drug species. In turn, this requires knowledge of the drug's interactions with the components of the gastrointestinal tract and careful assessment of the performance of the dosage form in controlling and manipulating these interactions to the best advantage. The important

Table I. Factors affecting rate and extent of drug absorption.

Physical Parameters	Physiological Parameters
solubility	regional and local pH
dissolution rate	drug binding and
molecular size	complexation
partition coefficient	intestinal permeability
sensitivity to chemical	drug metabolism - lumenal,
hydrolysis	mucosal, hepatic
delivery system	gastric and intestina:
	transit time

variables can be conveniently separated into physical and physiological parameters as shown in Table I. This review will concentrate on the latter, discussing the physical parameters only where they impinge on the biology of the process.

THE GASTROINTESTINAL TRACT

The gastrointestinal tract represents a hostile environment for any drug or drug dosage form. The stomach has, as its principal role, the storage and trituration of foodstuff prior to its release in a form which the small intestine can further process for absorption of components of nutritional value. In principle the stomach is not an absorbing organ, although, because of its low pH, it may play some role in the absorption of weak acids which are less highly charged under these conditions. The principal absorption sites are to be found in the small intestine - duodenum, jejunum and ileum, the total length of which is approximately 150 cm in the human. The pH ranges from 1-3 (or greater) in the stomach, through 4-5 in the duodenum to 7 and greater in the ileum. The transit through the small intestine is complex, consisting of many different modes of muscular activity which propel, mix and retropel the boli of fluid which have been released from the stomach.

The gi tract is lined with a covering of mucous consisting mainly of glycoprotein mucin but also containing dead cells and cell debris. This layer, which

can vary in thickness from 5 to 500 μm, is in a state of
constant turnover as it is degraded and abraded on its
lumenal side and replenished by secretion of new mucin
from the goblet cells of the gastric and intestinal
walls. The mucous layer is highly hydrated and probably
offers little resistance to the passage of small molecular
weight compounds (Sarosiek et. al., 1983) although the
possibility of ionic and hydrophobic binding must be
considered.

The absorption processes are numerous and varied,
consisting of simple passive diffusion, facilitated,
saturable transport and active, energy-dependent
processes. Enzymes in the gastric and intestinal juices,
bound in the glycocalyx, on the surface of the mucosal
cells, and within the cells themselves add further
barriers to the penetration of drug molecules into the
systemic circulation.

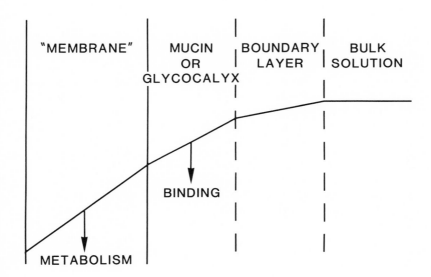

Fig. 1. Diagramatic representation of the barriers to
drug absorption.

A schematic representation of the intestinal barrier to drug absorption is shown in figure 1 where the composite structure is shown as a series of resistances which impede, to a greater or less extent, the passage of a molecule from the intestinal lumen to the systemic circulation.

The gastric and intestinal mucosae are capable of secreting acid and base and, thus, have the capability of either lowering or raising the pH within their microenvironments (Garner et. al., 1984). Evidence for this comes from a number of studies including direct measurement of the pH gradient in the gastric mucous layer (Bahari et. al., 1982), calculations of the effect of the mucin layer on the distribution of hydrogen ions in the environment of the stomach wall (Engel et. al., 1984) and measurement of the intestinal wall pH under conditions of different pH in the solution perfusing rat small intestine (Hogerle and Winne, 1983). Thus, knowledge of the pH in the intestinal lumen may not be sufficient to define the pH at the surface of the absorbing microvilli. Nevertheless, it is clear that more information regarding the nature of the gastrointestinal barrier can be obtained from in situ and in vitro experiments than can be procured from conducting only in vivo drug administration where so many of the key variables are both uncontrolled and indeterminate. It is in the context of this framework that studies can be conducted to assess the effects of

Table II. In situ and in vitro methods to estimate drug absorption.

In situ
    Perfused intestinal sections - animals, humans

    [Can be supplemented with sampling of appropriate fluids, e.g. portal blood or lymph in animal studies, blood and urine in human studies].

In vitro
    Everted intestinal sacs
    Everted intestinal rings
    Isolated mucosal cells
    Intestinal brush-border vesicles

structural and formulation variables on the absorption process.

Over the years a number of experimental procedures have been developed to examine the transport of drugs across the intestinal wall (Table II). Their potential applications and some examples of their use are discussed.

IN SITU INTESTINAL PERFUSION

Of all the methods available, this technique best allows control of the experimental variables such as lumenal pH, ionic composition, drug concentration etc. while still maintaining the intestine in a condition as close as possible to that pertaining in vivo. A number of different variations of the technique are available but single pass perfusion at relatively low flow rates to examine the absorption of small peptides has been chosen to illustrate the value of the method. The experimental set up is shown in figure 2. Two small synthetic peptides, believed to be stable in the gi tract were used: MK421 (enalapril), a pro-drug for MK422, a potent inhibitor of angiotensin converting enzyme (Sweet et. al., 1981), and L-363,586 a cyclic hexapeptide which is a very potent somatostatin analog (Veber et. al., 1981).

Enalapril is relatively well absorbed (50-60%) in a number of animal species including man (Tocco et. al., 1982) and is converted, probably in the liver, to MK422, the active inhibitor, which is itself poorly absorbed (Tocco et. al., 1982). The absorption profile of enalapril demonstrates rapid uptake (peak within 1-2 hours) with apparently little or no further absorption thereafter (Ulm et. al., 1982). An examination of the structure of the compound shows it to be a zwitterion with an isoelectric point at approximately pH 4.2. We postulated therefore that, since the pKa's of the acidic and basic groups are relatively close (3.0 and 5.4), optimum absorption might occur at the isoelectric point where the concentration of uncharged species would be significant and greatest. Since this pH is present only in the upper small intestine it was postulated that preferential absorption of the compound might occur in this region, accounting for the sharp in vivo absorption profile. The

in situ intestinal perfusion technique was considered
appropriate to address the pH-dependence of enalapril
absorption. Since this clearly involved perfusion of
intestinal segments in the acidic pH range, it was
necessary to carefully validate the technique particularly
with respect to water transport and the integrity of the
perfused intestinal tissue. Water transport was assessed
by three methods; weight of samples, and use of [³H] PEG
4000 or phenol red as non-absorbed markers. All three
techniques gave similar results and in subsequent experiments [³H] PEG and/or weights were used routinely. These
values were used to correct the effluent concentrations
for alterations due to fluid absorption or secretion (Selk
et. al., 1983). Histological examination of the tissue

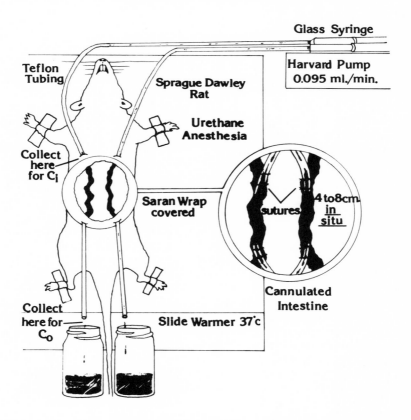

Fig. 2. In situ rat intestinal perfusion technique.

following two-hour perfusions under the prescribed
conditions showed that the tissue was not affected in the
pH range 4.0 to 9.0 but that at or below a lumenal pH of
3, significant damage was evident (Selk et. al., 1983).
No attempts were made to determine the exact wall pH, but
the buffer capacity of the solutions were maintained as
high as possible, consistent with isotonicity (which was
controlled by additional sodium chloride). Under these
conditions and using the data of Hogerle and Winne (1983)
it is probably that the wall pH approached that of the
lumenal solution.

Preliminary in vitro experiments indicated that
the partition coefficient of enalapril in an n-octanol/
aqueous buffer system was pH- but not concentration-
dependent, showing a ten-fold increase over the pH range
7.0 to 4.5 (Frederick and Gardner, unpublished data). The
in situ perfusion experiments using (^{14}C)-labelled MK421
gave the results shown in figure 3 (Selk et. al., 1983)
indicating a clear pH dependence of the absorption process
with a maximum in the pH 4-5 range. These results may
explain the absorption profile of enalapril and may also
explain why the zwitterion has much better bioavailability
than the diacid MK422.

The situation with L-363,586 was considerably more
complex. In vivo this compound shows extremely low
bioavailability (approximately 1-2%) despite its apparent
stability and the fact that a number of other peptide-like
compounds of higher molecular weight are reportedly well
absorbed (e.g. Beveridge et. al. 1981). Since L-363,586
is also zwitterionic with an isoelectric point near pH 10
(both ionizable groups have pKa's in this region) it was
postulated that absorption might be improved at higher
pH's (Gardner et. al., 1984). Since L-363,586 is well
cleared by the liver and is excreted in bile, cannulation
of the bile duct provided a convenient method to determine
if loss from the intestinal perfusate was really due to
absorption of the drug. Perfusions were run using pH 9
pyrophosphate buffers. In the presence of an intact bile
duct, there was little loss of (^{14}C)-labelled L-363,586
from the perfusate, and analysis of the effluent by HPLC
was also indicative of little absorption or metabolism of
the drug. Experiments run with cannulated bile ducts
indicated slightly greater, but still small, losses of

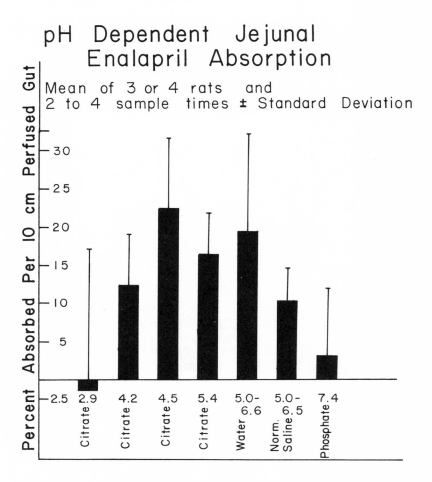

Fig. 3. Loss of MK421 (^{14}C) from in situ intestinal
        perfusate as a function of pH.

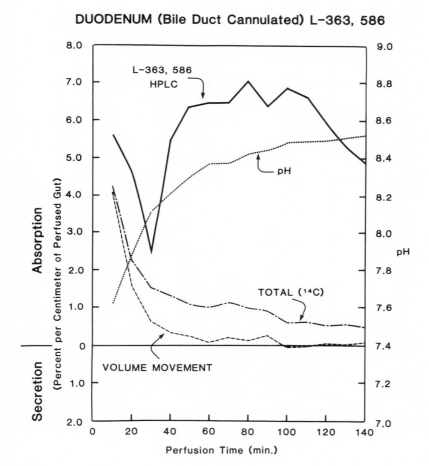

Fig. 4. HPLC and radioisotope analysis of loss of
L-363,586 from in situ intestinal perfusates.

(^{14}C) from the perfusate with appearance of similar
amounts of material in the bile. By contrast, when the
effluent was analyzed for drug content by HPLC, there was
very significant loss of material (figure 4). Radio-
isotopic analysis of the HPLC fractions showed that
^{14}Carbon was present in two major fractions, one
corresponding to intact drug, and another whose identity

is unknown. Subsequent in vitro incubations of labelled drug with perfusates in the presence or absence of bile revealed that there was time-dependent breakdown of the parent compound when bile was absent but that this metabolism was essentially absent when bile was present or when fresh buffer was used. The agent which causes this degradation remains undetermined as yet, but the data indicate the need to use independent methods of analysis even when putatively stable peptide analogs are being examined. Experiments with natural peptides which are good substrates for intestinal enzymatic activity are even more complex to conduct and interpret.

Since small peptides are likely to occur with increasing frequency as drugs of the future it will be necessary to understand the mechanisms whereby they are processed and absorbed by the gi tract. Such information may be of critical importance to the medicinal chemists who attempt to synthesize orally absorbed peptide analogs.

IN VITRO ABSORPTION TECHNIQUES

While providing useful information on the absorption of drug molecules the in situ perfusion technique is time-consuming and is unsuitable for control of all the variables or for study of the biochemical processes involved. For this reason, we have examined a number of in vitro techniques to determine their usefulness in predicting in vivo data and in understanding the mechanisms of drug absorption and pre-systemic metabolism at the cellular and sub-cellular levels.

Numerous investigators have attempted to use everted intestinal sacs and the limitations, in terms of absorption pathway and time-dependent tissue degradation, are well documented (Levine et. al., 1970). Everted intestinal rings have also been used on occasion, particularly for peptide-absorption studies (Matthews et. al., 1974). In this case, in contrast to the everted sacs, the time of exposure in the incubating solutions is much shorter, and hence the potential for loss of viability much less. Isolated intestinal mucosal cells, and brush border vesicles prepared from them, have also been utilized in absorption studies but their use has been restricted

essentially to uptake of ions, amino acids, sugars and
other nutrients which are transported via active
mechanisms (Sepulveda et. al., 1982; Murer and Kinne,
1980). To our knowledge there have been few attempts to
examine such techniques systematically for their potential
in rapidly assessing drug absorption processes.

Rat intestinal mucosal cells were isolated by two
published techniques (Weiser, 1973; Hartmann et. al.,
1982) and their properties determined to demonstrate
viability of the system (Osiecka et. al., 1984). In our
hands the procedure of Weiser (1973) yielded cells of
better morphological viability and they were used in all
subsequent experiments. Brush border vesicles were
prepared from the isolated cells by known techniques
(Kessler et. al., 1978) and were used either fresh or
after storage at -80°C.

In both systems, cells and vesicles, it was possible
to demonstrate uptake of glucose analogs as a stereoselective process and to show the inhibition of the facilitated
process by phlorizin, a compound known to inhibit glucose
transport in vivo (Alvarado and Crane, 1962).

The cells were also observed to display enzymatic
activities consistent with their identity as villus cells
or crypt cells and to take up amino acids and incorporate
them into proteins. These data clearly demonstrated that
the cells were capable of transporting nutrients in a
manner compatible with retention of functional viability.

A series of drug substances was chosen for study,
spanning a wide range of in vivo absorption properties,
and the uptake of these compounds measured in cells and
brush border vesicles (Osiecka et. al., 1984). The uptake
of these substances proved much more difficult to
determine accurately and reproducibly than had been the
case with sugars and amino acids.

In particular the kinetics of the process were so
rapid that use of centrifugation techniques proved
difficult while filtration methods gave variable results
largely due to difficulties in correcting for entrapped
incubation medium which contributed a significant but
variable amount to the total drug accumulation on the

Table III. Comparison of oral absorption data (rats) and
in vitro uptake in isolated mucosal cells and everted
intestinal rings for a series of drugs displaying a range
of in vivo bioavailability. The data are normalized so
that theophylline has a value of 100 in all three systems.

Drug	In Vivo	Isolated Mucosal Cells	Everted Intestinal Rings
Theophylline	100	100	100
Salicylate	29	52	61
α-Methyldopa	25	14	17
Cefoxitin	3	30	0

The oral bioavailability of theophylline in rats was 75 ±
2.1% (SEM) (n = 6) (compared to i.v. administration).

filters. Despite these difficulties, results were
obtained which demonstrated a fairly good correlation
with in vivo absorption of the same compounds (Table
III). Currently, the use of intestinal mucosal cells in
studying pre-systemic metabolism of drug compounds is
being investigated.

In contrast to the difficulties encountered with
cells and vesicles, the use of everted intestinal rings
or segments proved extremely valuable.

As in the case of the intestinal perfusions it was
necessary to demonstrate the integrity of the intestinal
segments and to determine the time frame in which the
tissue was morphologically and functionally viable. While
the tissue retains its viability well at 0°C, incubation
at 37°C leads to significant deterioration by 10-20
minutes. In all subsequent studies, uptake studies were
limited to 5 minutes or less (Osiecka et. al., 1984).

Of particular interest to us was the nature of the
uptake of α-methyldopa (Aldomet™). This drug, a major
antihypertensive agent, is an amino acid analog and
is known to have poor and highly variable absorption

in humans and animals. It has been postulated that
α-methyldopa might be absorbed via the large neutral amino
acid transport system (Young and Edwards, 1966) although
the evidence for this is conflicting (Wass and Evered,
1971). On the other hand it is fairly clear that the drug
is transported into the central nervous system via such a
carrier process (Markovitz and Fernstrom, 1977).

Studies were conducted to compare the absorption
properties of L-α-methyldopa with L-phenylalanine using
everted intestinal rings so that the appropriate variables
could be carefully controlled. All uptake data were
corrected for drug accumulation in the extracellular
tissue spaces using (^{14}C)-inulin as a marker. The results
are summarized in Table IV (Osiecka et. al., 1984; Osiecka
et. al, in preparation). Both compounds were accumulated
by saturable processes having apparent half-maximal rates
around 5 mM, the range reported in many studies for
α-amino acid transport (Finch and Hird, 1960). Uptake was
greater in the jejunum than in the duodenum or ileum but
the differences were not dramatic. The effect of fasting
was interesting: rings from fasted rats (48 hours)
accumulated both compounds much more rapidly than was
observed in fed animals.

Table IV. Comparison of uptake of L-phenylalanine and
L-α-methyldopa into everted intestinal rings

Property	L-phenylalanine	L-α-methyldopa
saturable uptake	yes	yes
concentration for 1/2 max rate	4.8 mM	5.6 mM
site dependent	yes	yes
fasting/fed uptake rate	1.9	3.0
temp dependent (37°/0°) ratio	4.5	4.7
% inhibition by other amino acids (5 or 10 mM)	50-95%	30-40%
% inhibition by ouabain (2 mM)	87%	55%
% inhibition in absence of:		
glucose	76%	73%
sodium	94%	94%

Uptake of α-methyldopa and phenylalanine was highly temperature dependent, the rate at 0-4°C being only approximately 20% of the rate at 37°C while uptake at 25°C was intermediate.

These data suggest that uptake of α-methyldopa occurs via a saturable process whose characteristics are similar to those of the L-phenylalanine transport system. If absorption occurs via this mechanism in vivo then varia- bility of the lumenal contents may well be responsible for the variation seen in Aldomet bioavailability.

One potential problem with the use of everted intestinal rings is the fact that both the serosal and mucosal surfaces are exposed to the incubating medium thereby permitting entry of drug from the "ablumenal" as well as the "lumenal" side. Two experiments were conducted to determine the magnitude of the uptake from the "serosal" side and the extent of drug accumulation in non-mucosal cells. In the first of these uptake of L-phenylalanine and L-methyldopa was compared in three systems: everted rings, tissue everted over a rod so that only the mucosal surface was exposed to the incubation solution; and tissue similarly mounted so that only the serosal surface was exposed. The results are shown in Table V. Clearly the uptake into the everted rings more closely mimicked the uptake when the mucosal surface was exposed than when only the serosal surface was available.

In a second series of experiments uptake into the rings was allowed to proceed and after termination of the uptake process, the mucosal cells were scraped off the underlying tissue and the drug content of the cells and the muscular tissue determined separately. In this case between 80 and 95% of the total drug uptake was found associated with the mucosal cells. These experiments demonstrate that the process being examined is uptake from the lumenal surface into the mucosal cells of the small intestine.

If used carefully with appropriate attention to tissue viability and identification of the uptake site, everted intestinal rings can provide a rapid means of assessing the mechanism of drug accumulation by the intestinal mucosa and of studying some of the variables in

Table V. Dependence of uptake of L-phenylalanine and L-α-methyldopa on availability of serosal or mucosal surfaces.

Preparation	Uptake (pmoles/mg.min)	
	L-phenylalanine	L-α-methyldopa
Everted intestinal rings	500 ± 51 (100%)	556 ± 60 (100%)
Everted intestinal sac (mucosal surface exposed)	450 ± 72 (81%)	378 ± 49 (68%)
Intestinal sac (serosal surface exposed)	69 ± 15 (12%)	156 ± 30 (28%)

this process. They appear to be superior to the use of everted intestinal sacs, brush border vesicles or isolated mucosal cells although the latter may find use in studying various aspects of pre-systemic drug metabolism.

GI TRANSIT TIME

To a large extent drug bioavailability is controlled by the physicochemical properties of the drug and its interactions with the components of the gi tract. However, as newer technologies are used to control the rate of release of drugs into the gastrointestinal system, another important physiological parameter comes into play - namely the gi transit time. It is well recognized that the small intestine provides the major absorptive surface for most drugs but there are a number of unanswered questions concerning the extent of absorption in the stomach or the colon, or the existence of "absorption windows" in the small intestine. The answers to these questions are clearly drug-dependent, but are important in defining the usefulness of a controlled-release device, and indeed, in designing the dosage form which is most appropriate for each drug substance. In this regard an understanding of the physiology of gastric emptying and intestinal transit is extremely important.

During the last ten to fifteen years the patterns of gastric emptying have been uncovered and it is clear that there are two major phases - (i) emptying of food and (ii) emptying patterns in the fasted state (Kelly, 1981).

We have investigated the effect of feeding patterns on gastric retention of a non-disintegrating capsule (the Heidelberg capsule, Connell and Waters, 1964) of similar size to a standard dosage form (Mojaverian et. al., in press). This device is capable of measuring the pH in its vicinity and signaling the information via a radio transmitter to a receiver and decoder strapped around the subject.

The data are shown in Table VI. In the fasted state in dogs or humans the device was rapidly eliminated from the stomach. In human subjects, one meal, depending on its size and/or caloric content, was capable of preventing exit of the capsule for a period of several hours. A normal daily eating pattern resulted in gastric retention of the device for more than 16 hours in most of the human subjects and for greater than 8 hours in all the dogs.
The pattern of eating clearly has an effect on the performance of enteric-coated dosage forms. Bogentoft et. al. (1978) have demonstrated that feeding has very little effect on the appearance of salicylate in plasma following administration of conventional tablets or enteric-coated microparticulates (1 mm) which leave the stomach independent of the state of feeding. On the other

Table VI. Effect of fasting and fed regimens on gastric retention of a Heidelberg capsule.

Subjects	Gastric Retention Time (hrs)	
	Fed	Fasted
Beagle Dogs	>8 (n = 8)	2.6 ± 0.7 (n = 8)
Human volunteers	>16 (8/10) 13.5 (1/10) 4 (1/10)	0.48 ± 0.12 (n = 10)
Human volunteers (breakfast only)	4.8 ± 0.6 (n = 6)	1.2 ± 0.3 (n = 6)

hand, feeding dramatically moves the plasma time profile to the right when enteric-coated aspirin tablets are given in the fed state. The explanation probably lies in the fact that the enteric-coated tablets exit the stomach rapidly in the fasted state but are retained for several hours when taken with food. Since they have acid-resistance coats there is a consequent delay before the drug is released by the neutral or alkaline environment in the intestine.

The implications for any controlled-release formulation are considerable. If these devices are given to fasting individuals or if meals are not consumed on a regular basis, the residence time of the delivery system in the stomach and small intestine is likely to be only a few hours. Depending on the site of absorption of the drug being released, the duration of effective delivery may be very much shorter than that built into the device and hence efficacy of the product may be severely affected.

CONCLUSIONS

There are many variables which affect the bioavailability of an orally administered therapeutic agent. By a series of in vitro, in situ and in vivo experiments it may be possible to identify the effects of some of these parameters and to devise structural or formulation alterations which can overcome some of the problems or take advantage of some of the physiological and biochemical properties of the gi tract. As we move into an era where drug substances are designed to be more specific in their actions we should also be prepared to take into account at an early stage the properties which will maximize the availability of the compound. This will be particularly true for small peptides which are likely to be a major source of new drugs of the future.

Controlled release of active agents can have many benefits in terms of reduced side effects, patient compliance etc. However, the role of the physiology of the gi tract in modifying the performance of such devices should not go ignored or it may produce some unpleasant surprises for the unprepared.

ACKNOWLEDGEMENTS

In addition to the references citing their work the author would like to acknowledge the contributions of the following individuals to the illustrative examples used in this presentation: I. Osieska, R. Borchardt, J. Fix, P. Porter, S. Selk, M. Cortese, R. Shaffer, K. Engle, L. Caldwell and L. Frost.

REFERENCES

Alvarado, F. and Crane, R. K., Phlorizin as a competitive inhibitor of the active transport of sugars by hamster small intestine in vitro, Biochim. Biophys. Acta., 56 (1962) 170-172.

Bahari, H. M. M., Ross, I. N. and Turnberg, L. A., Demonstration of a pH gradient across the mucus layer on the surface of human gastric mucosa in vitro, Gut, 23 (1982) 513-516.

Beveridge, T., Gratwohl, A., Michet, F., Niederberger, W., Nuesch, E., Nussbaumer, K., Schaub, P. and Speck, B., Cyclosporin A: Pharmacokinetics after a simple dose in man and serum levels after multiple dosing in recipients of allogeneic bone marrow grafts, Curr. Therap. Res., 30 (1981) 5-18.

Bogentoft, C., Carlsson, I., Ekenued, G. and Magnusson, A., Influence of food on the absorption of acetylsalicylic acid from enteric-coated dosage forms, Eur. J. Clin. Pharmacol., 14 (1978) 351-355.

Connell, A. M. and Waters, T. E., Assessment of gastric function by pH telemetering capsule, Lancet ii (1964) 227-230.

Engel, E., Peskoff, A., Kauffman, G. L., and Grossman, M. I., Analysis of hydrogen in concentration in the gastric gel mucus layer, Am. J. Physiol., 247 (1984) G321-G338.

Finch, L. R. and Hird, F. J. R., The uptake of amino acids by isolated segments of rat intestine. II. A survey of affinity for uptake from rates of uptake and competition for uptake, Biochim. Biophys. Acta., 43 (1960) 278-287.

Gardner, C. R., Selk, S., Cortese, M. and Higashi, T., In situ peptide absorption studies - uptake, binding or metabolism? Presented at Higuchi Research Seminar, 17th Annual Meeting, Lake Ozark, MO, March 1984.

Garner, A., Flemstrom, G., Allen, A., Heylings, J. R. and
McQueen, S., Gastric mucosal protective mechanisms: Roles
of epithelial bicarbonate and mucus secretions, Scand. J.
Gastroenterol., 19 (suppl 101) (1984) 79-86.

Hartmann, F., Owen, R. and Bissell, D. M., Characterization of isolated epithelial cells from rat small
intestine, Am. J. Physiol., 242 (1982) G147-G155.

Hogerle, M. L. and Winne, D., Drug Absorption by the rat
jejunum perfused in situ, Nannyn-Schmiedeberg's Arch.
Pharmacol., 322 (1983) 249-255.

Kelly, K. A., Motility of the stomach and gastroduodenal
junction, in Johnson, L. B. (Ed) Physiology of the
gastrointestinal tract, Raven Press, New York, 1981,
pp 393-410.

Kessler, M., Acuto, O., Storelli, C., Murer, H., Muller,
M. and Semena, G., A modified procedure for the rapid
preparation of efficiently transporting vesicles from
small intestinal brush border membranes. Biochim.
Biophys. Acta., 506 (1978) 136-154.

Levine, R. R., McNary, W. F., Kornguth, P. J. and LeBlanc,
R., Histological re-evaluaton of everted gut technique for
studying intestinal absorption, Eur. J. Pharmacol., 9
(1970) 211-219.

Markovitz, D. and Fernstrom, J. D., Diet and uptake of
Aldomet by the Brain: Competition with natural large
neutral amino acids. Science 197 (1977) 1014-1015.

Matthews, D. M., Addison, J. M. and Burston, D., Evidence
for active transport of the dipeptide carnosine
(β-alanyl-L-histidine) by hamster jejunum in vitro, Clin.
Sci. Mol. Med., 46 (1974) 693-705.

Mojaverian, P., Ferguson, R., Vlasses, P., Riley, L.,
Rocci, M., Oren, A., Fix, J., Caldwell, L. and Gardner,
C., Gastric emptying of a non-disintegrating solid:
Influence of feeding frequency and meal composition
in human volunteers, Gastroenterology, in press.

Murer, A. and Kinne, R., The use of isolated membrane vesicles to study epithelial transport processes, J. Memb. Biol., 55 (1980) 81-95.

Osiecka, I., Borchardt, R. T., Fix, J. A., Gardner, C. R. and Porter, P. A., A comparison of intestinal rings, isolated mucosal cells and brush border membrane vesicles as models for in vivo drug absorption, Fed. Proc., 43 (1984) 1779 (abstract no. 2122).

Sarosiek, J., Slomiany, A. and Slomiany, B. L., Retardation of hydrogen ion diffusion by gastric mucus constituents: Effect of proteolysis, Biochem. Biophys. Res. Comm., 115 (1983) 1053-1060.

Selk, S. H., Gardner, C. R. and Caldwell, L. J., Evaluation of an in situ intestinal perfusion model for drug absorption studies, presented at the 130th meeting of the APhA, New Orleans, LA, April 1983.

Sepulveda, F. V., Burton, K. A. and Brown, P. D., Relation between sodium-coupled amino acid and sugar transport and sodium/potassium pump activity in isolated intestinal epithelial cells, J. Cell. Physiol., 111 (1982) 303-308.

Sweet, C. S., Gross, D. M., Arbegast, P. T., Gaul, S. L., Britt, P. M., Ludden, G. T., Wertz, D. and Stone, C. A., Antihypertensive activity of N-[(S)-1-(ethoxycarbonyl)-3-phenylpropyl]-L-Ala-L-Pro (MK421), an orally active converting enzyme inhibitor, J. Pharmacol. Exp. Ther., 216 (1981) 558-566.

Tocco, D. J., deLuna, F. A., Duncan, E. W., Vassil, T. C. and Ulm, E. H., The physiological disposition and metabolism of enalapril maleate in laboratory animals, Drug Met. Disp., 10 (1982) 15-19.

Ulm, E. H., Hichens, M., Gomez, H. J., Till, A. E., Hand, E., Vassil, T. C., Biollay, J., Brunner, H. R., and Schelling, J. L., Enalapril maleate and a lysine analogue (MK521): Disposition in man, Br. J. Clin. Pharmac., 14 (1982) 357-362.

Veber, D. F., Freidinger, R. M., Perlow, D. S., Paleveda, W. J., Holly, F. W., Strachan, R. G., Nutt, R. F., Arison, B. H., Homnick, C., Randall, W. C., Glitzer, M. S., Saperstein, R. and Hirchmann, R., A potent cyclic hexapeptide analogue of somatostatin, Nature, 292 (1981) 55-58.

Wass, M. and Evered, D. F., Transport characteristics of the amino acid analogues cycloserine and α-methyldopa, using rat small intestine in vitro, Life Sci., 10 (1971) 1005-1013.

Weiser, M. M., Intestinal epithelial cell surface membrane glycoprotein synthesis, J. Biol. Chem., 248 (1973) 2536-2541.

Young, J. A. and Edwards, K. D. G., Competition for transport between methyldopa and other amino acids in rat gut loops, Am. J. Physiol., 210 (1966) 1130-1136.

STRATEGIES FOR DRUG DELIVERY THROUGH THE BLOOD-BRAIN
BARRIER

William M. Pardridge

Department of Medicine/UCLA School of Medicine

Los Angeles, California   90024

ABSTRACT

Traditional approaches to circumventing the blood-
brain barrier (BBB) involve intrathecal administration of
neuropharmaceuticals; however, this results in drug
distribution only to the surface of the brain. Another
approach to circumventing the BBB involves drug latentiation
or the conversion of water soluble substances to lipid
soluble compounds. This approach portends a vast promise
for the neuropharmaceutical industry, which has yet to be
realized for a wide variety of chemotherapeutic agents.
However, studies with the lipid soluble peptide, cyclosporin,
indicate that drug latentiation may not be a particularly
promising approach for the delivery of systemically
administered neuropeptides to brain. A new strategy,
called transport-directed drug delivery to brain, involves
coupling of the neuropharmaceutical agent to a peptide
(e.g., insulin) that is normally transported through the
BBB by a peptide specific transport system.

INTRODUCTION

The capillaries in virtually all vertebrate brains are
characterized by unique morphologic properties which include
epithelial-like high resistance tight junctions that
literally cement adjacent brain capillary endothelial cells

83

together (Brightman, 1977). There is also a paucity of
pinocytosis or transendothelial channels in brain
capillaries, although these structures are abundant in
peripheral capillaries (Brightman, 1977). Owing to the
presence of these unique anatomical features, circulating
substances may gain access to brain interstitial space by
only one of four mechanisms: (a) pore-mediation, which
allows for the transport of water through water-specific
pores in the BBB (Pardridge, 1984); (b) lipid-mediation,
which allows for the free diffusion of lipid soluble
substances such as the steroid hormones or many lipid
soluble drugs through the BBB (Oldendorf, 1974); (c) carrier-
mediation, which allows for the transport of circulating
water soluble nutrients through the BBB via the action of
nutrient-specific carrier systems localized in the lumenal
and antilumenal membranes of brain capillaries (Pardridge
and Oldendorf, 1977); (d) receptor-mediated transcytosis of
circulating peptides via peptide-specific receptor systems
localized on both the lumenal and antilumenal membranes of
brain capillaries (Pardridge, et al., 1985a). Owing to the
presence of these active mechanisms for transport in the
BBB, this membrane system plays a dynamic role in controlling
the flux of substances between the brain and the systemic
circulation.

The traditional view that the BBB plays a more or less
passive role in brain function is not only old fashioned,
but also imparts the idea that the permeability properties
of the BBB are relatively inert and cannot be circumvented
by specific pharmacologic strategies. This review will
emphasize the view that an understanding of the basic
physiology of BBB transport processes can lead to the design
of new strategies for delivery of neuropharmaceuticals to
brain. Table 1 lists the five basic strategies for
delivery of neuropharmaceuticals to the central nervous
system, and the transport-directed approaches in strategy 5
(Table 1) represent the newest strategies for drug delivery
to brain.

Circumventricular Organs

About a half-dozen tiny areas of brain around the
ventricles called the circumventricular organs (CVOs) lack
a BBB (Weindl, 1973). The capillaries perfusing these small
areas constitute less than 0.5% of the total capillary

TABLE 1. Strategies for Pharmaceutical Delivery through
          the Blood-Brain Barrier

---

1. circumventricular organs
2. intrathecal (intranasal) administration
3. hyperosmolar opening of the blood-brain barrier
4. latentiation (liposomes)
5. transport-directed drug delivery
   a. nutrient carrier systems
   b. peptide transcytosis
   c. plasma proteins

---

surface area in brain, and have open inter-endothelial
junctions and abundant pinocytosis (Brightman, 1977).
Substances as large as horseradish peroxidase (M.W. = 40,000)
readily gain access to the interstitial space of the CVOs
following systemic administration. Table 2 lists the CVOs.
The most prominent CVO is the choroid plexus. The choroid
plexus and the other CVOs make up the blood-cerebrospinal
fluid (CSF) barrier. The blood-CSF barrier is composed of
tight junctions joining the ependyma or epithelial cells
that line the ventricular surface at each respective CVO
(Brightman, 1977). Circulating substances may distribute
to nerve endings terminating in the interstitial space of
CVOs, but the tight junctions at the ependyma prevent the
rapid diffusion of these substances into the immediate
ventricular space.

TABLE 2. The Circumventricular Organs (CVO)

CVO	Contiguous Brain Region
choroid plexus	ventricles
median eminence	arcuate nucleus, hypothalamus
OVLT	preoptic nucleus, hypothalamus
subfornical organ	roof of third ventricle
area postrema	base of fourth ventricle

OVLT = organum vasculosum lamina terminalis

Intrathecal Administration

Most of the CSF in brain is secreted by the ependyma of the CVOs, and this secretion causes CSF to flow over the surface of brain. Owing to the deep convexities of the human brain surface, no parts of the brain are more than 0.5-1.0 cm away from the CSF. However, these distances are still quite large for the diffusional movement of molecules. Accordingly, the intrathecal administration of neuropharmaceuticals allows for only delivery of the drug to the meningeal surfaces of the brain (Collins and Dedrick, 1983). Although greatly limited, this approach has found success in some diseases which have a predilection for meningeal involvement, such as the infectious meningitides or CNS leukemia, where the intraventricular injection of methotrexate has caused a marked reduction in CNS leukemia (Freeman, et al., 1983). Owing to the caudal flow of CSF, the intralumbar injection of neuropharmaceuticals is generally not beneficial (Poplack, et al., 1981). Intracisternal or intraventricular administration of drugs is necessary. This approach requires the implantation of a cannula into the ventricular system and is obviously not an approach that will be used widely.

One variation of the intrathecal administration of neuropharmaceuticals is the administration of the agent via an intranasal spray. Recent studies have shown that lipid soluble substances such as progesterone achieve higher CSF levels following the intranasal administration as compared to an intravenous administration of the agent (Kumar, et al., 1982). This observation can be explained on the basis of recent physiological data which are compatible with the continuation of cerebral perivascular spaces and subarachnoid space of olfactory lobes with the submucous bases of the nose (Bradbury, et al., 1981). Since the intranasal administration of drugs is routine, this approach is deserving of further investigation as a general approach for the delivery of neuropharmaceuticals to the ventricular space of brain. Although promising, two caveats should be born in mind. First, it is unlikely that water soluble substances will gain access to the CSF following intranasal administration and secondly, the intranasal administration of agents, like any intrathecal approach, allows for distribution of the agent to the surface of the brain, but will probabaly not allow for substantial neuropharmaceutical action within the bulk of the brain.

Hyperosmolar Opening of the BBB

Owing to the limitations of intrathecal administration of neuropharmaceuticals in delivering the agent to areas deep within the brain, more heroic measures have been introduced which involve toxicologic opening of the BBB in a transient and apparently reversable way with hyperosmolar agents. The intracarotid infusion of 1-2M solutions of osmotically active substances (e.g., mannitol) results in osmotic disruption of the BBB (Neuwelt, et al., 1981). This strategy has been used to mediate the delivery of certain enzymes to brain in experimental animals, such as hexoseaminidase A, the enzyme that is deficient in Tay-Sachs disease. However, this approach for delivery of enzymes to brain appears to be very limited. First, the enzyme must be administered immediately after the intracarotid bolus of the osmotically active agent and the enzyme must be administered directly into the carotid artery. Secondly, less than 1% of the administered enzyme reaches the brain substance (Neuwelt, et al., 1981). A more successful approach for the delivery of enzymes to brain may be via coupling of the enzyme to a peptide that normally crosses the BBB (see below).

Drug Latentiation (Liposomes)

A highly rational yet rarely investigated approach for drug delivery to brain is latentiation, or conversion of water soluble molecules into lipid soluble substances (Verbiscar and Abood, 1970). The permeability of the BBB to a given substance drops by one log order for every hydroxyl group added to the parent molecule (Pardridge and Mietus, 1979). One hydroxyl group forms two hydrogen bonds in water and this substituent results in a ten-fold drop in BBB permeability. Blockade of hydrogen bond-forming functional groups on the parent molecule results in log order increases in penetration of the drug through the BBB. The classic example of drug latentiation is the conversion of morphine into diacetylmorphine or heroin. The acetylation of the two hydroxyl groups on morphine removes four hydrogen bonds from the parent molecule and increases the permeability of the BBB to the compound by two log orders of magnitude (Oldendorf, et al., 1972). Thus, heroin is rapidly transported through the BBB on a single pass, whereas morphine is slowly transported on one pass. After several systemic circulations, a substantial amount of systemically

administered morphine does gain access to brain. In this
regard, the relatively slow metabolism of morphine allows
for drug efficacy despite the relatively low permeability
of the BBB to morphine. Were morphine rapidly metabolized
by hepatic or renal tissues, then the low first pass
extraction by brain would greatly restrict the central
activity of the compound. Some of the most inventive
strategies for drug latentiation of substances such as the
catecholamines (e.g., dopamine), or substances such as
quaternary ammonium salts have been devised by Bodor and
colleagues (Bodor, et al., 1975; Bodor and Simpkins, 1983).
The strategies for drug latentiation employed by Bodor
parallel the morphine-heroin model, in that the latentiated
compound, once inside the brain, is metabolized back to
the parent compound. For example, in the case of heroin,
this substance is rapidly de-acetylated in brain back to
morphine (Inturrisi, et al., 1984), presumably by capillary
pseudocholinesterase (Renkawek, et al., 1976). Conversion
of the latentiated compound to the parent molecule is
necessary because it is likely that the latentiated form
of the drug will have a much reduced biological potency.

The question arises as to whether small neuropeptides,
which are highly water soluble and do not normally cross the
BBB (Pardridge, 1983a), can be latentiated to a lipid
soluble derivative that may cross the brain capillary. A
prototype example of a lipid soluble peptide is cyclosporin
(Fig. 1). Cyclosporin is an eleven amino acid, cyclic
peptide that is highly lipid soluble (Wenger, 1982). The
octanol/Ringer's partition coefficient of cyclosporin is
approximately 1,000, which makes this substance as lipid
soluble as a steroid hormone such as testosterone (Cefalu
and Pardridge, 1985). The high lipid solubility of cyclosporin can be attributed to three major sets of chemical
properties of this molecule. First, the peptide is cyclized
which allows for the closure of the terminal amino and
carboxyl groups which result in the loss of hydrogen bond-
forming functional groups. Second, the amino acids
comprising the peptide are all of the aliphatic variety, and
include alanine, leucine, and valine derivatives. Third,
and most important, all amide hydrogen bond forming
functional groups in cyclosporin are either directly or
indirectly closed off (Fig. 1). For example, three of the
amide nitrogens form internal hydrogen bonds within the
structure of the molecule. Moreover, all other amide
nitrogens which are potential hydrogen bond forming functional

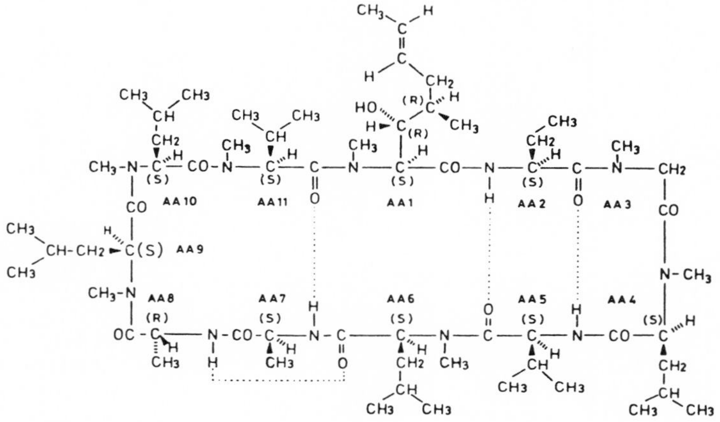

Fig. 1. Structure of cyclosporin A

groups have a methyl moiety; that is, N-methyl amino acids
are the precursors of the synthesis of this novel peptide.
Because of these features there are few groups in the
peptide which are open for hydrogen bonding with water.
Therefore, it is probably not possible to synthesize a
peptide that is more latentiated than is cyclosporin. Indeed,
the high lipid solubility of this substance attests to the
excellent job nature has done in synthesizing a latentiated
lipid soluble peptide. Despite these features, we have found
that the transport of ^{3}H-cyclosporin through the BBB is
disappointingly slow. For example, in the presence of serum
proteins, the first pass extraction of ^{3}H-cyclosporin
through the rat brain is on the order of 2% (Cefalu and
Pardridge, 1985). It is likely that in the course of
transport of cyclosporin through the biological membrane,
the four internal hydrogen bonds are broken and exposed to
water as the molecule undergoes conformational changes in
the transport process. Whatever the mechanism, there is a
major diffusion restriction of this peptide through the BBB
despite its very high lipid solubility.

A variation on drug latentiation for delivery of
substances to brain is the use of liposomes, or the encapsulation of the water soluble neuropharmaceutical agent in
a lipid sphere (Patel, 1984). However, liposomes have not
sustained the initial enthusiasm of this approach for the

delivery of substances to brain. This is because liposomes are not cleared through continuous capillaries such as those which exist in brain, but are selectively taken up by endothelia in the reticuloendothelial system of liver and spleen (Patel, 1984). Thus, liposomes provide an excellent approach for delivery of drugs to liver and spleen but appear not to offer much promise for drug distribution to tissues such as the brain.

Transport-Directed Drug Delivery to Brain

In this approach, strategies for delivery of drugs to the CNS emanate from an understanding of the basic physiology of transport processes at the BBB for nutrients, plasma proteins, and peptides. With regard to nutrients, is is known that neutral amino acids in the blood gain access to brain interstitium via transport by a neutral amino acid specific carrier system localized in the BBB (Pardridge and Oldendorf, 1977). This transport system is a leucine or L-preferring system that is sodium independent and insulin insensitive, and mediates the bidirectional or equilibrative movement of neutral amino acids between blood and brain. A variety of neuropharmaceuticals happen to be neutral amino acids. These drugs include α-methyl-dopa, L-dopa, α-methyl-tyrosine, and phenylalanine mustard or melphalan. All four of these agents gain access to brain despite being very water soluble. This is because these α-amino acid-drugs are transported through the BBB by the neutral amino acid transport system. Indeed, these drugs are probably transported into all tissues via a neutral amino acid system localized on the cell membrane. However, an understanding of the physiology of BBB amino acid transport leads to new insights as to how the distribution of these drugs in brain may be selectively enhanced relative to that of other organs. The affinity of the BBB transport system is much higher for neutral amino acids than are the transport systems in other tissues of the body. That is, the Km of neutral amino acid transport is set down near the plasma level of amino acids in the 50-100 μM range (Pardridge, 1983b). Conversely, the Km of neutral amino acid transport in virtually all other tissues of the body is in the 1-10 mM range, or even greater (Pardridge, 1983b). Since competition effects in vivo do not occur unless the Km of the transport system is set near the physiologic concentration of plasma amino acids, it can be predicted that tissues other then brain will not be sensitive to competition effects in the

physiologic range. That is, the development of hyperaminoacidemia, such as after a protein meal, will lead to
a decrease in the brain uptake of amino acid drugs whereas
it is likely that no decrease in uptake of the amino acid
drug will occur in peripheral tissues. Indeed, Fernstrom
et al., (1980) have shown that the brain uptake of α-methyl-
dopa can be predicted from information on the plasma amino
acid profile for neutral amino acids. The development of
hypoaminoacidemia via insulin, such as after a carbohydrate
meal, results in enhanced brain uptake of α-methyl-dopa.
Similarly, a high protein meal inhibits the uptake of drugs
such as L-dopa and this dietary induced decrease in the
uptake of L-dopa by brain may underlie the on-off phenomena
in the treatment of Parkinson's disease (Mena and Cotzias,
1975). Other drugs such as α-methyl-ρ-tyrosine (Pardridge,
1977) or melphalan (W.M. Pardridge, unpublished observations)
are also known to be transported through the BBB by the
neutral amino acid transport system. In summary, it
would be expected that the development of insulin-induced
hypoaminoacidemia would allow for the enhanced delivery of
these drugs to the brain in a specific way, without
causing any increase in the uptake of the drug by peripheral
tissue. This strategy may be most important for the
administration of melphalan, which is a highly toxic
substance and is often used in very high concentrations
particularly for the treatment of brain tumors (Lazarus, et
al., 1983). If intravenous melphalan therapy was coordinated
with insulin-induced hyperaminoacidemia in the acute period
during drug administration, then the brain uptake of the
drug can be selectively enhanced. This would allow for
greater drug efficacy in brain with the minimization of side
effects of the drug in peripheral tissues such as bone marrow.

With regard to peptide delivery, the preceeding section
indicated that latentiation of peptides will unlikely prove
to be successful in enhancing the delivery of these agents
to brain, at least insofar as the results with cyclosporin
are concerned. However, a physiologic based approach for
neuropeptide delivery to brain would involve covalent
coupling of the neuropeptide agent to another peptide that
normally crosses the BBB via a peptide specific transport
system. That is, not all neuropeptides in circulation have
a specific transport system at the BBB. For example,
substances such as enkephalin or CCK (Pardridge et al., 1985b)
appear not to have a specific transport system at brain
capillaries. However, other peptides in the circulation

such as insulin, or the insulin-like growth factors (IGF)
I and II (also called somatomedin-C and multiplication-
stimulating activity, respectively) appear to have specific
transport systems in brain capillaries (Pardridge, et al.,
1985; Frank, et al., 1985). The uptake of peptides such as
insulin or the IGFs by cells occurs via receptor-mediated
endocytosis. Similarly, the export of these peptides
from cells occurs via receptor-mediated exocytosis (Bar,
et al., 1983). In this scheme, the sequential endocytosis
of the circulating peptide at the lumenal aspect of the
BBB is followed sequentially by the exocytosis of the
peptide in its unmetaboized form at the antilumenal aspect
of the BBB. There are several pieces of data which lend
support to the validity of this scheme. First, the
concentration of insulin or the IGFs, particularly IGF-II,
in CSF is unusually high and is approximately ten-fold
higher than would be expected if these peptides gained
access to CSF only via the nonspecific routes open to all
plasma proteins, i.e., slow transport through the CVOs
(Pardridge, 1983a). Since there is no evidence that insulin
or the IGFs are synthesized in the brain, the high CSF
levels of these substances suggest a specific transport
system is operative either at the BBB or the blood-CSF
barrier. Secondly, we have shown, using isolated capillaries
from human brain, that insulin is taken up by capillaries
via receptor-mediated endocytosis and is also exported
unmetabolized by these capillaries (Pardridge, et al., 1985a).
Moreover, using affinity cross-linking techniques with
radiolabeled insulin or IGFs, we have shown that the insulin
receptor or IGF receptor found in peripheral tissues is
also present in the plasma membrane of isolated brain
capillaries (Pardridge, et al., 1985a; Frank, et al., 1985).
Given this basic physiologic information, one can then
devise strategies whereby the peptide or other neuropharmaceutical agent of choice is covalently coupled to a peptide,
such as insulin, that normally crosses the BBB. It would
then be hoped that (a) the peptide-insulin complex is still
transported through the BBB, and (b) the peptide-insulin
complex is still active at its receptor sites once within
the central nervous system. A side effect of this therapy
is insulin-induced hypoglycemia (Poznansky, et al., 1984),
since it is likely that the pharmaceutical-insulin complex
is still active at insulin receptor sites in the periphery.
Such side effects can be eliminated by using peptides other
than insulin that also cross by specific peptide transport
systems.

Finally, an additional strategy is coupling of the neuropharmaceutical to a variant of albumin that has been rendered basic by coupling of polylysine (Shen and Ryser, 1978), or other positively charged moieties to the albumin molecule. It has been shown that albumin, which normally slowly enters the CSF, does so at a much higher rate when the albumin molecule is modified from its normal isoelectric point of 3.9 to a more basic isoelectric point of 8.5 (Griffin and Fiffels, 1982). Apparently, the basic albumin has a greater affinity for negatively charged sites in the glycocalyx of capillaries, and this may enhance the fluid-phase endocytosis of the albumin by the cell. Whether this process of uptake of basic albumin occurs at the ependyma of the blood-CSF barrier or at the brain capillary endothelia comprising the BBB is at present not known. However, it is clear that basic albumins are more rapidly taken up by brain and coupling of a neuropharmaceutical to a basic albumin could allow for enhanced drug delivery via piggyback of the agent to the basic albumin.

It is hoped that this last section of transport-directed drug delivery to brain will convince the reader that an understanding of the basic physiology of blood-brain barrier transport processes leads quickly to the design of new strategies, and possibly new opportunities for the enhanced delivery of neuropharmaceuticals to brain.

ACKNOWLEDGEMENTS

This research was supported by NIH grant R01-NS-17701, R01-AM-25744, and RCDA-AM-00783. The author is indebted to Jody Eisenberg and Jing Yang for excellent technical assistance, and to Dawn Brown for superb preparation of the manuscript.

REFERENCES

Bar, R.S., DeRose, A., Sandra, A., Peacock, M.L., and Owen, W.G. Insulin binding to microvascular endothelium of intact heart: a kinetic and morphometric analysis. Am. J. Physiol. 244:E447-E452, 1983.
Bodor, N, Shek, E., and Higuchi, T. Delivery of a quaternary pyridinium salf across the blood-brain barrier by its dihydropyridine derivative. Science, 190:155-156, 1975.

Bodor, N. and Simpkins, J.W. Redox delivery system for
   brain-specific, sustained release of dopamine.
   Science 221:65-67, 1982.
Bradbury, M.W.B., Cserr, H.F., and Westrop, R.J. Drainage
   of cerebral interstitial fluid into deep cervical
   lymph of the rabbit. Am. J. Physiol. 240:F329-F336,
   1981.
Brightman, M.W. Morphology of blood-brain interfaces.
   Exp. Eye Res. Suppl:1-25, 1977.
Cefalu, W.T. and Pardridge, W.M. Restrictive transport of
   a lipid soluble peptide (cyclosporin) through the
   blood-brain barrier. Clin. Res. 33:in press, 1985.
Collins, J.M. and Dedrick, R.L. Distributed model for drug
   delivery to CSF and brain tissue. Am. J. Physiol. 245:
   R303-R310, 1983.
Frank, H.J.L., Pardridge, W.M., Morris, W.L., and Rosenfeld,
   R.G. Binding and processing of insulin-like growth
   factors by blood-brain barrier. Clin. Res. 33:in press,
   1985.
Freeman, A.I., Weinberg, V.,Brecher, M.L., et al. Comparison
   of intermediate-dose methotrexate with cranial
   irradiation for the post-induction treatment of acute
   lymphocytic leukemia in children. N. Engl. J. Med.
   308:477-484, 1983.
Griffin, D.E. and Giffels, J. Study of protein characteristics
   that influence entry into the cerebrospinal fluid of
   normal mice and mice with encephalitis. J. Clin. Invest.
   70:289-295, 1982.
Inturrisi, C.E., Mitchell, B.M., Foley, K.M., Schultz, M.,
   Seung-Uon, S., and Houde, R.W. The pharmacokinetics
   of heroin in patients with chronic pain. N. Engl. J.
   Med. 310:1213-1217, 1984.
Kumar, T.C.,A., David, G.F.X., Sankaranarayanan, A., Puri, V.
   and Sundram. Pharmacokinetics of progesterone after
   its administration to ovariectomized rhesus monkeys by
   injection, infusion, or nasal spraying. Proc. Natl.
   Acsd. Sci. USA 79:4185-4189, 1982.
Lazarus, H.M., Herzig, R.G., Graham-Pole, J., et al.
   Intensive melphalan chemotherapy and cryopreserved
   autologous bone marrow transplantation for the
   treatment of refractory cancer. J. Clin. Oncol. 1:359-
   367, 1983.
Mena, I. and Cotzias, G.C. Protein intake and treatment of
   Parkinson's disease with levodopa. N. Engl. J. Med.
   292:181-184, 1975.

Neuwelt, E.A., Barranger, J.A., Brady, R.O., Pagel, M., Furbish, F.S., Quirk, J.M., Mook, G.E., and Frenkel, E. Delivery of hexosaminidase A to the cerebrum after osmotic modification of the blood-brain barrier. Proc. Natl. Acad. Sci. USA 78:5838-5841, 1981.

Oldendorf, W.H. Blood-brain barrier permeability to drugs. Ann. Rev. Pharmacol. 14:239-248, 1974.

Pardridge, W.M. Cerebrovascular permeability status in brain injury, In: NIH Central Nervous System Trauma Report (D.P. Becker and J.T. Povlishock, eds.) in press. 1984.

Pardridge, W.M. Kinetics of competitive inhibition of neutral amino acid transport across the blood-brain barrier. J. Neurochem. 28:103-108, 1977.

Pardridge, W.M. and Oldendorf, W.H. Transport of metabolic substrates though the blood-brain barrier. J. Neurochem. 28:5-12, 1977.

Pardridge, W.M., Eisenberg, J., and Yamada, T. Rapid sequestration and degradation of somatostatin analogues by isolated brain microvessels. J. Neurochem. in press 1985b.

Pardridge, W.M., Eisenberg, J., and Yang, J. Human blood-brain barrier insulin receptor. J. Neurochem. in press 1985a.

Pardridge, W.M. and Mietus, L.J. Transport of steroid hormones through the rat blood-brain barrier. Primary role of albumin-bound hormone. J. Clin. Invest. 64: 145-154, 1979.

Pardridge, W.M. Neuropeptides and the blood-brain barrier. Ann. Rev. Physiol. 45:73-82, 1983a.

Pardridge, W.M. Brain metabolism: a perspective from the blood-brain barrier. Physiol Rev. 63:1481-1535, 1983b.

Patel H.M. Liposomes: bags of challenge. Biochem. Soc. Trans. 12:333-335, 1984.

Poplack, D.G., Bleyer, A.W., and Horowitz, M.E. Pharmacology of antineoplastic agents in cerebrospinal fluid. In: Neurobiology of Cerebrospinal Fluid (J.H. Wood, ed.), Plenum Press, New York, 1981.

Poznansky, M.J., Singh, R., Singh, B, and Fantus, G. Insulin: Carrier potential for enzyme and drug therapy. Science 223:1304-1306, 1984.

Renkawek, K., Murray, M.R., Spatz, M. and Klatzo, I. Distinctive histochemical characteristics of brain capillaries in organotypic culture. Exp. Neur. 50: 194-206, 1976.

Shen, W.C. and Ryser, J.P.H. Conjugation of poly-L-lysine
    to albumin and horseradish peroxidase: a novel method
    of enhancing the cellular uptake of proteins. Proc.
    Nat. Acad. Sci. USA 75:1872-1876, 1978.
Sved, A.F., Goldberg, I.M., and Fernstrom, J.D. Dietary
    protein intake influences the antihypertensive potency
    of methyldopa in spontaneously hypertensive rats.
    J. Pharmacol. Exp. Ther. 214:147-151, 1980.
Verbiscar, A.J. and Abood, L.G. Carbamate ester latentiation
    of physiologically active amines. J. Med. Chem. 13:
    1176-1179,1970.
Weindl, A. Neuroendocrine aspects of circumventricular
    organs. In: Frontiers in Neuroendocrinology (W.F.
    Ganong and L. Martini, eds.), Oxford University Press,
    New York, 1973.
Wenger, R. Chemistry of cyclosporin. In: Cyclosporin A
    (D.J.G. White, ed.), Elsevier Biomed. Press, New York,
    1982.

THE DERMAL BARRIER TO LOCAL AND SYSTEMIC DRUG DELIVERY

W. I. Higuchi,* J. L. Fox,* K. Knutson,*
B. D. Anderson,* and G. L. Flynn**

*Department of Pharmaceutics, The University
of Utah

Salt Lake City, Utah 84112

**College of Pharmacy, The University of
Michigan

Ann Arbor, Michigan 48109-1065

I am honored and grateful to the Organizing
Committee to have been invited to participate in this
Symposium honoring Tak. It may be especially so because
my assignment is to talk about drug transport in skin
and my first job after receiving my Ph.D. in 1956 was to
study factors influencing drug transport across skin at
the University of Wisconsin under a Defense Department
contract directed by Tak and Dale Wurster.

This presentation will attempt to review some
recent research activities at the University of Michigan
and the University of Utah in the area of drug transport
across skin having particular bearing on how drug
molecule factors and vehicle formulation factors may
influence dermal or transdermal delivery. As will be
seen, there are more new questions than answers but,
taken altogether, there has been much progress with new
insights in the area of percutaneous drug transport.

SKIN COMPONENT	HUMAN SKIN	HAIRLESS MOUSE SKIN
Stratum Corneum	10 - 50 μ	10 - 40 μ
Viable Epidermis	100 - 200 μ	10 - 30 μ
Dermis	1000 - 2000 μ	500 μ

TABLE 1. Physical Model for Solute Transport in
          Skin

FULL-THICKNESS SKIN AND WHEN THE STRATUM CORNEUM
IS RATE-LIMITING AND WHEN IT IS NOT.

Table 1 provides some typical data on the
thicknesses of the stratum corneum, epidermis and dermis
in hairless mouse skin and human skin. The stratum
corneum is made of densely packed, dead, partially
dessicated, keratinized epidermal cells (1). The cells
are actually cell remnants that are flattened, highly
proteinaceous material surrounded by lipid-rich
intercellular material (2). The epidermis is rapidly
proliferating nucleated cells and the dermis is
essentially a noncellular collagenous hydrogel. All of
this suggests a three-layer transport model as shown in
Figure 1 which is a schematic illustration of a two-
chamber cell diffusion experiment.

For the situation in Figure 1, we may write

$$J = P (C_D - C_R)$$ Equation 1

where J is the transport rate per unit area, P is the
permeability coefficient and C_D and C_R are the donor and
receiver concentrations, respectively, for the drug. In
most experimental situations, $C_R \simeq 0$ (sink conditions);
so we may write

$$J = PC_D$$ Equation 2

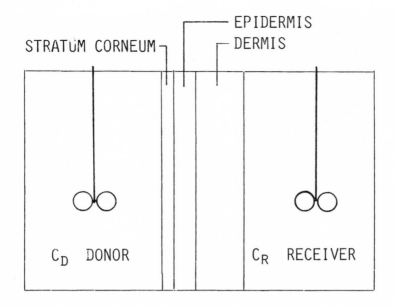

PER UNIT CROSSECTIONAL AREA,

$$J = P \ (C_D - C_R)$$

WHICH, FOR C_R = 0 (SINK CONDITIONS)

$$J = PC_D$$

FIGURE 1.   Illustration of the Two-Chamber Cell
Experiment

Now, for the three-layer model

$$P = \frac{1}{\frac{1}{P_{SC}} + \frac{1}{P_E} + \frac{1}{P_D}} \qquad \text{Equation 3}$$

Where P_{SC}, P_E and P_D are the permeability coefficients
for the three layers.

Equation 3 is a very useful relationship because, together with the appropriate transport experiments, we may investigate the nature of the stratum corneum, the epidermis and the dermis. For example, by tape-stripping hairless mouse skin, we can remove the stratum corneum (3). Equation 3 then becomes

$$P = \frac{1}{\frac{1}{P_E} + \frac{1}{P_D}} \qquad \text{Equation 4}$$

The dermis may be isolated by dermatoming (4) or by removal of the epidermal membrane after heat treatment (5). In this case, we have

$$P = P_D \qquad \text{Equation 5}$$

Thus it is seen that by appropriate techniques the drug transport behavior of the three principal components of skin may be studied via equations 3-5.

Figure 2 is taken from a recent study by Flynn et al. (3) on the influence of tape-stripping on the transport behavior of the normal alkanols. It is seen that, with removal of the stratum corneum, the chain-length effect is lost. The loss of chain length effect means that the residual epidermis/dermis barrier for the alkanols is largely aqueous in this experimental situation as water was the solvent in both chambers. On further analysis, we note that the limiting permeability coefficient for the alkanols is of the order of $P = 0.10$ cm/hr which corresponds to $P \simeq 3 \times 10^{-5}$ cm/sec. For a homogeneous membrane,

$$P = \frac{KD}{h} \qquad \text{Equation 6}$$

Where D is the diffusivity, K is the partition coefficient, and h is the thickness. Assuming that the epidermis/dermis is a hydrogel and when water is the solvent, then it is reasonable to have $K \simeq 1$. Taking $h = 0.05$ cm (Table 1), we find that

$$D \simeq 2 \times 10^{-6} \text{ cm}^2/\text{sec}$$

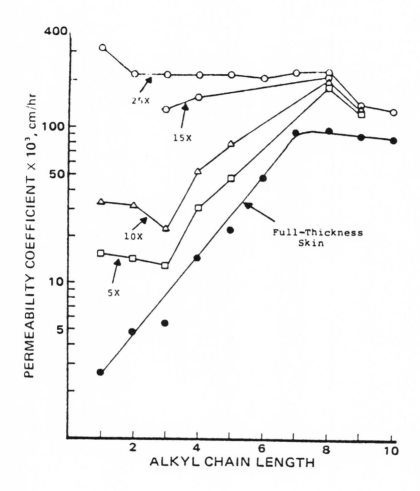

FIGURE 2.   Semilog Plot of Permeability Coefficients for Stripped Hairless Mouse
Membranes and Normal Hairless Mouse
Skin as a Function of Alkyl Chain
Length.   All Data were Obtained at
37°.   The Skin was Stripped 5, 10, 15
and 25 Times.   Taken from Flynn <u>et</u> <u>al</u>
(3).

which is a reasonable value for a hydrogel (water itself would be the order of 1-2 X 10^{-5} cm^2/sec).

The practical significance (e.g., in design of transdermal patches) of this limiting P-value is the following. It approximately represents the maximum possible P-value for most low-to-medium molecular weight compounds. Thus, together with equation 2 when $C_D = C_S$, where C_S is the solubility, this P-value permits estimating the maximum possible flux for any drug. Such maximum possible P-values and maximum fluxes may be achieved, for example, by (a) tape-stripping, (b) heat treatment of hairless mouse skin at 60°C and above (6, 7), (c) pretreatment of hairless mouse skin with 100% DMSO (8) or (d) pretreatment with an aqueous Azone emulsion (9).

Figure 3 is taken from the work of Smith and Flynn (10). These results show that the 21-n-alkyl esters of hydrocortisone show essentially the same behavior as the normal alkanols. With intact stratum corneum, there is a substantial chain-length effect with the P-values increasing 2- to 3- fold per methylene group as was found with the normal alkanols. With the stratum corneum removed, however, the chain length effect (and the lipophilic character of the barrier) is lost. One notes here, also, that approximately the same limiting P-value is obtained, i.e., P $\simeq$ 0.10 cm/hr.

Another important outcome of the data in Figures 2 and 3 is the following. For intact full-thickness skin, there is a maximum limiting P-value reached as the lipophilicity of the homologous series is increased. For the normal alkanols, this limiting P-value is reached around n- octanol; for the hydrocortisone esters, it is around the C_6 ester. The practical significance of this in dermal delivery drug design is that little may be gained on the P-value above a certain lipophilicity. The data in Figures 2 and 3 and other unpublished data also suggest that the limiting P-value attained with intact stratum corneum is the same as the limiting P-value when the stratum corneum barrier is abolished by tape-stripping, solvent action (100% DMSO) or through use of an effective penetration enhancer such as Azone.

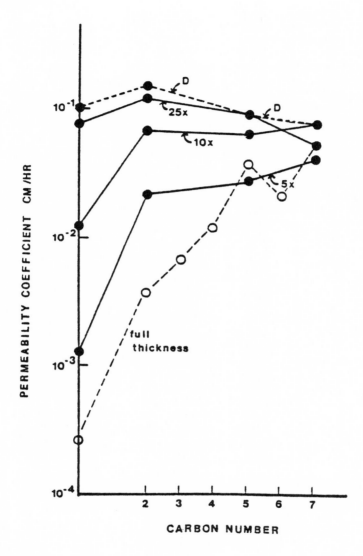

FIGURE 3. Permeability Coefficients for the
Hydrocortisone Ester Series for
Stripped Skin and Isolated Dermis.
The skin was stripped 5, 10, 15 and
25 times. Taken from Smith and Flynn
(10).

Figure 4 schematically illustrates what we have from the stand point of concentration gradients for this situation. When stratum corneum dominates as the barrier, we have what is illustrated by the upper diagram in this figure. The lower diagram applies to the situation where the stratum corneum is not important, either because the drug molecule is highly lipophilic or because the stratum corneum's barrier is abolished by tape-stripping, heat-treatment or penetration enhancer treatment. As a side note, we see that when the stratum corneum barrier is reduced, the steady-state epidermis concentrations of the drug are increased. As will be discussed later, this effect directly leads to the prediction that the efficacy of topically applied drug should be improved under these conditions.

Before we leave this topic, let us look (see Figure 5) at the data taken from Michaels et al. (1) on human cadaver skin permeability coefficients for drugs over a wide range of lipophilicity and note the tendency for a limiting P-value for the highly lipophillic drugs (nitroglycerin, estradiol and fentanyl). The limiting P-value for this set of data is lower (by about a factor of ten) than the P ≃ 0.10 cm/hr seen in Figures 2 and 3. Although it is speculative, one could suggest that this lower limiting P-value may be the result of the human epidermis/dermis being thicker (Table 1) on the average and that these studies were conducted at 30°C instead of 37°C. Comparative experiments (i.e. using the same compounds and same temperatures) are needed to resolve this important question.

"STRUCTURE/ACTIVITY" RELATIONSHIP

The data presented in Figures 2, 3 and 5 also suggest that, at least in the polar molecule region (i.e. where the stratum corneum is rate-limiting), there is a simple relationship between lipophilicity and the P-values. However, there is evidence that such may not be the case. Table 2 presents some recently obtained data on the permeability coefficients for the 5'-mono ester prodrugs of vidarabine with hairless mouse skin. These results point up the remarkably modest dependence upon lipophilicity for this homologous series. While

FOR POLAR SOLUTES: $P_{SC} \ll P_E$ OR P_D

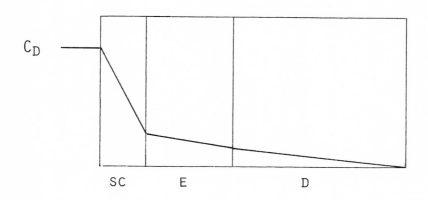

FOR NONPOLAR SOLUTES: $P_{SC} \gg P_E$ OR P_D

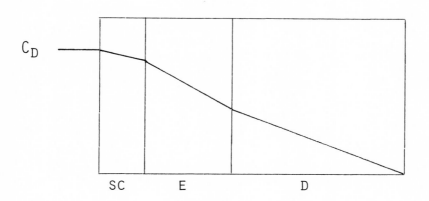

FIGURE 4. Concentration Gradients when Stratum Corneum is Rate-Limiting and when it is not

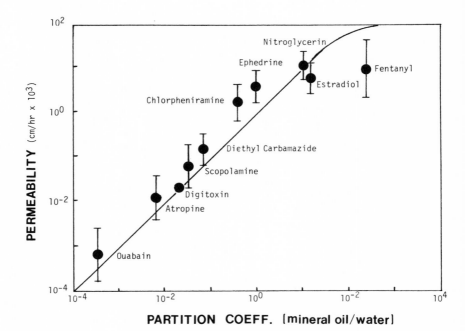

FIGURE 5.   Variation of Transdermal Permeability
            with Partition Coefficient. (Taken
            from Reference 1)

Mouse number	Permeability coefficient $\times 10^8$ (cm/sec)				
	ara-A	A-ara-A	V-ara-A	O-ara-A	Ester/ara-A
0621797	0.74	0.90	--	--	1.21
0621798	0.93	1.18	--	--	1.26
0714802	0.81	0.97	--	--	1.20
0714803	0.65	0.84	--	--	1.30
0621797	0.74	--	1.39	--	1.87
0621798	0.93	--	1.92	--	2.06
0714802	0.81	--	1.47	--	1.81
0714803	0.65	--	1.34	--	2.07
0621797	0.74	--	--	3.22	4.33
0621798	0.93	--	--	3.37	3.61
0714802	0.81	--	--	3.42	4.22
0714803	0.65	--	--	3.01	4.65

TABLE 2.   Permeability Coefficients of Ara-A,
Ara-A-5'-Acetate (A-ara-A), Ara-A-5'-
Valerate (V-ara-A) and Ara-5'-
Octanoate (O-ara-A) Through Whole Skin.

around a hundred-fold increase in the P-value was
expected between the P-value for the 5'-acetate and that
for the 5'-octanoate, the effect was only around 3-
fold. Results such as those in Table 2 may be
suggestive of a change in mechanism (i.e. change in
pathways) for highly polar molecules such vidarabine and
its esters and that this may be molecular weight
dependent.

There is also the question of what is the
microenvironmental nature of the rate-limiting
pathways. First, is the microenvironment lipoidal like
mineral oil or is it lipoidal like octanol or some other
lipophilic medium. Secondly, is the microenvironment
liquid-like or no-so-liquid like? Clearly more well-
designed studies are needed before we can begin to
answer these questions.

SOLID-VS. LIQUID-LIKE NATURE OF THE STRATUM-CORNEUM LIPID
BARRIER

Scheuplein et al. (11) and Michaels et al. (1) have
suggested that the extremely low diffusivities are
calculated from data such as those in Figures 2, 3 and 4
using equation 6, $K \simeq 1$ (polar drug molecules) and h $\simeq$
10 to 50 rm. For example, for hydrocortisone, $P \simeq 5$ x
10^{-4} cm/hr $\simeq 10^{-7}$ cm/sec. Taking $K \simeq 1$ and h $\simeq 20\,\mu$m, we
have from equation 6

$$D = \frac{Ph}{K} = \frac{10^{-7} \times 2 \times 10^{-3}}{1} \simeq 2 \times 10^{-10} \text{ cm}^2/\text{sec}$$

which is around four to five orders of magnitude lower
than for diffusion in water and is suggestive of a high
degree of solid-like nature or lipid structuring in the
microenvironment where transport is occurring.

Figures 6 and 7 are taken from the work of Elias et
al. (2) showing the authors concept of the lipid
structure in the intercellular region and an actual
electron micrograph (Figure 7) of the intercellular
region in neonatal mouse stratum corneum. The
photograph reveals the multiple lipid bilayer
structures which may be responsible for the "solid-like"
nature for these lipids.

Lambert et al. have recently (12) obtained some
interesting data on the influence of temperature on the
transport of hydrocortisone across full-thickness
hairless mouse skin. Figure 8 shows the data which
demonstrate the remarkable effect temperature has upon
the transport barrier. There is almost a 1 X 10^{4}-fold
effect upon P when the temperature is increased from
around 30°C to 60°C where from the previous discussion
we learned that the importance of the stratum corneum
barrier is completely eliminated. The data in Figure 8,
as Lambert et al. have suggested, are consistent with
the idea that, at least up to around 50°C, the fluidity
of the stratum corneum barrier increases significantly
with increasing temperature making the barrier more
liquid-like at the higher temperatures.

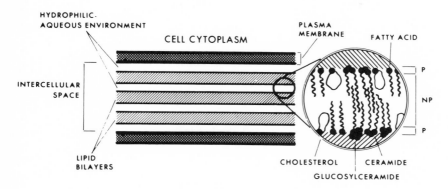

P. Polar Region of Bilayer
NP. Non-Polar Region of Bilayer

FIGURE 6. Diagram Illustrating a Possible Arrangement of Lipids Forming Intercellular Bilayers in the Stratum
Corneum. Though Phospholipids are not
Present, Polar Moieties of Neutral
Lipids and Ceramides along with Gluco-
sylceramides are Hypothesized to Maintain the Observed Bilayer Arrangement.
(Taken from Reference 2)

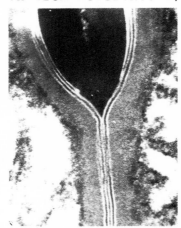

FIGURE 7. Thin Section Image of Neonatal Mouse
Stratum Corneum Cell Membrane Region.
Image Reveals the Intercellular Spaces
to be Full of Broad Lamellar Sheets.
(Taken from Reference 2)

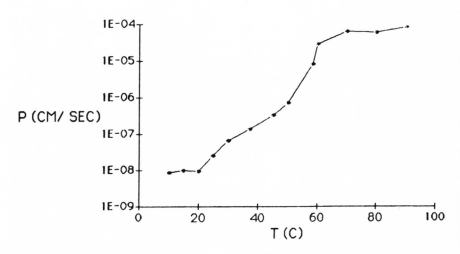

FIGURE 8.   The Influence of Temperature on the
            Permeability Coefficient of Hydro-
            cortisone in Hairless Mouse Skin.

VEHICLES THAT ALTER INTRINSIC PROPERTIES OF THE STRATUM CORNEUM

When a membrane is not altered intrinsically by the
solvent (Figure 1) in contact with it, we may write

J = constant   Equation 7

for all saturated solutions independent of the
solubility. I believe Tak was the first to present this
fundamental thermodynamic truth in its application to
percutaneous drug delivery.

The key issue as to whether equation 7 should hold
is whether the rate-limiting region (e.g., stratum
corneum) is altered in any way by the vehicle. Several
examples follow where the vehicle (solvent) does alter
the stratum corneum and therefore

J ≠ constant   Equation 8

Jones and his collaborators have discovered the

"sponge effect" (13). An important example of this phenomenon is when the solvent is a mixture of propyleneglycol and water and the drug is fluocinonide. In this system, there is significant uptake of solvent by the stratum corneum which is accompanied by significantly enhanced partitioning of the drug into the stratum corneum. Figure 9 is taken directly from the work of Jones and Raykar. It shows that J $\neq$ constant for these saturated solutions and, very interestingly, the rates are directly proportional to the solubility of fluocinonide in the stratum corneum. One caution in the interpretation of these data is that the flux data are from full thickness skin and the solubility data are with isolated human stratum corneum.

Another interesting system is the DMSO/water solvent case. Kurihara (8) working with Flynn showed that the hairless mouse skin stratum corneum is essentially unaltered up to 50% DMSO. Beyond 50% DMSO, however, the solvent significantly alters the stratum corneum properties, and at 100% DMSO, the barrier properties of the stratum corneum is essentially completely eliminated. A good example of the DMSO/H_2O system is given in Figure 10 which is for vidarabine as the drug. Up to 50% DMSO, the P-value for vidarabine decreases monotonically and approximately inversely (8) to vidarabine's solubility in the solvents. This is in accord with equation 7. Beyond 50% DMSO, however, the P-values begin to increase instead of continuing to decrease as expected if equation 7 were to hold. Thus, the stratum corneum barrier does not remain inert to the solvent beyond 50% DMSO. Finally at 100% DMSO, it is found that the P-value is essentially the same as that for tape-stripped skin (14). The barrier properties of the stratum corneum is eliminated.

The last example is that of Azone (9). The dramatic effect of pretreating hairless mouse skin with 3% Azone emulsion in 0.10% Tween 20 on the transport of 2', 3'-diacetate of vidarabine is seen in Figure 11. The rates observed after the pretreatment were 100-to 1000-fold greater than with no pretreatment and correspond to P-values close to that for stripped skin. Again, the stratum corneum barrier was

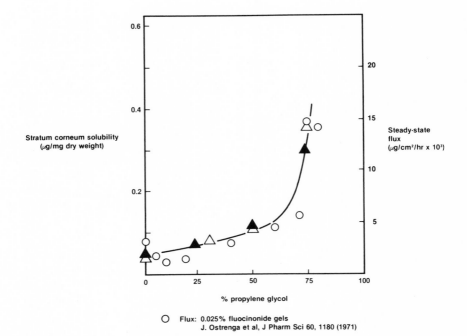

FIGURE 9.   Comparison of Stratum Corneum Solu-
            bility of Fluocinonide with Steady-
            State Flux from Saturated Solution
            through Full-Thickness Human Skin
            In Vitro (Figure Taken from the Work
            of Jones and Raykar, Reference 13)

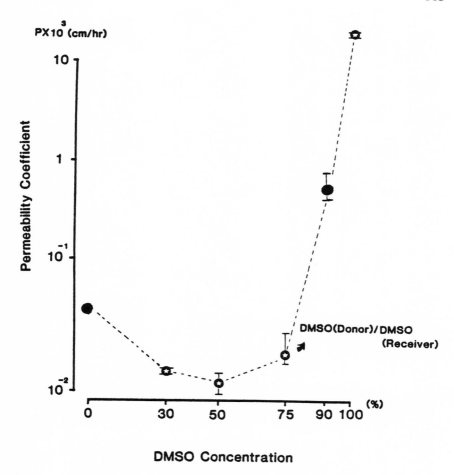

FIGURE 10. Permeability Coefficients of Vidarabine through Fresh Hairless Mouse
Skin in DMSO-Water Mixture

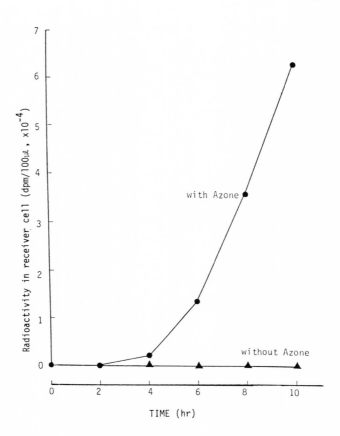

FIGURE 11.   Total Radioactivity Transported
              across Full-Thickness Skin in a Two-
              Chamber Cell Experiment. Donor Cell
              Contained Radiolabeled 2', 3'-Ara-
              A-Diacetate and 3% Azone as an Aque-
              ous Emulsion with 0.1% Polysorbate
              20.

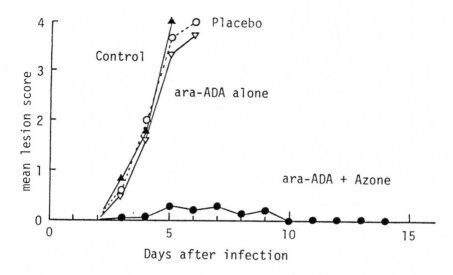

FIGURE 12. Effect of Ara-Ada With and Without
Azone in the Topical Treatment of
Cutaneous HSV-1 Infections of Hair-
less Mice (Lesion Score)

essentially completely eliminated by this agent. As a
side note, Figure 12 shows the remarkable effects of
Azone on the antiviral efficacy of 2, 3-diacetate of
vidarabine against cutaneous HSV-1 infections in
hairless mice. These dramatic in vivo results are
clearly consistent with predictions (9) based on
calculated concentration profiles such as those shown in
Figure 4 when Azone was present and when it was absent
in the formulations.

REFERENCES

(1) A.S. Michaels, S.K. Chandrasekaran and J. E. Shaw,
     A. I. Ch. E. J., 21,985 (1975).

(2) P.M. Elias, Int'l. J. Derm., 20,1 (1981).

(3) G.L. Flynn, H.H. Durrheim, W.I. Higuchi, J. Pharm.
     Sci., 70,52 (1981).

(4) C.D. Yu, J.L. Fox, N.F.H. Ho, W.I. Higuchi, J.
     Pharm. Sci., 68,1347 (1979).

(5) R.J. Scheuplein, J. Invest. Derm., 48,79 (1967).

(6) G.L. Flynn, C.R. Behl, K.A. Walters, O.G.
     Gatmaitan, A. Wittkowsky, T. Kurihara, N.F.H. Ho,
     W.I. Higuchi, C.L. Pierson, Burns, 8,47 (1980).

(7) W.J. Lambert, K. Knutson, P.K. Banerjee and W.I.
     Higuchi, unpublished data.

(8) T. Kurihara, Ph.D. Thesis (1982), The University of
     Michigan.

(9) W.M. Shannon, L. Westbrook, W.I. Higuchi, K.
     Sugibayashi, D.C. Baker, J.L. Fox, G.L. Flynn,
     N.F.H. Ho, R. Vaidyanathan, J. Pharm. Sci., in
     press.

(10) W.M. Smith, Ph.D. Thesis (1982), The University of
     Michigan.

(11) R.J. Scheuplein, I.H. Blank and D.J. MacFarlane, J.
     Invest. Derm., 49,582 (1967).

(12) W.J. Lambert, K. Knutson, P.K. Banerjee and W.I.
     Higuchi, Abstract No. 50, 37th National Meeting of
     the Academy of Pharmaceutical Sciences,
     Philadelphia, October, (1984).

(13) R.F. Jones, unpublished data. See also, P. Raykar
     and R.E. Jones, Abstract No. 40, 35th National
     Meeting of the Academy of Pharmaceutical Sciences,
     Miami Beach, November (1983).

(14) C.D. Yu, W.I. Higuchi, N.F.H. Ho, J.L. Fox and G.L. Flynn, <u>J. Pharm. Sci.</u>, <u>69</u>,770 (1980).

C. PHYSICAL-CHEMICAL APPROACHES TO DIRECTED DRUG DELIVERY

A PHYSICAL APPROACH TO DRUG DELIVERY

Felix Theeuwes, D.Sc.
ALZA Corporation
950 Page Mill Road
P.O. Box 10950
Palo Alto, Ca 94303-0802

INTRODUCTION

Tak Higuchi (1963) found the elegant analytical expression for the release rate of the diffusional matrix system more than 20 years ago, and this expression is the basis for many systems that are even claimed to be new today. This development was a milestone in area of physical pharmacy and dosage form development. Tak has been a driving force in the field of pharmacy: he gave people a mission and has been a source of inspiration. I was a low temperature physicist before I met Tak, and he convinced me that osmosis was a phenomenon under utilized in the field of pharmacy.

In this presentation I would like to place into perspective some contributions that can be made by the physical approach to systemic drug delivery, review some dosage form-biological interface issues that need to be understood for successful product design, and use as an example, oral dosage forms for systemic treatment.

It can probably be said for all drugs, that a concentration of drug at some site in the body, as a function of time, relates to the therapeutic effect of that drug. The effect exerted by the drug has, in general, the appearance

of a spectrum that includes possible modification of the
symptoms of the disease, possible interference with the
progression of the disease, or it may create additional
effects--such as side-effects. There is not necessarily
a one-to-one correspondance between the effect and a known
concentration in a particular site of the body; however,
there are some drugs for which we know that systemic
effects relate to the concentration in the systemic circulation. The concentration in a particular site in the body
as a function of time is, as we know from pharmacokinetics,
a function of the absorption, distribution, and in excretion rates.

A medicament, shown in Table 1, can be thought of as
coming about by two approaches: the chemical approach (the
synthesis of the drug substance) and the physical route
(the dosage form design part). The contributions made by
these approaches are listed in the two right columns of the
table. To the patient, however, only a few of the entries
in this table are important. They are the spectrum, or
more importantly, the particular effects that can be
selected, the duration and route of administration, and the
external appearance. It is not possible just to add up the
different entries in each column that relate to the value
to the patient, and to add the value based on a count. It
can be seen, however, that there is substantial value in
the physical approach.

As shown in Table 2, one can divide the different
aspects of dosage form design in categories dealing with
the design of the dosage form, the issues relating to the
interface between the dosage form and the body, and the
issues relating to the effect or the concentrations to be
achieved in the body. Dr. Zaffaroni (1971) described the
building elements of the therapeutic system (module, platform, and program). The module comprises the energy source
for delivery, a rate-controlling element that limits the
output of the dosage form, the drug reservoir, and the
delivery portal. The platform issues that he identified
relate to the quality of the interface between the dosage

Table 1:   Approach to Design and Implication
of a Medicament

Medicament		
Approach	Chemical	Physical
Composition	Drug Substance	Dosage Form
Effect	Spectrum	Selection
Concentration	Absorption (t)	Absorption (t): duration
	Distribution (t)	Site in the body
	Excretion (t): duration	
Prescription	Route of administration	Route of administration
		External appearance

form and the body, and the program through which the dosage
form contributes its effect relates to the outcome and its
effect and concentration into the body. The aspects of the
biological interface between dosage form and body include
the boundary conditions that the interface creates and its
effect on the functionality of the dosage form, the imped-
ance to drug absorption that is created by the body (that
includes resistance to drug absorption and metabolism), and
the duration of absorption allowed by gastrointestinal
transit.

Table 2:   Issues to be Addressed in Dosage
            Form Design for System Treatment

Dosage Form	Interface	Body
Module		
Energy source	Boundary conditions	Effect
Rate controller	Duration of absorption	Concentration
Reservoir	Resistance to absorption	
Portal		
Platform		
Program		

THE ORAL DOSAGE FORM

There are, as shown in Table 3, a wide variety of oral
dosage forms that one can distinguish based on their
energy source or mechanism of operation: polymer relaxation
controlled systems, systems based on ion exchange, dissolution controlled dosage forms, and also osmotic systems.
One can further distinguish them by their module or basically their internal structure, be it matrix forms, powders,
liquids, tablets, pill forms, etc. as for example for dissolution controlled forms. Although some of these systems
are primitive from a rate control point of view, nevertheless, one can still identify the various subcomponents in
the module that speak to the delivery of those particular
dosage forms. For osmotic systems, the three different
structures that have been published are the mini-osmotic
systems, the elementary osmotic pump (EOP), and push-pull

Table 3: Oral Dosage from Classification

Mechanism	Osmotic	Dissolution	Ion Exchange	Polymer Relaxation/
Energy source				Dissolution
Module				
Rate controller	mini-osmotic	powder	matrix	matrix
Energy source	EOP	liquid	matrix/membr.	
Reservoir	push-pull	tablet		
Portal		matrix		
		membr. res.		
		pill		
Appearance				
Platform	Single unit	single	multiple	multiple(capsule)
Portal	Single orifice	multiple	(capsule)	single
	Multiple orifice	(capsule)		
	Multiple units			

systems (P-P). The appearance of the dosage forms to the body relate to platform and portal. Each type can have the form of multiples in a capsule, or single units. For the osmotic systems in addition, there are issues relating to the number and placement of the orifice.

It is useful to consider the theoretical rate M_o as a function of time in order to identify the variables that affect the release rate, and also to understand the sensitivity of the rate to production parameters and the parameters of its environment--the GI tract.

In general, one can say that the theoretical rate is a function of the physical/chemical mechanism that underlies the operation of the form, the internal structure of the form that relates to how the energy source is positioned relative to the rate-controlling element, and also the boundary conditions that are placed on the dosage form. For example, one can write that the release rate from the diffusional reservoir system, as given by Equation (1)

$$\dot{M}_o = K \cdot D \cdot A \cdot \frac{C_o}{h} \tag{1}$$

in which K is the partition coefficient of the drug substance between the membrane and the reservoir; D, the diffusion of the drug substance in the membrane; A, the area of the membrane; C_o the concentration inside of the reservoir; and h, the membrane thickness. The release rate from all diffusion control systems, of course, is not the same and depends on the structure of the dosage form given for a matrix by Higuchi's (1963) Equation:

$$\dot{M}_o (t) = \frac{A}{2} \left[D \frac{\varepsilon}{\tau} (2 C_o - \varepsilon C_s) C_s \right]^{-\frac{1}{2}} \cdot t^{-\frac{1}{2}} \tag{2}$$

wherein the release rate is shown to be proportional to the square root of time with the parameters as indicated.

A: Total external surface area of the matrix

D: Diffusion coefficient of drug in the matrix structure

C_s: Solubility of drug in the matrix channels

t: Time

ε: Porosity of the matrix

τ: Tortuosity of the maxtrix

Osmotic systems of various types have been made that are very suitable as oral dosage forms. The elementary osmotic pump (Theeuwes and Higuchi, 1974; Theeuwes, 1975) is the most simple form, shown in Figure 1. The drug with or without an osmotic driving agent is in tablet form, surrounded with a membrane that is semipermeable, with a delivery orifice. Water from the environment is absorbed through the membrane to dissolve the substance, which is pumped out in solution through the orifice. The release rate from these systems is predictable as shown by the Equations (3) and (4).

$$\frac{dm}{dt} = \frac{dV}{dt} \cdot C \tag{3}$$

$$\frac{dV}{dt} = \frac{A}{h} \cdot L_p \ [\sigma \Delta \pi - \Delta P] \tag{4}$$

The mass release rate (dm/dt) is given by the volumetric pumping rate (dV/dt) and the concentration of the drug in solution (C). The volumetric rate in turn can be calculated from the hydraulic permeability coefficient of the membrane L_p, and the driving force. This force is equal to the reflection coefficient (σ), times the osmotic pressure ($\Delta \pi$), minus the back pressure (ΔP) generated by the flow of liquid from inside to the outside. By proper dosage form

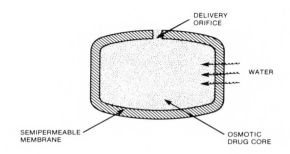

Figure 1:   Cross-section of a typical oral
elementary osmotic pump

design, one can make the orifice so that this pressure (ΔP)
is zero and arrive at a very simple expression, as given in
Equation 5 for the zero-order rate.

$$\left(\frac{dm}{dt}\right)_Z = \frac{A}{h} \cdot k \cdot \pi \cdot S \qquad (5)$$

with A, the membrane area; h, the membrane thickness; k,
the osmotic membrane permeability; and S, the drug solubility. Also, the non-zero-order rate has been predictable, but less important, as the non-zero-order fraction is
usually small. Equation (6) contains the internal volume
of the system (V), and the time where the zero-order period
ends (t_z).

$$\frac{dm}{dt} = \frac{(dm/dt)_Z}{\left[1 + \frac{1}{S \cdot V} \left(\frac{dm}{dt}\right)_Z (t - t_Z)\right]^2} \qquad (6)$$

One of the first examples made of this system was the
system delivering potassium chloride, shown in Figure 2,
where the solid line is the calculated rate compared to
the range of experimental data obtained with 5 systems.

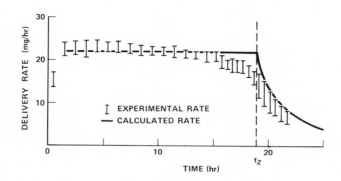

Figure 2: In vitro release rate of potassium chloride from elementary osmotic pumps in water at 37°C. Key: $\underline{\text{I}}$, range of experimental data obtained from five systems.

The rate that is ultimately important to achieve the concentration and effect, however, is the absorption rate $\dot{M}_3$. So there is quite a distance between the theoretical rate and the absorption rate and that link needs to be understood (Theeuwes, in press). $\dot{M}_0$ is the theoretical rate, $\dot{M}_1$, the in vitro rate or the output of the dosage form in a particular environment in vitro. $\dot{M}_2$ is the output of the dosage form in the in vivo environment, and finally $\dot{M}_3$ the absorption rate. In order to have reproducible medicine, one then must know the link between the quality that one controls $\dot{M}_1$ and the absorption rate. By selecting the boundary conditions in vitro to be analogous to the biological environment, one can expect that the in vivo rate is equal to the in vitro rate if, in vivo, the same mechanism is operational and no new mechanisms are turned on, the structure of the dosage form behaves the same, and if the boundary conditions in vivo are the same as in vitro.

THE GASTROINTESTINAL TRACT AS INTERFACE

It is therefore important to know the boundary conditions that are created in vivo for oral dosage forms, such as temperature, motility, pH, enzymatic activity, osmolality, peristaltic pressure.

Some of these variables are known from the Geigy Scientific Tables (Lentner, 1981). The temperature is very constant, ranging between 36° and 37°C. The pH, on the other hand, is very variable and can range between 1 and 7 in the stomach of man. In the intestine it is fairly constant between 6 and 8. The tonicity is very constant between 285-292 mmol/kg. The stirring rate is another highly variable entity as can be seen from some of the flow rates that have been observed in man. Flow in the jejunum is about 2 ml/min, while in the ileum, 0.7 ml/min. It is known that the stomach, being either in a fed or fasting mode, can have periods of total quiescence or high activity. Based on the pragmatic approach, the Food and Drug Administration prefers to have stirring rates in the U.S.P. apparatus measured between 0 and 75 rpm, since those rates have been found to be most analogous to the conditions seen in the GI tract. It is then wise to select a dosage form for which the release rate depends only on variables that are fairly constant in the intestinal tract--temperature and tonicity--and independent of the others. Osmotic systems are such systems.

When the release rate in vivo is different from the release rate in vitro, very often it is that the release rate is sensitive to a variable (X_i) in the intestinal tract. In this case a factor Q can be written to express the difference between the rate in vitro and rate in vivo as equation (7).

$$\dot{M}_2 = Q \ \dot{M}_1 \tag{7}$$

If Q exists, as is shown in Equation (8),

$$Q = 1 + \frac{1}{M_1} \ \frac{\partial \dot{M}_1}{\partial X_i} \ \Delta Xi \tag{8}$$

because one has not selected the conditions in vitro to be
close enough to the conditions in vivo, $\Delta X_i \neq 0$, then one
can adjust these and obtain the value of Q, that is 1. If
on the other hand, Q exists because the dosage form release
rate is sensitive to variables in the GI tract (X_i variable), then it becomes very difficult to validate the
performance of such a dosage form because the conditions in
the GI tract are unpredictable. It is therefore more
advantageous to pick a dosage form that has a release rate
which is insensitive to variables in the GI tract,
$\partial M_1 / \partial X_i = 0$.

Figure 3 shows the cumulative mass from an elementary
osmotic pump delivering oxprenolol succinate (Theeuwes
et al., in press) at a rate of 16 mg per hour for a total
content of 260 mg. The mass rate is shown in normal saline,
artificial gastric fluid, and artificial intestinal fluid
without enzymes. The release rate is no different in any
of these environments. The average release rate during
hours 2 to 12 in the zero-order portion is shown to be
independent of stirring, the stirring conditions 25 to 75
rpm in saline (pH = 7), and in gastric fluid (pH = 1.2) as
shown in Figure 4.

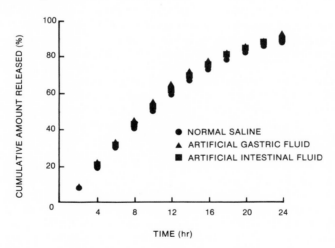

Figure 3: Cumulative amount released from
OROS® (oxprenolol succinate) 16/260.

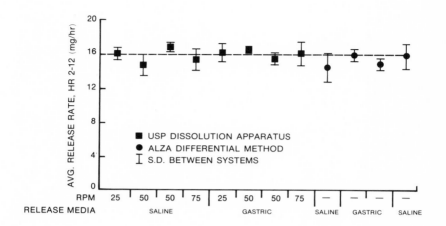

Figure 4: Average release rates for a single batch of
OROS® (oxprenolol) 16/260 determined in USP dissolution
under different test conditions.

As a consequence of the insensitivity of the release
rate to the conditions in the GI tract, Figure 5 shows that
the cumulative amount of metoprolol released in the GI
tract of dogs (Fara et al., in press) is the same as the
release rate in vitro and equal to the theoretical rate
shown by the solid line. Data of this type are obtained in
dogs by dosing the animals at regular time intervals with
systems of known content. The systems are retrieved when
the animal is sacrificed, and from the residual content and
initial content, the difference released is measured and
plotted as shown in Figure 5.

The duration of absorption that one can achieve with
oral dosage forms cannot be longer than the residence time
in the GI tract. It must be realized that the total duration of efficacy achieved depends on the duration of absorption and duration of excretion. For conventional dosage
forms, the efficacy period is more substantially dependent
on the excretion half-life. In addition, for a delivery
system, one can depend on the absorption time, and the sum
of the two can carry the total dosing period of the

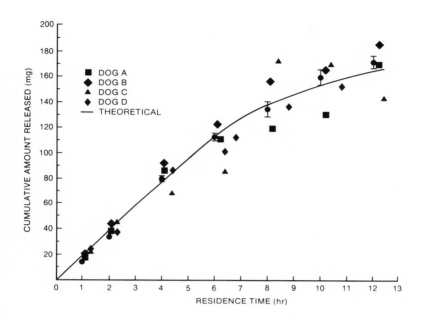

Figure 5: Mean cumulative amounts of drug released in vivo and in vitro from OROS® (metoprolol) 19/190 systems. The vertical bars for the in vitro data represent standard errors of the mean.

dosage form. If the plasma half-life is relatively long, the absorption time does not have to be long. For a compound with a very short halflife the maximum duration of absorption is desired.

A substantial amount of work in the area of gastrointestinal physiology has been carried out to demonstrate useful absorption times that can be expected from the GI tract. Some of this work was published by Fara (1982), and recently Davis and co-workers have generated several papers on that subject (Davis, 1983; Davis et al., in press). This information is summarized in Table 4.

TABLE 4:   Residence Time in the Gastrointestinal Tract in Man

Motility State of Intestine	Fasting		Fed	
Pellet size	A	B	A	B
Gastric emptying (t_{50})	1.9	2.1	3.75	>10 hr
Arrival at caecum (t_{50})	5.6	5.1	8.1	>10 hr

A: Spherical size: diameter 0.7 to 1.2 mm (Davis, 1983)

B: Cylindrical size: length 25mm; diameter 8mm (Davis
et al., 1984)

Adhesion has been recognized as one of the mechanisms
to retard dosage forms through the GI tract, Table 4 shows
the duration of absorption under conditions without
adhesion.

It is now well known that the intestinal tract can
work under two modes--fasting and fed (Fara, 1982). Certain residence times can be identified during both conditions. These residence times are now understood to be a
function of the size of the object, as reflected by the
Table 4 half-times of transition. In the fasting state
when transit time is the shortest, John et al. (in press)
stated that measurements in six studies indicated that, for
45 systems recovered, 5 (or 11%) had a total transit time
of less than 22 hr, and the median recovery time was 27 hr
with two-thirds of the data falling between 22 and 33 hr.
In the fed condition, residence times will be longer in the
stomach. Davis et al. (in press) showed recently that all
OSMET™ modules were maintained in the stomach during the
fed mode for a period of 10 hr. The absorption time in
some cases is only a fraction of the transit time, depending on limits to absorption or the absorption window. It
appears that the minimum absorption time is 6 to 8 hr for
drugs that are only absorbed in the upper tract and the

maximum practical absorption time for drugs that are well
absorbed throughout the total intestinal tract is 24 hr.

To understand conditions of adhesion in the GI tract,
Swisher et al., (in press) recently measured the adhesive
forces exerted by the GI tract on a number of dosage forms.
The data depicted in Figure 6 indicate that the osmotic
systems experience an adhesive force that, after one minute
of soaking, is about an order of magnitude lower than that

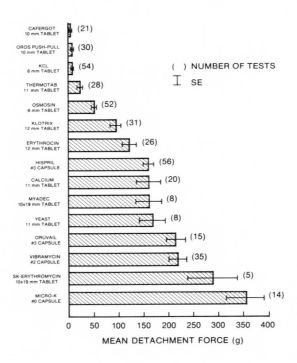

Figure 6: Mean force required to detach various oral
products from isolated dog esophagus one minute after
placement. All products, except yeast and SK-Erythro-
mycin, were tested in at least two preparations.

which is found with some gelatin capsules. The adhesive
force measured for OSMOSIN® systems derives from an hydroxy-
propyl-methylcellulose overcoat. When this coat dissolves,
the adhesive force subsequently drops another order of
magnitude. The adhesive force is then negligible and no
different from an uncoated tablet. The average transit
times that one can expect with osmotic systems are therefore not different from what has previously been found in
literature for inert objects (Hinton et al., 1969).

The absorption rate $(\dot{M}_3)$, relates to the output of the
dosage form in the GI tract $(\dot{M}_2)$ as shown by Equation (9).

$$\dot{M}_3 = F \cdot \dot{M}_2 \tag{9}$$

The degree of system control exerted by the dosage form can
be defined by X and can be expressed both in terms of rates
or in terms of total amount, as shown in Equations (10) and
(11).

$$X = \frac{\dot{M}_3}{\dot{M}_1} \tag{10}$$

$$X = \frac{\int_0^t \dot{M}_3 \, dt}{\int_0^t \dot{M}_1 \, dt} = \frac{M_3}{M_1} = F \cdot Q \tag{11}$$

M_3 is the integral up to time t of $\dot{M}_3$, and M_1 is the cumulative output of the dosage form in vitro up to time t.
For a dosage that has an in vitro rate equal to the in vivo
rate Q, Equation (11) is one, and the relationship between
the in vitro rate and the in vivo rate is then given by the
factor F, which conventionally is measured in bioavailability studies. In order to ascertain the absorption rate in
the population of interest, one must conduct the study in
that population and under conditions of use.

A study on OROS® metoprolol systems by Godbillon and co-workers (in press) reports the absorption rate as a function of time, compared to the in vitro release rate as shown in Figure 7. This figure shows that both rates are identical, as the two curves can be superimposed, however, the in vivo rate was displaced to the left by one hour, indicating that there was a lag time of absorption. The ratio of the amounts absorbed to released at any time is one, indicating that for this drug, system control by the dosage form is constant over the total GI tract up to 24 hr.

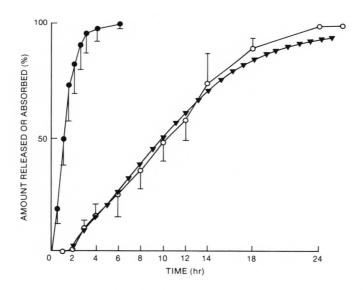

Figure 7: Comparison of the mean apparent in vivo absorption (o), and in vitro (▼) profiles for the OROS® (metoprolol) 19/285. The in vivo profile for a conventional tablet formulation (●) also is shown. The vertical bars represent 1 S.D.

A multiple-dose study with OROS® metoprolol systems
indicates that plasma concentration can be controlled very
well at steady state up to 24 hr, as shown in Figure 8
(Grainger et al., in press). After the initial rise, the
plasma concentration remains constant at steady state,
shown on day 8, compared with 100 mg metoprolol tartrate
tablets administration twice a day. The OROS® system
releases 285 mg metoprolol fumarate, which is equivalent to
300 mg metoprolol tartrate.

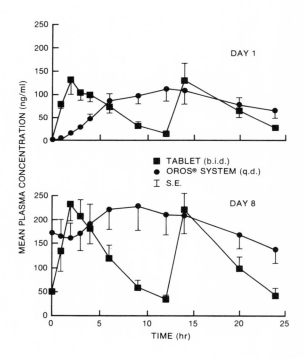

Figure 8: Mean plasma concentration/time profiles
after single and multiple dosing with 100 mg conventional metoprolol tablets twice daily (■) and OROS®
(metoprolol fumarate) 19/285 once daily (●).

There is data to indicate a close relationship between plasma concentration and excerise heart rate, as shown in Figure 9. The exercised heart rate falls and rises inversely proportional to the drug concentrations in the plasma following administration of the tablets. With the OROS® system regimen, the heart rate can be suppressed and maintained constant over 24 hr. This is done without compromising the effects on the mean blood pressure, as shown in Figure 10 (Grainger et al., in press).

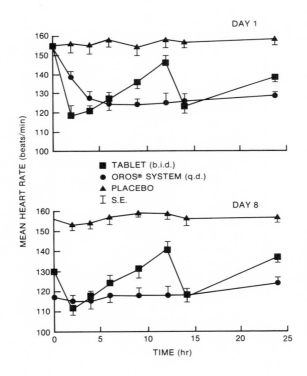

Figure 9: Mean exercise heart rates on days 1 and 8 of treatment with placebo, 100 mg conventional metoprolol twice-daily, and OROS® (metoprolol) 19/285 once-daily.

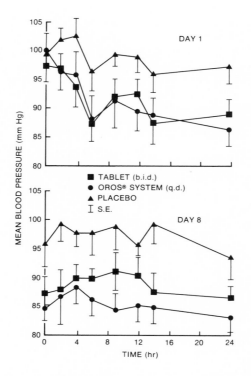

Figure 10: Mean blood pressure profiles on days 1 and 8 of treatment days with placebo, 100 mg conventional metoprolol twice-daily, and OROS® (metoprolol) 19/285 once-daily.

FUTURE DEVELOPMENT

It has been a challenge to deliver very soluble and insoluble compounds via osmotic dosage forms. To that end, the push-pull system (Figure 11) was invented (Theeuwes, 1981). With the push-pull system, the drug is formulated in a drug reservoir separate from the osmotic push compartment, shown in the lower section of the figure. The membrane is semipermeable and encapsulates the reservoir. The delivery orifice is positioned through the membrane into

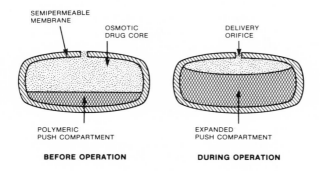

SEMIPERMEABLE
MEMBRANE
OSMOTIC
DRUG CORE
DELIVERY
ORIFICE
POLYMERIC
PUSH COMPARTMENT
EXPANDED
PUSH COMPARTMENT
BEFORE OPERATION   **DURING OPERATION**

Figure 11:   Cross-section of the push-pull
osmotic pump

the drug reservoir. For a highly soluble drug, the drug
itself is the osmotic driving agent and is solubilized by
the influx of water into the top compartment. The push
compartment continuously expels the drug solution so that
the solid drug phase can be maintained throughout the total
lifetime of the system, thereby giving rise to delivery of
high zero-order fractions. The more interesting application of the push-pull system is the delivery of insoluble
drugs. In this case the drug is mixed with an osmotic
driving agent and a suspending agent in the drug reservoir.
By this combined action--the pulling in of water in the
drug compartment (creating a suspension) and the pushing
action of the push compartment--the drug is delivered. The
release rate of this system can be predicted from the
osmotic volume imbibition rates into both compartments:
(F) the drug compartment and (Q) the push compartment. The
rate can be written as Equation (12)

$$dm/dt = (F + Q) \cdot C \qquad (12)$$

where C is the concentration of drug of the dispensed
formulation.

Despite the significant advances in dosage form design that have been achieved over the last 15 years, the same pharmacodynamic issues still remain: What drugs benefit from a controlled drug delivery profile? What is the ideal drug program? What will be the therapeutic value?

In order to answer these questions without having to resort to developing a dedicated dosage form, the ALZET® system was designed for animal use. This pump (Theeuwes and Yum, 1976) is an empty dosage form that can be filled with any drug substance and programmed essentially at any mass rate by the researcher. Although the pump's volumetric rate is programmed, the mass rate can be changed by varying the concentration of drug in the dosage form. Such systems have been used extensively in animal testing and more than 900 research papers have appeared in print (Urquhart et al., 1984). In addition to this system, there now exists a category of systems (OSMET™) that can deliver the drug content over a 24-hr period for studies in man. Both the ALZET® and OSMET™ modules are available with an internal volume of 200 µl and 2 ml. The small pumps can be used as a simulator for zero-order oral dosage forms, and the large ones can be used as a simulator for rectal dosage forms. To study the pharmacodynamics of a drug substance, one can use either form or approach for studies that lead to the selection of an oral form as the commercial system.

Figure 12 shows the normalized in vitro release rate from such OSMET™ systems and shows that these profiles are in quality no different from those for the long duration 1 and 2 week ALZET® systems.

Pioneering work using the OSMET™ modules in the area of pharmacokinetics-pharmacodynamics has been carried out under the direction of Dr. Breimer in Leiden. In Figure 13 he shows that the rectal route is a very dependable way to achieve controlled plasma levels (De Leede et al., 1981). The plasma concentrations achieved are very comparable to those achieved with I.V. infusions.

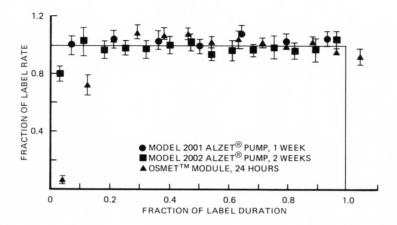

Figure 12: In vitro performance of OSMET™ drug delivery module and ALZET® mini-osmotic pump.

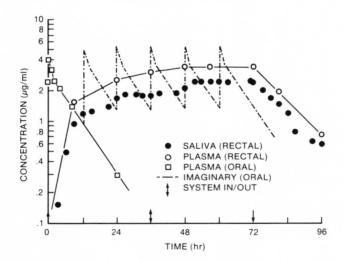

Figure 13: Comparison of an oral solution and a rectal infusion of theophylline in one subject.

CONCLUSIONS

It can stated that in the last 15 years, significant
progress has been made in the area of system design. This
has led to the development of oral dosage forms that can
deliver any drug substance at controlled rates. The bio-
logic dynamic interface -- the GI tract -- has been studied
extensively and we have learned, to a great extent, the
opportunities and limitations for oral controlled drug
absorption. Given those limitations for most drugs, a
twice-a-day, or most often a once-a-day dosage form should
be possible. The area of greatest opportunity for the
future definitely lies in the identification of the compounds that can benefit from controlled delivery, and the
identification of the needed drug program that will allow
the achievment of the optimal therapeutic value of each
drug.

ACKNOWLEDGEMENT

I would like to express my sincere thanks to
Manuela Henry and Jim Yuen for their editorial assistance
in the preparation of the manuscript.

REFERENCES

Davis, S. S, The use of scintigraphic methods for the
    evaluation of drug dosage forms in the gastrointest-
    inal tract. In Topics in Pharmaceutical Sciences
    1983. Proceedings of the 43rd International Congress
    of Pharmaceutical Sciences of F.I.P., Montreux,
    Switzerland, 5-9 September 1983.

Davis, S. S., Hardy, J. G., Taylor, M. J., Whalley, D. R.
    and Wilson, C. G., The effect of food on the gastroin-
    testinal transit of pellets and an osmotic device
    (OSMET). Int. J. Pharm. 21 (1984) 167-177.

De Leede, L. G. J., De Boer, A. G., Van Velzen, S. L.,
and Breimer, D. D., Rectal infusion of drugs in
man with an osmotic delivery system. In Aiache, J. M.
and Hirtz, J. (Eds) Biopharmaceutics, Technique et
Documentation, Paris, 1981, 239-243.

Fara, J. W., Gastrointestinal transit of solid dosage
forms. Drug Dvlpmt. Ind. Pharm., 8 (1982) 22-26.

Fara, J. W., Myrback, R. E., and Swanson, D. R., Evaluation
of oxprenolol and metoprolol OROS systems in the dog:
comparison of in vivo and in vitro drug release, and
of drug absorption from duodenal and colonic infusion
sites. Br. J. Clin. Pharmacol., in press.

Godbillon, J., Gerardin, A., Richard, J., Leroy, D., and
Moppert, J., Osmotically controlled delivery of metoprolol in man: in vivo performance of OROS systems
with different durations of drug release. Br. J.
Clin. Pharmacol., in press.

Grainger, S. L., John, V. A., and Smith, S. E., Pharmacokinetic and pharmacodynamic evaluation of conventional
and 19/285 OROS formulations of metoprolol after
single and multiple dosing. Br. J. Clin. Pharmacol.,
in press.

Higuchi, T., Mechanism of sustained-action medication.
J. Pharm. Sci., 52 (1963) 1145-1149.

Hinton, J. M., Lennard-Jones, J. E., and Young, A. C.,
A new method for studying gut transit times using
radioopaque markers. Gut, 10 (1969) 842-847.

John, V. A., Shotton, P. A., Moppert, J., and Theobald, W.,
A short report on the gastrointestinal transit of OROS
drug delivery systems in healthy volunteers. Br. J.
Clin. Pharmacol., in press.

Lentner, C. (Ed), Geigy Scientific Tables, Volume 1. Units
of Measurement, Body Fluids, Composition of the Body,
Nutrition, 8th Ed., Ciba-Geigy Corp., West Caldwell,
NJ, 1981.

Swisher, D. A., Sendelbeck, S. L., and Fara, J. W.,
   Adherence of various oral dosage forms to the esophagus. Int. J. Pharm., in press.

Theeuwes, F., The elementary osmotic pump. J. Pharm. Sci.
   64 (1975) 1891–1897.

Theeuwes, F., Novel drug delivery systems. In Prescott,
   L. F., and Nimmo, W. S. (Eds) Drug Absorption, ADIS
   Press, Balgowlah, Australia, 1981, 157–176.

Theeuwes, F., Validation of rate-controlled dosage forms.
   In Prescott, L. F. and Nimmo, W. (Eds) Drug Absorption, Churchill Livingstone, Edinburgh, in press.

Theeuwes, F. and Higuchi, T. U.S. Patent 3,845,770,
   "Osmotic Dispensing Device for Releasing Beneficial
   Agent," Issued 5 November 1974.

Theeuwes, F., Swanson, D., Guittard, G., Ayer, A., and
   Khanna., S., Osmotic delivery systems for the
   β-adrenoceptor antagonists metoprolol and oxprenolol:
   design and evaluation of systems for once-daily administration. Br. J. Clin. Pharmacol., in press.

Theeuwes, F. and Yum, S. I., Principles of the design and
   operation of generic osmotic pumps for the delivery of
   semisolid or liquid drug formulations. Ann. Biomed.
   Eng., 4 (1976) 343–353.

Urquhart, J., Fara, J. W., and Willis, K. W., Rate-controlled delivery systems in drug and hormone research.
   Ann. Rev. Pharmacol. Toxicol., 24 (1984) 199–236.

Zaffaroni, A., New approaches to drug administration. In
   Abstracts of the 31st International Congress of Pharmaceutical Sciences, Washington, D.C., 7–12 September
   1971, 19–20.

MICROPARTICULATE DRUG CARRIERS

R. L. Juliano, Ph.D.

Department of Pharmacology

University of Texas Medical School
Houston, Texas   77025

Introduction

Several type of microparticulate carriers have been
employed in recent years in conjunction with a wide
variety of drugs and a broad range of therapeutic goals.
One of the most salient characteristics of microparticulate materials as drug carriers is that, in general, the
drug-carrrier complex must be administered parenterally,
usually by intravenous injection. Thus, an understanding
of the in vivo behavior of the drug carrier and its
interaction with a number of critical biological systems
becomes an important aspect of designing therapeutic
strategies relying on microparticulate carriers. In this
chapter I will briefly describe the physical characteristics and preparation of several types of microparticulate
drug carrier complexes. I will then go on to consider
their interaction with the vasculature and the reticuloendothelial system and how this affects behavior in
vivo. Finally, I will discuss selected therapeutic
applications which seem consonant with the biological
properties of microparticulate carriers. Many of the
issues discussed in this chapter have been reviewed at
greater length elsewhere (Poznanski & Juliano, 1984;
Juliano, 1984).

Preparation and Characteristics of Microparticulate Carriers

a) Liposomes

Phospholipids dispersed in water spontaneously form liposomes, which are closed structures with internal aqueous compartments bounded by phospholipid bilayer membranes (Bangham 1972). A variety of amphiphilic compounds are used in conjunction with glycerophospholipids to make liposomes; thus sterols (e.g. cholesterol), sphingolipids, glycolipids, long chain fatty acids and even membrane proteins can be used (Juliano & Layton, 1980; Juliano 1983). Non phospholipid compounds including sterol esters and even certain amphiphilic polymers (Fendler & Schupp 1984) can also form vesicle structures which resemble phospholipid liposomes. Thus a variety of amphiphilic substances can be used in the formulation of liposomes. The charge, stability, chemical reactivity and biological properties of the liposome preparation will be influenced by the choice of chemical constituents.

A simple technique for preparing drug containing liposomes involves drying a solution of lipids in an organic solvent on to the wall of a flask or tube, hydrating the lipid, dispersing it by adding buffer, and vortexing. Water soluble drugs to be incorported into the liposome are included in the buffer, while non polar drugs are included in the organic solvent. A fraction of the water soluble drug will be trapped in the internal aqueous compartment of the liposome while hydrophobic drugs dissolve in the lipid and become intercalated into the liposome membrane (Juliano & Stamp 1979). Free and liposome bound drug can then be separated by gel filtration chromatography. The liposomes formed in this manner are heterogeneous in size (about 0.1-3 microns), have several concentric layers of membranes and are termed MLVs (multi-lamellar vesicles). MLVs encapsulate only a small fraction (up to 5%) of the available water soluble drug. The amount of lipid soluble (hydrophobic) drug entrapped depends on the amount of lipid and on the degree of drug induced destabilization of the liposome which can be tolerated - usually about 5-10 mol % drug can be successfully incorporated (Juliano & Stamp 1979; Lee 1978). A large variety of drugs have been successfully incorporated into liposomes including anti tumor agents, polyene antibiotics, anti bacterial drugs and anti parasitic agents (Juliano 1983).

Over the last ten years a large number of refinements of the technique of liposome preparation have been introduced (Szoka & Papahadjopoulos 1980). Most of these refinements have had one of two goals; either to increase the size uniformity of the liposome preparation, or to increase the fraction of drug which is entrapped in the liposome. Thus sonication or solvent dilution techniques can be used to prepare rather uniform SUVs (small unilamellar vesicles) with diameters in the 300-500 angstrom range; unfortunately these preparations are very inefficient in trapping water soluble compounds. Other groups have prepared LUVs (large unilamellar vesicles) of about 1 micron diameter using reverse emulsion techniques or other approaches; these vesicles are extremely efficient in terms of trapping water soluble drug (up to 40-60% entrapment) but seem to be somewhat less stable than other vesicle types.

It should be noted that use of emulsions, rather than liposomes, may result in the preparation of drug carrier complexes which share some of the biological behavior of liposomes, but which present formulation problems more familiar to the pharmaceutical industry (Davis 1981).

There has been considerable concern about the problem of the lack of stability of drug containing liposomes during prolonged storage in vitro (Fildes 1981). However, the problem of liposome stability seems to have been solved to a considerable degree; thus storage for periods in excess of one year has been claimed by a number of investigators. In general liposomes containing cholesterol and/or composed of long chain saturated lipids are highly stable, while use of sphingomyelin rather than phosphatidylcholine has also been reported to increase stability (Gregoriadis et al, 1983). Details of liposome preparations and their physical and chemical properties can be found in several excellent reviews of these topics (Juliano 1983; Szoka & Papajopoulos 1980; Deamer & Uster 1982; Gregoriadis et al, 1983).

b) Microspheres

There is substantial interest in using protein or polymer based microspheres as drug carriers (for review see Widder et al 1982). We shall call particles ranging between 100 nm and a micron or so as "microspheres" (the smaller ones are also sometimes termed "nanoparticles"). One common approach involves coacervation of a protein solution and subsequent desolvation and hardening of the colloidal particles formed (Oppenheim 1980). A second widely used approach involves a phase separation emulsion technique. Here proteins or polymers in water are emulsified by sonication into an organic phase. The polymeric particles are chemically crosslinked or hardened by heat treatment and the residual organic phase is removed. Water soluble drug molecules can be incorporated into the microspheres by including them in the polymer solution. Up to 10% w/w drug can sometimes be trapped in the microparticles in this way (Widder et al 1972). The general approach described here has been used to make albumin or gelatin microspheres (Kramer 1974), protein microspheres coated with polymers (Longo et al, 1982), acrylic microspheres containing immobilized protein (Arturson et al, 1983; Edman & Sjoholm 1983), and even magnetically "steerable" protein microspheres containing magnetite (Widder et al, 1982). In contrast to the case of liposomes, there has been little concern about the in vitro stability properties of protein or polymer microspheres. Characteristics of some of the common microparticulate carriers are summarized in Fig. 1.

Nature of the Carriers

Type	Composition	Size Range
Liposomes	phospholipid sterols surfactants proteins	suv-300-500A ○ luv-0.2-2.0u ○ mlv-0.2-2.0u ◎
Microspheres	polydextrans proteins polyacrylamide	1000A-100u
Emulsions	surfactants oils polymers	microns

In Vivo Determinants of Microparticulate Distribution

The microparticulate drug carriers are usually injected into the systemic circulation and must find their way from the bloodstream to the target site. Working against this are a number of barriers which constrain the in vivo distribution and kinetic behavior of injected microparticles. In general, these barriers will be the same or at least similar for liposomes, microparticles and emulsions. Thus in order for a therapeutic strategy utilizing microparticulate carriers to be successful, it must take into account the existence of these various barriers. The problem of avoiding or overcoming these barriers is, as we shall see, a rather difficult proposition at present; thus only therapeutic approaches which are consistent with the limitations imposed by these in vivo barriers will be likely to succeed. We will discuss two of the major barriers to the in vivo distribution of microparticulates, namely (a) the endothelial barrier of the vasculature, and (b) the phagocytic cells of the reticuloendothelial system.

The lumen of a blood vessel is bounded by a layer of endothelial cells which demarcate the vascular and extra vascular compartments and which regulate the flow of solutes, including macromolecules and microparticles, between these compartments. Most solute exchange takes place in the capillaries rather than in the larger vessels. This is largely based on surface area since the total area of the systemic capillary bed is enormous (in man about 60 M2) (Simionescu & Simionesco 1983). One must also keep in mind the fact that the characteristics of the endothelium differs in different tissues. Thus in liver and spleen sinusoidal vessels, both the endothelial cell layer and the underlying basement membrane are "fenestrated", that is, they have small gaps or openings (Freudenberg, et al, 1983). An endothelium of this type will thus allow the egress of small microparticles (dia 1000A) into the tissue spaces of these organs. The most common capillary barrier, however, is a continuous endothelium where the cells closely abut one upon another, are joined by tight occluding junctions and are subtended by a continuous basement membrane of 200-500A thickness. Although the cellular lining of a continuous type capillary will clearly prevent the exit of particles with a dia in excess of 1000A, it is also clear that macromolecules of more modest dimensions can cross this barrier. Most recent evidence supports the view that macromolecules cross the capillary endothelial cell layer by riding in a system of vesicles which engulf fluid and solutes on the luminal side of the capillary and release their contents on the tissue side (Simionescu & Simionescu, 1983). Using electron microscopic tracer techniques, investigators have shown that macromolecules ranging in size from cytochrome C (30A) to ferritin or glycogen (300A) cross the endothelial cell enclosed within endosomal vesicles via a process which has been called "transcytosis". One should also keep in mind the fact that macromolecules which have moved across the endothelial cell will still have restricted diffusion because of the presence of the basement membrane layer which subtends these cells (Martinez 1981).

In summary then, while macromolecules up to a diameter of several hundred angstoms can cross the capillary endothelial barrier by "transcytosis", larger particles such as liposomes, most microspheres, and emulsion particles will be excluded from the transcytosis vesicles. Thus these microparticulate carriers will either remain impacted upon the luminal side of the capillary endothelium, or may exit from the circulation in specialized (fenestrated) sites such as the sinusoidal vessels of liver and spleen.

Fig. 2   The Endothelial Barrier

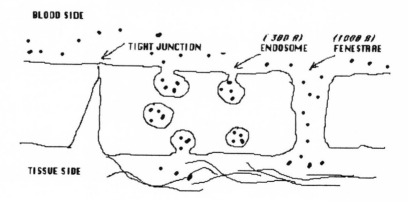

TRANSCAPILLARY TRANSPORT

The reticuloendothelial (RE) system consists of a set of mononuclear phagocytic cells which originate from precursors in bone marrow, enter the bloodstream as monocytes and then pass into various tissues and differentiate into macrophages (Meuret 1981). Macrophages are an essential part of the defense functions of the body; thus they are involved in antibody production via antigen processing and presentation to T lymphocytes (Unanue 1981); they are also responsible for secreting certain factors (lymphokines) which regulate the functions of lymphoid cells. Finally, macrophages are themselves effector cells for host defense since, under certain circumstances, they can acquire the ability to attack and destroy both pathogens and tumor cells (Adams 1982).

A crucial function of the macrophages of the RE system is to remove and engulf circulating pathogens, tissue debris and damaged macromolecules from the bloodstream (Altura & Saba, 1981). Likewise the RE system cells will very effectively capture foreign microparticulate drug carriers and clear them from the circulation. The cells most involved with foreign particle clearance are the macrophage-like Kupffer cells of the liver and the splenic macrophages. The non-specific phagocytic capabilities of macrophages are highly developed and these cells readily take up a variety of microparticles including liposomes (Kao & Juliano, 1981; Hsu & Juliano, 1982), microspheres (Arturson et al, 1983), as well as other colliodal particles (Altura & Saba, 1981). In addition, macrophages possess specific, receptor mediated endocytotic mechanisms including surface receptors for the Fc domain of IgG (Steinman et al, 1983), for complement components (Lambris & Ross, 1982), for mannosyl/fucosyl terminated glycoproteins (Stahl & Gordon, 1982) and for fibronectin (Hsu & Juliano, 1982). Particle uptake via these specific systems can often exceed basal uptake by a factor of 100 or more. The specific receptor mediated endocytotic systems may come into play in the clearance of microparticulate drug carriers. For example, repeated use of a drug coupled to a protein microcarrier may elicit an immune response; the antibodies formed would then bind to the microparticle and promote rapid uptake via the Fc receptor of macrophages. Alternatively, microparticulates may simply adsorb certain serum proteins capable of interacting with macrophage receptors, thus promoting particle clearance.

Factors Affecting Particle Clearance

The chemical and physical characteristics of the carrier which affect behavior in vivo have been studied in most detail for liposomes. It has long been known that both particle size and charge can affect liposome clearance kinetics. Thus large liposomes are cleared more rapidly than small ones and negatively charged vesicles are cleared more far rapidly than neutral or positive ones of equivalent size (Juliano & Stamp, 1975). The chemical composition of the liposomes, particularly with respect to stabilization of the membrane against the disrupting effects of serum lipoproteins is also an important aspect of liposome behavior (Gregoriadis et al, 1982). Another important consideration is the dose or load of liposomes administered (Ellens et al, 1982; Kao & Juliano, 1981). As with other particles, the liposome clearance rate of the reticuloendothelial system is inversely related to the load of particles (Altura & Saba, 1981); thus the fractional rate of clearance of a large dose of liposomes is slower than for a smaller dose. One must also keep in mind changes in clearance due to possible toxicities of the liposomes (or other microparticles) to the reticuloendothelial system, although, the toxicities reported thus far have been rather minimal (Hart et al, 1981; Allen et al, 1984). The literature on factors controlling the in vivo behavior of drug containing microspheres is currently somewhat limited, although some analyses are beginning to appear (Arturson et al, 1983). An interesting recent development is the observation that coating microspheres with certain detergents can result in a markedly prolonged circulation lifetime (Illum & Davies 1984); however, one must keep in mind possible detergent toxicities to the reticuloendothelial system.

In summary, a variety of physical factors including particle size, surface charge, surface chemistry and the "load" of particle will all affect the particle clearance rate. Nonetheless the structure of the capillary endothelium and the phagocytic capabilities of the RE cells will tend to eventually cause the accumulation of most of the injected microparticles in organs such as liver and spleen where the endothelium is fenestrated and where macrophages are abundant.

The barriers affecting microparticulate clearance and distribution in vivo are summarized in Fig. 3.

Fig. 3

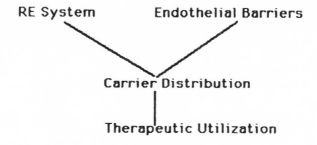

RE System   Endothelial Barriers

Carrier Distribution

Therapeutic Utilization

Selected Examples of Drug Delivery with Microparticulate Carriers

Microparticulate carriers have been used to deploy a wide variety of pharmaceutical agents in a number of different therapeutic situations; thus the literature on these topics is a rather vast and oftimes confusing one. We will confine ourselves to a discussion of certain applications where the characteristics of the carrier system seem very well matched to the intended therapeutic application. Some likely applications of microparticu-late drug carriers are summarized in Table 1.

Table I

SELECTED APPLICATIONS

1) Immunomodulation
a) Activation of Macrophages
b) Control of Metastases
c) Defenses against Pathogens

2) Treatment of Intracellular Pathogens
a) Obliqate intracellular parasites- *leishmaniasis*
b) Facultative intracellular pathogens- *salmonellosis*
c) Systemic fungal diseases- *candidiasis*

3) Cancer Chemotherapy
a) Toxicity buffering

a) Reduction of the Toxicity of Anti Tumor Drugs Using Liposomes

Some years ago liposomes were hailed as a major new strategy for the chemotherapy of cancer. This enthusiasm was mainly due to the concept that one might be able to "target" drugs to tumors using liposomal carriers. Although some success has been claimed in certain specialized instances, (Hashimoto et al, 1983), the overall picture of liposome enhanced therapy of solid tumors is rather dismal (reviewed by Kaye 1981). This may be due in part to the failure of most early investigators to appreciate the multiple barriers to liposome mediated drug delivery to tumors. As discussed at length above, the structure of the capillary endothelium, the action of the reticuloendothelial system, and the properties of most tumor cells (i.e non phagocytic) tend to prevent selective delivery of liposomal drugs to solid neoplasms. This would be true if one used conventional liposomes or liposomes coupled with a highly specific monoclonal antibody as a "targeting agent". This does not mean that the use of liposomes in tumor therapy is totally senseless, but rather that the attainable goals may be more limited than once hoped.

More recently, workers have made modest but valuable gains in chemotherapy by applying liposome technology, with appropriate understanding of its limitations, to the problem of reducing the toxicity of anti tumor drugs. Several workers have used hydrophobic drugs in liposomes; this would include alkylating agents (Kato et al, 1983; Babbage & Berenbaum, 1982), anti mitotic agents (Hildebrand et al, 1983), and most importantly anthracyclines such as Adriamycin (Rahman et al, 1980; Forssen & Tokes, 1981; Gabizon et al, 1982).

Strong evidence has accumulated showing that liposomal encapsulation of Adriamycin can reduce its dose-limiting toxicity to the myocardium without loss of antitumor potency (Forssen & Tokes, 1981; Herman et al, 1983). The mechanisms underlying these results are unclear, but may include low uptake of the drug by the myocardium (Forssen & Tokes, 1981; Olsen et al, 1982); however, a number of other possibilities may also be involved, including a reduction in immunosuppressive actions (Forssen & Tokes, 1983b), enhanced tumoricidal effects in certain organs such as the liver (Gabizon et al, 1983), or an enhanced membrane directed action of Adriamycin (Tritton & Yee, 1982). In any case, the considerable improvement in the therapeutic index of this important drug via liposome encapsulation deserves further study and development.

b) Anti tumor Drugs in Microspheres

The use of anti-tumor drugs in protein or polymer microspheres affords some of the same opportunities and is restricted by some of the same limitations as use of these drugs in liposomal carriers. Two rather distinct approaches have been used in this area. In the first approach, the microspheres are injected into the general circulation and thus may be expected to behave in the same way as liposomes or other circulating microparticulates; in the second approach the microspheres are administered directly to the tumorous organ by means of local intra-arterial injection.

The effects of the antineoplastic enzyme asparaginase when incorporated into polyacrylamide microspheres have been studied by Edman and his colleagues (Edman & Sjoholm, 1983; Arturson et al, 1983). When given either

systemically or by an intramuscular route these preparations reduced blood asparagine levels significantly more
effectively than did free asparaginase. This is an
example of the systemic use of microspheres as an anti
tumor agent. Kato and colleagues (Kato et al, 1980,
1980b, 1981) have used catheterization to deliver
mitomycin C containing ethylcellulose microspheres to
tumors in specific organs, especially renal carcinomas.
The microspheres employed were rather large (200 microns)
and contained up to 80% drug. Good localization of drug
in the kidney was found for up to six hours, with
relatively low systemic drug levels or systemic
toxicity. Magnetic microspheres have also been used for
antineoplastic therapy (Widder et al, 1982). Use of
intra-arterial infusion combined with high external
magnetic fields has achieved high levels of drug
localization, and has produced effective therapy of the
Yoshida rat tumor. An obvious limitation with this
approach is that it can only be applied to relatively
large, easily acessible tumors which can be catheterized
and subjected to localized magnetic fields. Thus it
really does not address the prime problem of
antineoplastic chemotherapy which is the treatment of
multiple small metastases.

Tokes and colleagues have explored the use of
anthracycline drugs coupled to polygluteraldehyde
microspheres (Rogers et al, 1983; Tokes et al, 1982,
Roger & Tokes, 1984). Most of this work has been with
neoplastic cells in vitro rather than in vivo and thus
some of the "barriers" to this type of therapy have not
yet been addressed. Nonetheless, this group has reported
some interesting effects including the ability of the
polymer conjugated drug to overcome anthracycline
resistance, and the conversion of an inactive
anthracycline derivative to an active agent by coupling
to the microsphere carrier (Rogers & Tokes, 1984).
Presumably the multiple repetative interactions of the
drug-polymer conjugate with the cell surface produces
novel opportunities for cytotoxicity.

c) Liposomal Immunomodulators

Lipid vesicles are readily taken up by macrophages
and thus can be used for the selective delivery of drugs
to these cells (Juliano & Layton, 1980; Alving 1983).

Among the functions of the macrophage is the ability, upon appropriate stimulation, to attack and destroy tumor cells, an aspect of macrophage activity which seems to be essential to the control of tumor metastasis (Fidler & Poste, 1982). Macrophages can be induced to tumoricidal competence in vitro by a number of immunomodulating agents including lymphokines, double stranded polynucleotides, and products or analogs of bacterial cell wall structures including lipopolysaccharide (LPS) and muramyl dipeptide (MDP). None of these agents is, however, suitable for in vivo stimulation of macrophage function because of inherent toxicities or due to low potency due to rapid degradation and/or excretion.

In order to contravene these problems, Fidler, Poste and their colleagues have explored the use of liposome encapsulated immunomodulators, both in vitro and in vivo (Poste et al, 1979; Fidler, 1980; Fidler et al, 1981). Among their most significant observations are: (1) the inclusion of lymphokine or of MDP into liposomes can markedly increase the potency of these substances in enhancing macrophage tumoricidal function; (2) liposomal MDP and lymphokines seem to act synergistically when used together; (3) in vivo use of liposomal MDP or lymphokine can protect mice against the metastatic spread of certain tumors. Recently a number of other workers have extended and elaborated upon these findings. Thus other agents such as poly I:C (Pidgeon et al, 1983) and C-reactive protein (Deodhar et al, 1984) incorporated into liposomes, have also been shown to cause macrophage activation. Liposomes containing the C-reactive protein have also been used to reduce the metastatic spread of disease in murine fibrosarcomas and adenocarcinomas (Deodhar et al, 1982). The strategy of liposomal activation of macrophage function has also been applied to the problem of macrophage defenses against herpes virus infection (Koff et al, 1983).

It seems clear, based on this growing body of observations, that liposomes can provide a useful means of delivering immunomodulating agents to macrophages. This will likely have important ramifications in the therapy of neoplastic and viral diseases.

d) Liposomal Drugs in the Therapy of Intracellular Pathogens

A number of important pathogens including brucella, salmonella, mycobacteria, rickettsia, chlamydia, various fungi and many protozoans, spend at least part of their time within the intracellular environment, oftentimes within macrophages (Alving 1983). Many commonly used antimicrobial drugs do not readily penetrate mammalian cell membrances (e.g. aminoglycosides), complicating the treatment of intracellular pathogens. Thus, the idea of using liposomes to convey antimicrobial agents to the intracellular (endosomal) compartment of macrophages is a sensible and natural one based on our understanding of liposome behavior in vivo.

The first important example of this type approach concerns the therapy of leishmaniasis, an obligate intracellular protozoan parasite common in sub-tropical areas (Alving et al, 1978; Black et al, 1977; New et al, 1978). The results were quite spectacular with a marked enhancement in the potency of the antimonial drugs used to treat this disease. Recently, liposome encapsulated antibiotics, either used singly or in combination, have also shown promise as highly efficacious therapy of salmonellosis (Desiderio & Campbell, 1983a,b), and of brucellosis (M Fountain et al submitted 1984).

A somewhat similar approach, although one in which the therapeutic effects cannot be fully attributed to "targeting" of the drug to macrophages, concerns the use of liposomal antifungal agents, particularly amphotericin B. Systemic fungal infections are primarily a problem in immunocompromised individuals, including cancer patients and transplant patients. For many years a mainstay for therapy for systemic fungal disease has been amphotericin B, a potent but extremely toxic polyene antibiotic. The multiple toxicities of amphotericin B prominently include severe nephrotoxicity as well as damage to the cardiovascular system and the CNS. Recently, it has been shown that incorporation of amphotericin B in liposomes results in a marked reduction in toxicity with no loss of antifungal potency. This is true for both cryptococcosis and candida infection (Graybill et al, 1982; Lopez et al, 1983). These effects seem to be based primarily on a basic change in the action of amphotericin B at the cellular level rather than a macrophage "targeting". Thus while free amphoB is toxic to both fungal cells and mammalian cells, the liposomal drug remains toxic to fungi but is no longer toxic to mammalian erythrocytes or other mammalian cells (Mehta et al, 1984). The antifungal effects of liposomal amphoB also occur in neutropenic animals (Lopez et al, 1984), indicating that a normal complement of monocytes and macrophages is not essential to the therapeutic effect.

SUMMARY

The inclusion of drugs in microparticulate carriers clearly holds significant promise for improvements in the therapy of several disease categories. One most keep in mind, however, that the behavior of all microparticulate carriers, be they liposomes, microspheres or emulsions, will be constrained by the same set of biological barriers, the most important of these being the impermeant walls of the microvasculature and the avid phagocytic cells of the RE system. With a clear understanding of the factors which regulate the clearance, disposition and degradation of microparticulates in vivo, one can then begin to select appropriate disease categories and appropriate strategies for therapy. As always in science, one must also expect the unexpected; although we are rapidly learning about the chemistry and biology of microparticulate carriers, and can begin to devise some general rules, we must also be prepared to be surprised. Thus there are hints that a drug carrier complex is more than the sum of its parts and that in some cases novel therapeutic mechanisms may be produced by joining the drug to the carrier moiety (eg. Roger & Tokes 1984, Mehta et al, 1984). This reviewer is confident that microparticle technology will take its place, along with other drug delivery technologies, in enhancing the effectiveness, convenience and general utility of new and existing drugs.

References

Adams, D.O., Macrophage activation and secretion.
Fed. Proc. 41 (1982) 2193-2197.

Allen, T.M., Murray, L., MacKeigan, S. and Shah, M.
Chronic liposome administration in mice:
effects on reticuloendothelial function and
tissue distribution. J. Pharmacol. Exp.
Ther. 229 (1984) 267-75.

Altura, B.M. and Saba, T.M., Pathophysiology of
the Reticuloendothelial System, Raven Press,
New York, 1981.

Alving, C.R., Steck, E.A., Chapman, W.L., Waits,
V.B., Hendricks, L.D., Swartz, G.M. and Hanson,
W.L., Therapy of leishmaniasis: superior
efficacies of liposome encapsulated drugs. Proc.
Natl. Acad. Sci. U.S.A. 75 (1978) 2959-2963.

Alving, C.R., Delivery of liposome-encapsulated
drugs to macrophages. Pharmacology and
Therapeutics 22 (1983) 407-424.

Arturson, P., Laakso, T. and Edman, P., Acrylic
microspheres In Vivo IX: blood elimination
kinetics and organ distribution of
microparticles with different surface
characteristics. J. Pharm. Sci. 72 (1983)
1415-1420.

Babbage, J.W. and Berenbaum, M.C., Increased
therapeutic efficiency of a lipid-soluble
alkylating agent incorporated in liposomes.
Br. J. Cancer 45(6) (1982) 830-834.

Bangham, A.D., Liposomes. Ann. Rev. Biochem. 41
(1972) 753.

Black, C.D.V., Watson, C.J. and Ward, R.J., Use of
pentostam liposomes in the chemotherapy of
experimental leishmaniasis. Trans. Royal
Soc. Trop. Med. & Hyg. 71 (1977) 550-552.

Davis, S.S., Emulsion systems for the delivery of drugs in optimization of Drug Delivery. H. Bundgaard, A.B. Hansen, H. Kofod (Eds) Munksgaard, Copenhagen, 1981.

Deamer, D.W. and Uster, P.S., Liposome preparation: methods and mechanism, in Liposomes. M. Ostro (Ed), Marcel Dekker, NY, 1982, pp. 27-51.

Deodhar, S.D., Gautam, S., Yen Lieberman, B. and Roberts, D., Macrophage activation and generation of tumoricidal activity by liposome-associated human C-reactive protein. Cancer Res. 44(1) (1984) 305-10.

Deodhar, S.D., James, K., Chiang, T., Edinger, M. and Barna, B.P., Inhibition of lung metastases in mice bearing a malignant fibrosarcoma by treatment with liposomes containing human C-reactive protein. Cancer Res. 41(12) (1982) 5084-5088.

Desiderio, J.V. and Campbell, S.G., Lipsome-encapsulated cephalothin in the treatment of experimental murine salmonellosis. J. Reticuloendothel Soc. 34(4) (1983) 279-87.

Desiderio, J.V. and Campbell, S.G., Intraphagocytic killing of Salmonella typhimurium by liposome-encapsulated cephalothin. J. Infect. Dis. 148(3) (1983) 563-70.

Edman, P. and Sjoholm, I., Acrylic microspheres in vivo VI: anti tumor effect of microparticles with immobilized L-asparaginase against 6C3HED lymphoma. J. Pharm. Sci. 72(6) (1983) 654-665.

Edman, P.D., Sjoholm, I., Prolongation of effect of asparaginase by implantation in polyacrylaride in rats. J. Pharm. Sci. 70 (1981) 684-85.

Ellens, H., Mayhew, E. and Rustum, Y.M., Reversible depression of the reticuloendothelial system by liposomes. Biochim. Biophys. Acta 714(3) (1982) 479-485.

Fendler J. and Schupp H., Acc. Chem. Res. 17(3) (1984).

Fidler, I.J. and Poste, G., Macrophage-mediated destruction of malignant tumor cells and new strategies for the therapy of metastatic disease. Springer Semin. Immunopathol. 5 (1982) 161-174.

Fidler, I.J., Sone, S. Fogler, W.E. and Barnes, Z.L., Eradication of spontaneous metastases and activation of alveolar macrophages by intravenous injection of liposomes containing muramyl dipeptide. Proc. Natl. Acad. Sci. USA 78(3) (1981) 1680-1684.

Fidler, I.J., Therapy of spontaneous metastases by intravenous injection of liposomes containing lymphokines. Science 208(4451) (1980) 1469-1471.

Fildes, Industrial aspects of liposomes in Liposomes: Physical Structure to Therapeutic Applications. G. Knight (Ed) Elsevier, Amsterdam, 1981.

Forssen, E.A. and Tokes, Z.A., Use of anionic liposomes for the reduction of chronic doxorubicin-induced cardiotoxicity. Proc. Natl. Acad. Sci. USA 78(3) (1981) 1873-1877.

Forssen, E.A. and Tokes, Z.A., Attenuation of dermal toxicity of doxorubicin by liposome encapsulation. Cancer Treat Rep. 67(5) (1983) 481-4.

Forssen, E.A. and Tokes, Z.A.: Improved therapeutic benefits of doxorubicin by entrapment in anionic liposomes. Cancer Res. 43(2) (1983b) 546-50.

Freudenberg, N., Riese, K.H. and Freudenberg,
M.A., The Vascular Endothelial System.
Gustav Fisher, Stuttgart, 1983.

Gabizon, A., Dagan, A., Goren, D., Barenholz, Y.
and Fuks, Z., Liposomes as in vivo carriers
of adriamycin: reduced cardiac uptake and
preserved antitumor activity in mice. Cancer
Res. 42(11) (1982) 4734-4739.

Gabizon, A., Goren, D., Ruks, Z., Barenholz, Y.,
Dagan, A. and Meshorer, A., Enhancement of
adriamycin delivery to liver metastatic cells
with increased tumoricidal effect using
liposomes as drug carriers. Cancer Res.
43(10) (1983) 4730-5.

Graybill, J.R., Craven, P.C., Taylor, R.L.,
Williams, D.M. and Magee, W.E., Treatment of
murine cryptococcosis with liposome-
associated amphotericin B. J. Infectious
Diseases 145(5) (1982) 748-752.

Gregoriadis, G., Kirby, C. and Senior, J.,
Optimization of liposome behavior in vivo.
Biol. Cell 47 (1983) 11-18.

Gregoriadis, G., Kirby, C., Large, P., Meehan, A.
and Senior, J., Targeting of Liposomes: study
of influencing factors. In Targeting of
Drugs, Gregoriadis, G., Senior, J. and
Trouet, A. (Eds) Plenum Publishing Corpn.
1982, pp. 155-184.

Hart, I.R., Fogler, W.E., Poste, G., Fidler,
I.J., Toxicity studies of liposome
encapsulated immunomodulators administered
intravenously to dogs and mice. Cancer
Immunol. Immunotherap. 10 (1981) 57-196.

Hashimoto, Y., Sugawara, M., Masuko, T. and Hojo,
H., Antitumor effect of actinomycin D
entrapped in liposomes bearing subunits of
tumor-specific monoclonal immunoglobulin M
antibody. Cancer Res. 43(11) (1983) 5328-34.

Herman, E.H., Rahman, A., Ferrans, V.J., Vick, J.A and Schein, P.S., Prevention of chronic doxorubicin cardiotoxicity in beagles by liposomal encapsulation. Cancer Res. 43(11) (1983) 5427-32.

Hildebrand, J., Ruysschaert, J.M. and Laduron, C., Antitumor activity of a water-insoluble compound entrapped in liposomes on L1210 leukemia in mice. JNCI 70(6) (1983) 1081-6.

Hsu, M.J. and Juliano, R.L., Interaction of liposomes with the reticuloendothelial system II non specific and receptor mediated uptake of liposomes by mouse peritoneal macrophages. Biochim. Biophys. Acta 720 (1982) 411-419.

Illum, L. and Davis, S.S., The organ uptake of intravenously administered colloidal particles can be altered using a non-ionic surfactant (Poloxamer 338). FEBS-Lett. 167(1) (1984) 79-82.

Juliano, R.L. and Layton, D., Liposomes as a drug delivery system. In Drug Delivery Systems, Juliano, R.L. (Ed), Oxford University Press, 1980, pp. 189-236.

Juliano, R.L. and Stamp, D., Interactions of drugs with lipid membranes. Biochim. Biophys. Acta 586 (1979) 137-145.

Juliano, R.L., and Stamp, D., Effects of particle size and charge on the clearance rates of liposomes and liposome encapsulated drugs. Biochem. Biophys. Res. Comm. 53 (1975) 651-58.

Juliano, R.L., Characteristics and Applications of Microparticulate Drug Carriers, in Controlled Drug Delivery. Robison, J. (Ed) 1984, in press.

Juliano, R.L., Interactions of proteins and drugs with liposomes. In Liposomes, Ostro, M. (Ed), Marcel Dekker, New York, 1983, pp. 53-86

Kao, Y.J. and Juliano, R.L., Interaction of liposomes with the reticuloendothelial system: effects of blockade on the clearance of large unilamellar vesicles. Biochim. Biophys. Acta 677 (1981) 453-461.

Kato, T., Nemoto, R., Mori, H., Iwata, K., Sato, S., Unno, K., Goto, A., Harada, M., Homma, M., Okada, M. and Minowa, T., An approach to magnetically controlled cancer chemotherapy. III. Magnetic control of ferromagnetic mitomycin C microcapsules in the artery. J. Japan Soc. Cancer Ther. 15 (1980) 28-32.

Kato, T., Nemoto, R., Mori, H. and Kumagai, I., Sustained-release properties, of microencapsulated mitomycin C with ethylcellulose infused into the renal artery of the dog. Cancer 46 (1980) 14-21.

Kato, T., Nemoto, R., Mori, H., Takahashi, M. and Tamakawa, Y., Transcatheter arterial chemoembolization of renal cell carcinoma with microencapsulated Mitomycin C. J. of Urology 125 (1981) 19-24.

Kaye, S.B., Liposomes-problems and promise as selective drug carriers. Cancer Treatment Reviews 8(1) (1981) 27-50.

Khato, J., del Campo, A.A. and Sieber, S.M., Carrier activity of sonicated small liposomes containing melphalan to regional lymph nodes of rats. Pharmacology 26(4) (1983) 23-40.

Koff, W.C., Showlater, S.D., Seniff, D.A. and Hampar, B., Lysis of herpesvirus-infected cells by macrophages activated with free or liposome-encapsulated lymphokine produced by a murine T cell hybridoma. Infect. Immun. 42(3) (1983) 1067-72.

Kramer, P.A., Albumin microspheres are vehicles for achieving specificity in drug delivery. J. Pharm. Sci. 63 (1974) 646-47.

Lambris, J.D. and Ross, C.D., Assay of membrane complement receptors with C3b and C3d coated fluorescent microspheres. J. Immunol. 128 (1982) 186-191.

Lee, A.G., Effects of charged drugs on the phase transition tempera ture of phospholipid lilayers. Biochem. Biophys. Acta 517 (1978) 95.

Longo, W.E., Iwata, H., Lindheimer, T.A. and Goldberg, E.P., Preparation of hydrophilic albumin microspheres using polymeric dispersing agents. J. Pharm. Sci. 71(12) (1982) 1323-28.

Lopez-Berestein, G. Hopfer, R.L., Mehta, R., Mehta, K., Hersh, E.N. and Juliano, R.L., Prophylaxis of candida albicans infections in neutropenic mice with liposome encapsulated amphotericin B. Antimicrob. Agents and Chemother. 25 (1984) 366-367.

Lopez-Berestein, G., Mehta, R., Hopfer, R.L., Mills, K., Kasi, L., Mehta, K., Fainstein, V., Luna, M., Hersh, E.M. and Juliano, R., Treatment and prophylaxis of disseminated infection due to Candida albicans in mice with liposome-encapsulated amphotericin B. J. Infect. Dis. 147(5) (1983) 939-45.

Martinez-Hernandez, A., The basement membrane in the microvasculature. In Microcirculation, Effros, R., Schmid-Shonben, H. and Ditzel, J. (Eds), Academic Press, New York, 1981, pp. 125-146.

Mehta, R., Lopez-Berestein, G., Hopfer, R., Mills, K. and Juliano, R.L., Liposomal amphotericin B is toxic to fungal cells but not to mammalian cells. Biochim. Biophys. Acta 770(2) (1984) 230-234.

Meuret, C., Kinetics of mononuclear phagocytes in man. Hematol. Bluttransfus. 27 (1981) 11-122.

New, R.R.C., Chance, M.L., Thomas, S.C. and Peters, W., Antileish manial activity in antimonials entrapped in liposomes. Nature 272 (1978) 55-56.

Olson, F., Mayhew, E., Maslow, D., Rustum, Y. and Szoka, F., Characterization, toxicity and therapeutic efficacy of adriamycin encapsulated in liposomes. Eur. J. Cancer Clin. Oncol. 18(2) (1982) 167-176.

Oppenheim, R.C., Nanoparticles, in Drug Delivery Systems, Juliano, R. (Ed), Oxford University Press, NY 1980, pp. 177-188.

Pidgeon, C., Schreiber, R.D. and Schultz, R.M., Macrophage activation: synergism between hybridoma MAF and poly(I). Poly(C) delivered by liposomes. J. Immunol. 131(1) (1983) 311-4.

Poste, G. and Kirsh, R., Site specific drug delivery in cancer therapy. Biotechnology 1 (1983) 869-878.

Poste, G., Kirsh, R., Fogler, W.E. and Fidler, I.J., Activation of tumoricidal properties in mouse macrophages by lymphokines encapsulated in liposomes. Cancer Res. 39 (1979) 881-892.

Poznansky, M.S. and Juliano, R.L., Biological approaches to the controlled delivery of drugs: a critical review. Pharm. Rev., 1984, in press.

Rahman, A., Kessler, A., More, N., Sikic, B., Rowden, G., Woolley, P. and Schein, P.S., Liposomal protection of adriamycin-induced cardiotoxicity in mice. Cancer Res. 40(5) (1980) 1532-7.

Rogers, K.E. and Tokes, Z.A., Novel mode of cytotoxicity obtained by coupling inactive anthracycline to a polymer. Biochem. Pharmacol. 33(4) (1984) 605-8.

Rogers, K.E., Carr, B.I. and Tokes, Z.A., Cell
    surface-mediated cytotoxicity of polymer-
    bound adriamycin against drug-resistant
    hepatocytes. Cancer Research 43 (1983)
    2741-2748.

Simionescu, N. and Simionescu, M.: The cardiovas-
    cular system. in Histology, Weiss, L. (Ed),
    Elsevier, N.Y., 1983, pp. 371-433.

Stahl, P. and Gordon, S., Expression of mannosyl/
    fucosyl receptor function for endocytosis in
    cultured primary macrophages and their
    hybrids. J. Cell Biol. 93 (1982) 49-54.

Steinman, R.M., Mellman, I.S., Muller, W.A. and
    Cohn, Z.A., Endocytosis and the recycling of
    plasma membrane, J. Cell Biol. 96 (1983)
    1-27.

Szoka, F. Jr. and Papahadjopoulos, D., Comparative
    properties and methods in preparation of
    lipid vesicles (liposomes). Ann. Rev.
    Biophys. Bioeng. 9 (1980) 467-508.

Tokes, Z.A., Rogers, K.E. and Hembaum, A., Synthe-
    sis of adriamycin-coupled polyglutaraldehyde
    microspheres and evaluation of their cytosta-
    tic activity. Proc. Natl. Acad. Sci. U.S.A.
    79 (1982) 2026-2030.

Tritton, T.R. and Yee, G., The anticancer agent
    adriamycin can be actively cytotoxic without
    entering cells. Science 217 (1982) 248-250.

Unanue, E., Regulatory role of macrophages in
    antigenic stimulation. Adv. Immunol. 31
    (1981) 1-121.

Widder, K.J., Senyei, A.E. and Sears, B.,
    Experimental methods in cancer therapeutics.
    J. Pharm. Sci. 71 (1982) 379-387.

BIODEGRADABLE POLY(ORTHO ESTERS) AS DRUG DELIVERY FORMS

J. Heller
Polymer Sciences Department
SRI International
Menlo Park, CA 94025

K. J. Himmelstein
INTERx Research Corporation
Merck, Sharp & Dome Research Laboratories
Lawrence, KA 66044

INTRODUCTION

Poly(ortho esters) are a polymer system containing backbone linkages that are stable in base, hydrolyze at very slow rates at the physiological pH of 7.4, and become progressively more labile as the pH is lowered. A major rationale for developing this system was a need for a polymer capable of a wide variety of erosion rates and where erosion could be confined to the surface of a solid device. Then, any selected, constant release rate can be achieved for therapeutic agents physically incorporated into the matrix by maintenance of an appropriate device geometry. Surface erosion and variations in delivery rates can be achieved by either stabilizing the interior of the polymer with a base so that erosion can take place only in the surface layers where the basic excipient is neutralized by the external medium or by using acidic excipients (Heller, 1980) incorporated into the typically highly hydrophobic matrix. In this latter case, surface erosion takes place only in the surface layer where the excipient is exposed to water.

In this chapter we describe polymer synthesis and characterization and the use of various excipients to achieve controlled release of compounds physically dispersed in the matrix.

171

POLYMER SYNTHESIS

Poly(ortho esters) can be prepared by means of a general synthesis that involves the addition of diols to ketene acetals (Heller et al., 1980). This general synthesis can be schematically represented as follows:

$$CH_2=\underset{\underset{OR}{|}}{C}-O-R'-O-\underset{\underset{OR}{|}}{C}=CH_2 \ + \ HO-R''-OH \ \longrightarrow \ \left[O-\underset{\underset{CH_3}{|}}{\overset{\overset{OR}{|}}{C}}-O-R'-O-\underset{\underset{CH_3}{|}}{\overset{\overset{OR}{|}}{C}}-O-R'' \right]_n$$

Poly(ortho ester)

The reaction is catalyzed by traces of acid, is exothermic, and proceeds to completion virtually instantaneously. Because no small molecule by-products are evolved, dense, crosslinked materials can be produced by using varying proportions of monomers having a functionality greater than two. Details of the synthesis of both linear and crosslinked polymers, their characterization, and preparation of devices has been described. (Heller et al., 1985a,b)

Two types of linear polymer and one crosslinked polymer were investigated. One type of linear polymer was prepared from 3,9-bis(methylene 2,4,8,10-tetraoxaspiro[5,5]undecane) (DMTOSU) and 1,6-hexanediol, (1,6 HD). The other type of linear polymer was prepared from 3,9-bis(ethylidene 2,4,8,10-tetraoxaspiro[5,5]undecane) (DETOSU), various ratios of trans-cyclohexanedimethanol (tCDM) and 1,6-hexanediol. In this latter case variations in the ratio of the two diols varied the glass transition temperature of the polymer from a low of 20°C to a high of 120°C. (Heller et al., 1983) The crosslinked polymer was prepared from a prepolymer formed by the reaction between a 3/2 mole ratio of 3,9-bis(ethylidene 2,4,8,10-tetraoxaspiro[5,5]undecane) and 2-methyl-1,4-butanediol (MBD) subsequently reacted with a 30 mol% excess of 1,2,6-hexanetriol (HT).

DRUG RELEASE STUDIES

During the performance of these studies, a number of different excipients were investigated to control release rates of therapeutic agents physically dispersed in the polymer. These were water-soluble salts, calcium lactate, magnesium hydroxide, and acid anhydrides.

Water-Soluble Salt Excipients

In studies of water-soluble salt excipients, a linear polymer prepared from 3,9-bis(methylene 2,4,8,10-tetraoxaspiro[5,5]undecane) and 1,6-hexanediol was used. To ascertain the effect of incorporated water soluble salts on erosion rates of the polymer, weight loss studies were conducted in a pH 7.4 buffer at 37°C. The effect of incorporated sodium carbonate and sodium chloride compared to pure polymer is shown in Figure 1 (Heller et al., 1981).

The pure polymer was essentially unaffected by water for about two months, after which rate of weight loss remained constant until about 55% weight loss occurred. At this point, the experiment was discontinued. Sodium chloride significantly accelerates polymer erosion, whereas no significant erosion occurs with sodium carbonate.

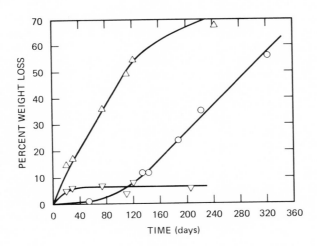

Fig. 1. Weight loss of DMTOSU/1,6HD polymer discs at pH 7.4 and 37°C. ○ neat polymer, ▽ polymer with 10 wt% Na$_2$CO$_3$, △ polymer with 10 wt% NaCl

These results indicate that a poly(ortho ester) at pH 7.4 and 37°C does undergo a slow rate of hydrolysis, but the pure polymer is so hydrophobic that no significant weight loss is noted until sufficient water permeates the matrix. In contrast, the polymer with incorporated sodium chloride undergoes hydrolysis without induction period at a rate comparable to, but somewhat higher than, that of the pure polymer. The lack of induction period and enhanced rate of hydrolysis is due to the osmotic imbibing of water into the hydrophobic polymer caused by the incorporated water-soluble salt (Fedors, 1980). Polymer containing incorporated sodium carbonate does not undergo erosion even though the water-soluble sodium carbonate drives water into the polymer. Lack of erosion is due to the basic nature of sodium carbonate, because poly(ortho esters) are stable in base.

Figure 2 shows rate of norethindrone release from disc-shaped devices containing dispersed 10 wt% norethindrone and 10 wt% Na_2CO_3 (Heller et al., 1983). As shown, release rate was linear for 240 days, at which time the experiment was discontinued. However, because at day 160 only 4% weight loss was measured, whereas about 13% of the drug had been released, rate of drug release was clearly not controlled by polymer erosion and was instead controlled by an osmotic imbibing of water driven by the incorporated water-soluble Na_2CO_3. The linearity of drug release was initially attributed to a uniform movement of a swelling front with resultant release of the drug from the swollen layer; however, it now appears more likely that the kinetics of release are principally determined by the rate of solubilization of the highly insoluble steroid. Because poly(ortho esters) are stable in base, the polymer swells without erosion.

Several studies were also performed with the neutral salts Na_2SO_4 or NaCl, which replaced the basic Na_2CO_3 salts. The results of drug release studies of a device containing 10 wt% norethindrone and 10 wt% NaCl are also shown in Figure 2. In this system, significant polymer erosion took place; at day 155, weight loss was 25%, with about 40% release of the incorporated drug. These results have previously been rationalized by a combined effect of polymer erosion and osmotically driven swelling.

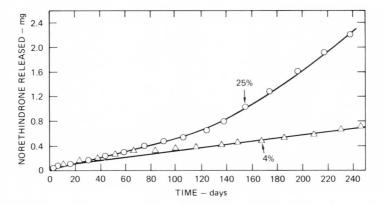

Fig. 2. Norethindrone release from DMTOSU/1,6HD polymer discs loaded with 10 wt% drug and various salts at pH 7.4 and 37°C. Disc thickness 1.2 mm (Arrows indicate weight loss). ◯ 10 wt% NaCl (4.0 mg drug) △ 10 wt% Na$_2$CO$_3$ (4.0 mg drug)

Although osmotically active, neutral salts have a significant accelerating effect on polymer erosion and drug release, the osmotically imbibed water leads to bulk erosion and rate of drug release is not dominantly controlled by the rate of polymer erosion. For this reason, other excipients were investigated.

Calcium Lactate Excipient

In these studies, the low water solubility, slightly acidic salt calcium lactate was used to lower the pH at the polymer-water interface. The polymer used in this study was a linear polymer formed from 3,9-bis(ethylidene 2,4,8,10-tetraoxaspiro[5,5]undecane) and a 65/35 mol% ratio of trans-cyclohexanedimethanol and 1,6-hexanediol. The glass transition temperature of this polymer was about 75°C. In a previous study, a calcium lactate loading of 2 wt% was established as optimum, with a levonorgestrel loading of 30 wt% (Heller et al., 1984).

Figure 3 shows cumulative release of levonorgestrel from 2.4 x 20 mm cylindrical devices containing 30 wt% levonorgestrel and 2 wt% calcium lactate. After an initial induction period, release rate remained constant

up to day 410, at which point the experiment was
discontinued. At that point, 7.4 mg or 23% of the drug
contained within the device had been released. Initial
release rate is about 10 mcg/day, which then accelerates
to a fairly constant 20 mcg/day.

The relationships between total weight loss of the
device determined gravimetrically and percent drug
release determined from residual drug measurements is
shown in Figure 4. After an induction period of about
40 days, polymer erosion rate accelerates and then
reaches a constant rate that is slightly higher than the
rate of drug release.

Results of a comparable in vivo study are shown in
Figure 5. In this study, weighed devices were implanted
subcutaneously into rabbits and explanted at two-week
intervals. Weight loss was determined gravimetrically
and residual drug was determined by HPLC analysis.
Because the data points are derived from measurements of
single devices, they are scattered, but they are
nevertheless in qualitative agreement with in vitro
studies in that polymer erosion also leads drug
release. Levonorgestrel release rate is about 33
mcg/day, which is considerably faster than the 20 mcg/day

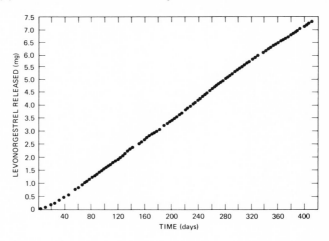

Fig. 3. Cumulative in vitro release of levonorgestrel from DETOSU/65,35
tCDM/1,6HD polymer rods, 2.4 x 20 mm containing 30 wt% drug and 2 wt%
calcium lactate. Total drug content 32.0 mg, pH 7.4 and 37°C

noted in the in vitro studies. However, polymer erosion appears to proceed at similar rates in both studies.

Figure 6 shows levonorgestrel blood plasma levels of rabbits with subcutaneously implanted devices. There is considerable scatter of points, partially because of errors in the radioimmunoassay measurements, which at the low levonorgestrel plasma concentrations operate at the limits of detection; however blood level is reasonably constant for about one year.

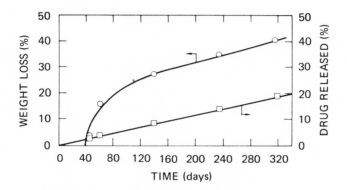

Fig. 4. In vitro cumulative weight loss (O) and cumulative release of levonorgestrel (□) from DETOSU/65,35 tCDM/1,6HD polymer rods, 2.4 x 20 mm containing 30 wt% drug and 2 wt% calcium lactate. Total drug content 32.0 mg, pH 7.4 and 37°C.

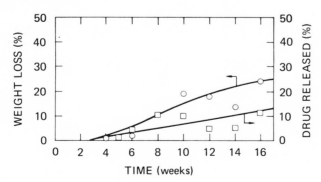

Fig. 5. In vivo cumulative weight loss (O) and cumulative release of levonorgestrel (□) from DETOSU/65,35 tCDM/1,6HD polymer rods, 2.4 x 20 mm containing 30 wt% drug and 2 wt% calcium lactate. Total drug content 32.0 mg, pH 7.4 and 37°C

Scanning electron microscopy examinations of devices
explanted from rabbits revealed the presence of large
voids surrounded by a foam-like layer. A typical SEM
photograph is shown in Figure 7. The appearance and
behavior of the devices has been rationalized as
follows: when placed in an aqueous environment, the
device will absorb water and will undergo a calcium-
lactate-catalyzed surface erosion process. As a
consequence of this erosion process, levonorgestrel is
released into the surrounding aqueous environment.
However, because the rate of polymer erosion exceeds the
rate at which levonorgestrel can solubilize, the drug
cannot be removed from the device at a high enough rate;
thus, polymer erosion into the device will continue
between dispersed levonorgestrel particles, producing the
foam-like layer surrounding the device.

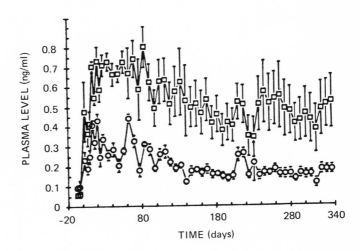

Fig. 6. Daily rabbit blood plasma levels of levonorgestrel from
DETOSU/65,35 tCDM/1,6HD polymer rods, 2.4 x 20 mm containing 30 wt% drug
and 2 wt% calcium lactate. Total drug content 32.0 mg.
    O 1 device/rabbit,   ☐ 3 devices/rabbit

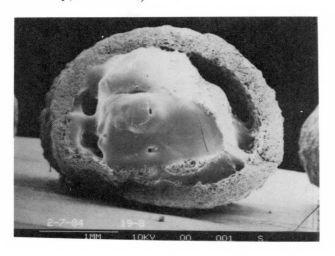

Fig. 7. Scanning electron micrograph of a DETOSU/65,35 tCDM/1,6HD polymer rod, 2.4 x 20 mm containing 30 wt% levonorgestrel and 2 wt% calcium lactate after 10 weeks in rabbit.

According to this mechanism, rate of drug release from these devices rapidly becomes determined entirely by the rate of solubilization of the highly water-insoluble levonorgestrel from the foam-like exterior of the device. It is likely that the pores of the foam are filled with a saturated water solution of levonorgestrel and that transport of the drug from the device to the outside environment takes place only from the outer layers. In this way, rate of drug release is directly proportional to the physical dimensions of the devices, an effect we have noted previously. The faster rate of drug release <u>in vivo</u> relative to <u>in vitro</u> is very likely due to the presence of lipophilic species in the surrounding tissue that facilitate levonorgestrel dissolution.

Magnesium Hydroxide Excipient

As shown in studies on the effect of incorporated water-soluble salts on rate of polymer erosion, in a sufficiently hydrophilic environment poly(ortho esters) undergo erosion at rates that are adequate for devices with a desired lifetime of many months. Because water permeability of a polymer above the glass transition

temperature is significantly higher than that of a
polymer below the glass transition temperature, it was of
interest to investigate release of levonorgestrel from
devices where the polymer is above its glass transition
temperature at body temperature. However, to ensure
dimensional stability of the implanted devices, we have
concentrated on crosslinked polymers. In addition,
poly(ortho esters) that can be converted from a viscous
liquid to a solid crosslinked device are of considerable
interest for the incorporation of sensitive therapeutic
agents such as polypeptides.

    Because water penetration into the matrix leads to
bulk erosion, we have prepared devices where the interior
has been stabilized with 7 wt% of magnesium hydroxide, a
slightly basic salt with a water solubility of only
0.8 mg/100 ml at 18°C.

    Figure 8 shows cumulative release of levonorgestrel
from 2.4 x 20 mm devices containing 30 wt% levonorgestrel
and 7 wt% magnesium hydroxide. The study was discontinued after 160 days, at which point about 1.4 mg or
4.5% of the incorporated levonorgestrel was released.

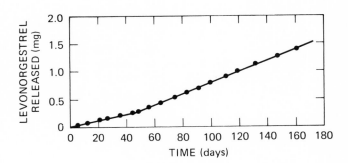

Fig. 8 Cumulative in vitro release of levonorgestrel from DETOSU/MBD/HT
polymer rods, 2.4 x 20 mm containing 30 wt% drug and 7 wt% Mg(OH)$_2$.
Total drug content 32.0 mg, pH 7.4 and 37°C

Figure 9 shows a plot of percent drug release and percent total weight loss of the devices as a function of time. Unfortunately, not enough data points were collected to define the initial portion of the total weight-loss line. Nevertheless, after 60 days, weight loss is a linear function of time for at least 140 days. However, rate of drug release is only 10 mcg/day, which is considerably slower than the 26.4 mcg/day required for concomitant erosion and drug release. Apparently, under this particular set of experimental conditions, levonorgestrel is not able to solubilize at a rate high enough to keep up with polymer erosion.

Results of in vivo experiments for rate of drug release and polymer erosion are shown in Figure 10. The data were obtained by implanting weighed devices subcutaneously into rabbits, explanting the devices at approximately two-week intervals, and determining weight loss and drug remaining in the devices. Because the data points are based on measurement with single devices, there is considerable scatter. Nevertheless, the data indicate that drug release and polymer erosion occur concomitantly for about 20 weeks, after which drug release may accelerate, even though polymer erosion rate remains constant. Because the experiment was discontinued after 25 weeks, it is not certain whether the values for percent drug release at weeks 22 and 25 are real or, more likely experimental error.

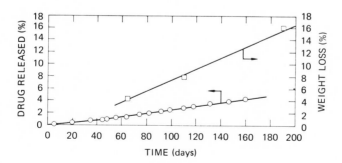

Fig. 9. In vitro cumulative weight loss (□) and cumulative release of levonorgestrel (○) from DETOSU/MBD/HT polymer rods, 2.4 x 20 mm containing 30 wt% drug and 7 wt% $Mg(OH)_2$. Total drug content 32.0 mg, pH 7.4 and 37°C

A comparison of Figures 9 and 10 shows that rate of
polymer erosion in vitro and in vivo are comparable in
that at day 196 (week 28) weight loss for the in vitro
device is about 16%, whereas that for the in vivo device
is about 12%. However, rate of drug release in vivo is
about 20 mcg/day, whereas that in vitro is only about
10 mcg/day. Apparently, as was the case for the linear
polymer devices, solubilization of levonorgestrel in an
in vivo environment also occurs more readily than in an
aqueous buffer, because of the presence of lipophilic
species at the implantation site.

Explanted devices did not contain voids, and
preliminary scanning electron microscopy examination of
the devices indicates a surface erosion process.

Acid Anhydride Excipients

The catalytic action of acid anhydrides depends on
reaction with water to yield a diacid, which then
catalyzes hydrolysis of the matrix (Shih et al., 1984;
Sparer et al. 1984). Polymer erosion, and hence rate of
drug release, can be controlled by the amount of
incorporated anhydride. As shown in Figure 11, rate of
release of the marker dye methylene blue from a
poly(ortho ester) disc is a linear function of the amount
of incorporated anhydride.

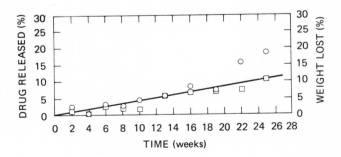

Fig. 10. In vivo cumulative weight loss (□) and cumulative release of
levonorgestrel (O) from DETOSU/MBD/HT polymer rods, 2.4 x 20 mm
containing 30 wt% drug and 7 wt% Mg(OH)$_2$. Total drug content 32.0 mg,
pH 7.4 and 37°C

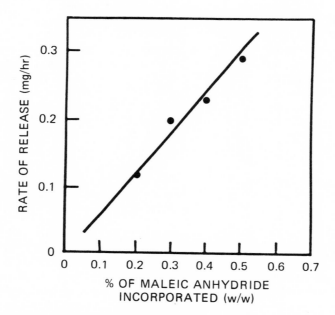

Fig. 11. Release rate of timolol maleate from a 7/3 blend of DETOSU/1,6HD and DETOSU/tCDM polymer discs at pH 7.4 and 37°C as a function of maleic anhydride content. Drug loading 2 wt%.

Because rate of hydrolysis of poly(ortho esters) increases as the pH of the surrounding medium decrease, rate of polymer erosion should be sensitive to the pKa of the corresponding acid of the incorporated anhydride. Figure 12 demonstrates the dependence on acid strength and amount. Over a given range, the release rate is proportional to the amount of anhydride incorporated. Above a particular concentration, increasing amounts of anhydride do not further accelerate the release rate, probably because diffusion of water into the reaction zone becomes rate limiting.

Convincing evidence of the mechanism of action of acid anhydrides and of a catalyzed surface erosion process is presented in Figure 13. The figure shows release rate of a methylene blue marker, release rate of $(1,4-^{14}C)$ succinic acid, and the rate of weight loss of a thin polymer disc containing dispersed methylene blue and ^{14}C-labelled succinic anhydride. The concomitant occurrence of all three events verifies that in an

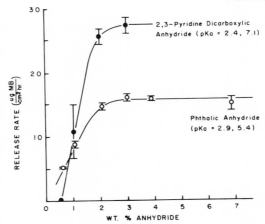

Fig. 12.   The effect of anhydride content and pKa on release rate of
methylene blue from DETOSU/35,65 tCDM/1,6HD polymer discs at pH 7.4 and
37°C.   Dye content 0.2 wt%.

initial step, the anhydride is hydrolyzed to the diacid,
which catalyzes polymer erosion with consequent device
weight loss and release of the incorporated marker dye
and excipient.

    The surface erosion nature of the anhydride-
catalyzed erosion and concomitant release of incorporated
drugs has been further verified by studying the effect of
drug loading and the effect of device geometry.

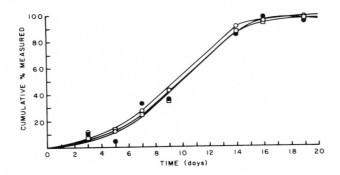

Fig. 13.   Cumulative release of methylene blue (O),   1,4-^{14}C succinic
acid (□) and polymer weight loss (●) from DETOSU/50,50 tCDM/1,6HD
polymer discs at pH 7.4 and 37°C.   Polymer contains 0.1 wt% 1,4-^{14}C
succinic anhydride and 0.3 wt% methylene blue.

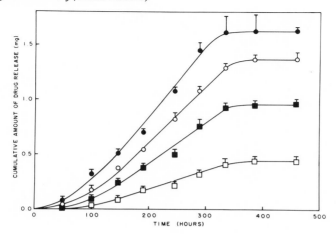

Fig. 14. The effect of loading on cumulative release of a drug from DETOSU/50,50 tCDM/1,6HD polymer discs containing 0.2 wt% sebasic anhydride at pH 7.4 and 37°C. Drug loading: 8 wt% ● , 6 wt% ○ , 4 wt% ■ , 2 wt% □ .

The effect of drug loading shown in Figure 14 clearly demonstrates that rate of release of the incorporated drug during the 14-day time span of the experiment is directly proportional to the loading; hence, release of the drug is indeed erosion controlled.

The effect of device geometry on rate and duration of drug release shown in Figures 15 and 16 is also entirely consistent with a surface erosion mechanism. Thus, release rate is directly proportional to the surface area and duration of release is directly proportional to device thickness.

CONCLUSION

Poly(ortho esters) combined with various acidic, basic or osmotic agents offer the possibility for the development of drug delivery systems with a wide range of erosion characteristics and rates. The utility of these systems for both short and long duration drug delivery regimes is considerably wider than previously developed erodible polymeric systems.

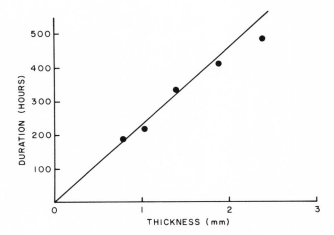

Fig. 15. The effect of disc thickness on duration of drug release from DETOSU/50,50 tCDM/1,6HD polymer discs containing 4 wt% drug and 0.2 wt% poly(sebasic anhydride) at pH 7.4 and 37°C

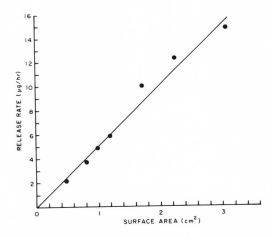

Fig. 16. The effect of disc surface area on rate of drug release from a DETOSU/50,50 tCDM/1,6HD polymer containing 4 wt% drug and 0.2 wt% poly(sebasic anhydride) at pH 7.4 and 37°C

ACKNOWLEDGEMENT

Work on poly(ortho esters) using the excipients Na_2CO_3, NaCl, calcium lactate, and $Mg(OH)_2$ was conducted at SRI International under sponsorship by the Contraceptive Development Branch, Center for Population Research, NIH, Contract No. NO1-HD-7-2826. Contributions were made by Mr. Bruce K. Fritzinger, Mr. Steven Y. Ng, and Mr. Donald W. H. Penhale. Work with anhydride excipients was performed at the Interx Research Corporation, Merck, Sharp and Dome, Research Laboratories with contributions by Dr. Randall V. Sparer, Dr. Chung Shih, and Ms. Cheryl D. Ringeisen. All polymers were synthesized at SRI International.

REFERENCES

Fedòrs, R. F., Osmotic effects in water adsorption by polymers. Polymer, 21 (1980) 207-212.

Heller, J., Controlled release of biologically active compounds from bioerodible polymers. Biomaterials, 1 (1980) 51-56.

Heller, J., Fritzinger, B. K., Ng, S. Y. and Penhale, D.W.H., In vitro and in vivo release of levonorgestrel from poly(ortho esters) I. Linear polymers. J. of Controlled Release, in press, a.

Heller, J., Fritzinger, B. K., Ng, S. Y. and Penhale, D.W.H., In vitro and in vivo release of levonorgestrel from poly(ortho esters) II. Crosslinked polymers. J. of Controlled Release, in press, b.

Heller, J., Penhale, D.W.H., Fritzinger, B. K. and Ng, S. Y., Controlled release of contraceptive agents from poly(ortho esters). In Zatuchni, G. I., Goldsmith, A., Shelton, J. D. and Sciarra, J. (Eds), Long Acting Contraceptive Delivery Systems, Harper & Row Publishers, Philadelphia, 1984, pp. 113-128.

Heller, J., Penhale, D.W.H., Fritzinger, B. K., Rose, J.
    E. and Helwing, R. F., Controlled release of
    contraceptive steroids from biodegradable poly(ortho
    esters). Contracept. Deliv. Syst., 4(1983) 43-53.

Heller, J., Penhale, D.W.H. and Helwing, R.F.,
    Preparation of poly(ortho esters) by the reaction of
    diketene acetals and polyols. J. Polymer Sci.
    Polym. Lett. Ed., 18 (1980) 619-624.

Heller, J., Penhale, D.W.H., Helwing, R. F. and
    Fritzinger, B. K., Release of norethindrone from
    poly(ortho esters). Polymer Eng. Sci., 21 (1981)
    727-731.

Heller, J., Penhale, D.W.H., Helwing, R. F. and
    Fritzinger, B. K., Controlled release of
    norethindrone from poly(ortho esters). In Roseman,
    T. J. and Mansdorf, S. Z. (Eds) Controlled Release
    Delivery Systems, Marcel Dekker, New York, 1983, pp.
    91-105.

Shih, C., Himmelstein, K. J. and Higuchi, T., Drug
    delivery from catalyzed erodible polymeric matrices
    of poly(ortho esters). Biomaterials, 5 (1984) 237-
    240.

Sparer, R. V., Shih, C., Ringeisen, C. D. and
    Himmelstein, K. J., Controlled release from erodible
    poly(ortho ester) drug delivery systems. J. of
    Controlled Release, 1 (1984) 23-32.

MACROMOLECULES AS DRUG DELIVERY SYSTEMS

Hitoshi Sezaki and Mitsuru Hashida

Faculty of Pharmaceutical Sciences, Kyoto University, Yoshidashimoadachi-Cho, Sakyo-Ku, Kyoto, 606 Japan

Introduction

The approach described in this chapter is an exploration of the possibility of using macromolecule-drug conjugate for directed delivery of therapeutic agents. Since active targeting such as antibody or receptor-mediated delivery will be mentioned in other chapters, discussions will be limited to the use of conjugates in which a drug is associated or covalently bound to a non-specific macromolecular carrier. Emphasis will be placed on the results of dextran-conjugated mitomycin C obtained in our laboratory because they serve nicely to illustrate important considerations in the design of macromolecular conjugate and appear be practical for use in human cancer chemotherapy.

Potential Utility of Macromolecule-Drug Conjugates

Drugs and hormones conjugated to natural and synthetic macromolecular carriers have numerous advantages and are receiving widespread attention (Gregoriadis, 1979; Juliano, 1980; Bundgaard et al., 1982; Gregoriadis et al., 1982; Venter, 1982; Goldberg, 1983). For chemotherapeutic agents, the possible reasons for the use of such macromolecular conjugates can be divided into the following categories.

A. Pharmaceutical
 1. Stabilization of the drug in its active form.
 2. Increased solubility, which facilitates the acceptability of the drug.
 3. Improving retention of drugs in vesicle carriers and prolonged release of the drug at some desired site.
 4. *In vitro* loading of drugs into cellular drug carriers.
B. Pharmacokinetic
 1. Increased circulation half-life by restricting the metabolic and immune attack and renal excretion of the drug.
 2. Confinement of the drug to a chosen compartment.
 3. Targeted distribution to the specific site, increasing the activity to the desired site and minimizing the exposure to other tissues.
C. Pharmacodynamic
 1. Cell-specific interaction and overcoming of drug transport barriers, which enables the achievements of ultimate specificity.
 2. Selective activation at the target site.
D. Others
 As a tool for drug mechanism studies such as "target site" and drug resistance studies.

In contrast to these advantages, there are objections and problems in their potential clinical usage. The most obvious one being the occurrence of adverse immunologic reactions. Prolonged or unwanted retention in the body is another serious problem. In the case of enteral administration, poor bioavailability often limites the clinical application of otherwise promising candidate macromolecular drugs. A general method of reducing, modifying, or eliminating the immunogenicity of normally immunogenic macromolecules should find many applications in immunology and medicine. The attachment of a sufficient amount of a non-immunogenic polymer to available groups on a normally immunogenic protein has been reported (Poznansky et al., 1982). The immunogenicity of asparaginase was reduced by the attachment of soluble dextran of molecular weight 10,000 and 70,000. The degree of the enzyme protection increased by increasing the molecular weight of the dextran attached. Poor bioavailability may be overcome by proper incorporation of absorption-enhancing agents or formulations. For the drugs targeted within the gastrointestinal

tract, poor absorption may serve as a kind of inverse
targeting by reducing side reactions which may occur after
absorption.

Design of Macromolecule-Drug Conjugate

The design and development of therapeutically active
macromolecule-drug conjugate require considerable precise
multidisciplinary knowledge. Since macromolecular carriers
greatly alter the *in vivo* disposition of parent drugs,
macromolecular conjugates have sometimes been tried without any sound rationale, in the hope that something unique
could be obtained in drug delivery. A general scheme showing a principal configuration of a macromolecule-drug
conjugate system is illustrated in Fig. 1. In this schematic
representation, the polymer backbone, which is mostly biodegradable and water-soluble, is modified by at least three
functional moieties. One area of the polymer is used to fix
the drug via a covalent linkage. A spacer arm may be
necessary to provide physical separation between drug and
polymer to improve configuration efficiency, and drug-

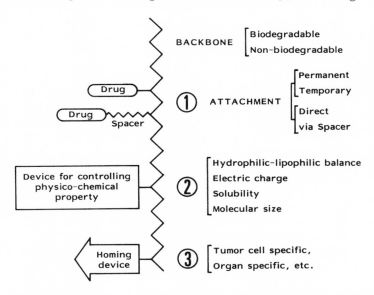

Fig. 1. Schematic representation of macromolecule-drug
conjugate.

receptor interaction efficiency, or improve the cleavability of polymer-drug linkage. The importance of a spacer
arm and the specific nature of the chemical linkage has
been well documented. In the case of polyamino acid-dauno-
rubicin conjugate, for instance, good correlation was
observed between the antitumor activity and the stability
of bonds formed between the drug and the carriers (Zunino,
F., 1984). Regeneration of the parent drug from the
conjugate may depend on the availability of enzymes and
other physicochemical properties such as the type of
chemical linkage, the presence of interactions with the
backbone, sites of attachment, and various cross-linking
reactions which govern the freedom of movement of the
attached drug. Sometimes, pharmacologic activity may be
conferred unintentionally on an inherently inactive polymer
carriers by a chemical fixation or substitution (Rogers and
Tökés, 1984). Target-specific moieties can be incorporated
in the conjugates as a device for actively directing the
therapeutic component to the target site. Another portion
of the conjugate can be utilized for controlling the
physicochemical properties of the conjugate molecule per
se. Occasionally, attempts have been made to non-covalently
associate macromolecular carriers with drugs. One of the
recent examples is our study of the lymphotropic delivery
of cationic bleomycin by ionic complex formation with
dextran sulfate via the colonic route of administration
(Yoshikawa et al., 1983).

Choice of Macromolecular Carrier

Numerous natural and synthetic polymers have been
tested as to their utility as macromolecular carriers for
drugs. Properties required for such carriers depend on the
intended clinical objectives and nature of drugs.
The criteria for choice of carriers are:

1. The carriers must be readily available.
2. The carriers should meet reasonable criteria of
   pharmaceutical formulation such as purity, solubility, and enough stability.
3. The carrier and its metabolic degradation products
   must be nonimmunogenic and should not adversely
   alter the antigenicity of the transported drugs.
4. The carrier and its metabolic degradation products
   lack all intrinsic toxicity.

5. The carrier and its metabolic degradation products must be biodegradable or at least should not show any serious accumulation in the body.
6. The carrier must have adequate functional groups for chemical fixation to attain high drug-carrying capacity.
7. The carrier-drug conjugate must retain the original activity of conveyed agent until it reaches the site of action or releases the transported drug in pre-designed manner.
8. The carrier-drug conjugate must retain the desirable specificity of the original carrier compound.

Occasionally carriers are classified as specific and non-specific; natural and synthetic; neutral, cationic, and anionic; and biodegradable and non-biodegradable. The majority of these have previously been reviewed (Sezaki and Hashida, 1984; Kato and Hara, 1983). Since one of the principal concepts and theoretical advantages of polymeric drugs is based on the idea that a portion of the complex can be utilized to target a second bioactive portion to specific cells or tissues, such specific carriers as antibodies, lectins and hormones have been extensively investigated.

Choice of Drugs

Drugs for preparing macromolecular conjugates usually possess such properties as (1) high pharmacologic activity, which can be used in therapy in accessible doses, (2) adequate functional groups in their molecular structure for chemical fixation, and (3) enough stability in the conjugated form until released. Besides molecular mechanism of action, chemical, pharmacokinetical, and clinical considerations are also important.

Behaviour of Macromolecular Conjugates *in Vivo*

This is closely related to the choice of route of administration. After the administration of a macromolecule-drug conjugate, a series of events takes place. In the case of intravenous administration, in which the largest number of investigations are involved, the distri-

bution and elimination properties are determinants for the
fate of conjugated drugs. They are usually confined to
the central compartment and are taken up principally by
cells identified with reticuloendothelial system (RES) and
are cleared by other elimination organs. Hence, in this
route of administration, passive or natural targeting makes
use of the inherent tendency of RES to incorporate macromolecules. Thus, like the most of the other particulate
delivery systems, the phagocytes are natural targets. In
the case of drugs like primaquine, anti-viral agents, and
many other anti-cancer agents, the target site of which
are the cell wall or within the cell, other important
steps are interaction and endocytosis of the polymer-bound
drug, followed by selective activation and release in the
intracellular milieu.

    Plasma half-life of macromolecule-drug conjugate per
se is governed primarily by its molecular weight, ionic
nature, configuration, and interacting tendencies in
physiological milieu. It is also influenced by the factors
limiting the permeability of biological membranes such as
pore size and electrostatic properties. Sometimes spacers
serve as secondary carriers of the drug after release of
the spacer-drug unit from the macromolecular carrier-spacer-
drug entity. Such secondary disposition of drug-carrier
entities may be important in understanding of the overall
fate of the original conjugate.

    The disease state markedly alters the clearance of
macromolecule-drug conjugate from the blood compartment.
In poorly perfused tumors such as carcinoma, extravascular
uptake of blood-borne substances is further hindered. In
such cases, increasing the blood flow rate and membrane
permeability selectively by a co-administered drug may have
beneficial effects. Inflammatory conditions, renal failure,
and experimental diabetic conditions increase capillary
permeability to macromolecules (Michels et al., 1982;
Zimmerman et al., 1984), which may in turn be utilized as
a means of delivering macromolecular conjugate through
leaky endothelia which are normally poorly accessible to
extravascular sites of action. Vessels lining the peritoneal cavities of some experimental animals bearing
ascites tumors display markedly greater permeability than
do the same vessels in control animals. Secretion of
permeability-increasing activity, an apparently common
feature of tumor cells (Senger et al., 1983), may contri-

bute to the extravascular directed delivery of macromolecular conjugates. It has recently been reported that
agents, such as high molecular weight dextrans, dextran
sulfates, and preparations of latex beads that activate
or depress the RES, depress cytochrome P-450 and related
hepatic drug metabolism (Peterson and Renton, 1984). The
secondary effects on drug metabolism by the intact polymer
conjugate and the remnant polymeric carriers require
further study.

Among compounds that exhibit activity after releasing
the parent drug, the active component is liberated either
during circulation or at or near the target site by means
of enzymatic or non-enzymatic cleavage reactions. However,
when the targets of therapy are extravascular and some
means of traversing the continuous endothelial barrier is
the prerequisite for the delivery of intact macromolecule-
drug conjugate, a freight container-like approach may be
utilized, as reported for liposomes loaded with macrophage-
activating agents (Alving, 1983). Thus, even active targeting using ligand or antibody is of little value when the
target cell is inaccessible. In order to circumvent such
transport barriers and to avoid possible side effect
accompanying systemic administration, compartmental targeting or local treatment modalities have been extensively
investigated and some of them attracted attention recently.

Mitomycin C-Dextran Conjugate

Mitomycin C (MMC) is an antitumor antibiotic that has
demonstrated activity against a number of human neoplasm.
In the following sections, emphasis will be placed on
dextran-conjugated MMC (MMCD). Dextrans are colloidal,
hydrophilic, water-soluble sunbstances, inert in biological
systems, and do not affect cell viability. It is the only
colloids that are approved by the FDA for prevention of
thromboembolic diseases in high risk surgical patients
(Ross and Angaran, 1984). These substances have proven to
be biopolymeric carriers for various biological active
compounds since they can be slowly hydrolyzed by dextranase
in vivo (Molteni, 1979). The major products being isomal-
tose and isomaltotriose units, which can then cross the
cell membrane.

MMC has shown to cross-link double helical DNA after

reduction to the corresponding hydroquinones. This process appears to be the main event lethal to tumor cells, although the generation of hydrogen peroxide by successive redox cycles of the DNA-bound MMC is also considered important. The positions 1a and 10 appear to be the alkylating sites of MMC, with their alkylating ability enhanced to give the indolohydroquinone. Consequently, it is considered that the substitution of the 1a position leads to the diminution of biological activity and this consideration is also applicable to dextran conjugates that show slight activity. Therefore, MMCD may represent a latent form or prodrug of MMC that supplies the parent drug with a special disposition behaviour resulting from polymerization. The molecular weight of dextrans, spacer arms, and the apparent charge of the macromolecules were varied to examine their effect on pharmacokinetic behaviour and activity after administration.

In the synthesis of cationic MMCD, dextran was activated with cyanogen bromide at pH 10.7 and MMC was coupled by a carbodiimide-catalyzed reaction at the 1a position via an amide linkage to a carbonyl group of ε-aminocaproic acid (C_6 spacer) which was introduced onto dextran as a spacer (Kojima et al., 1980). Concerning the linkage between the spacer and dextrans, three structures can be considered. Fig. 2 illustrates a representative isourea linkage, although structures such as N-substituted imido carbonate and carbamate are also probable. These structures may be at least partially responsible for the cationic charges of MMCD in a neutral pH range. Also the direct coupling of MMC to the BrCN-activated dextran could not be disregarded, but the MMC content and release characteristics of MMCD are obviously different from those of the direct conjugate with polysaccharide. All cationic conjugates (C_6 spacer) were estimated to contain MMC to an almost equal extent. The degree of substitution of dextrans by MMC was one molecule/14 to 17 glucose units. In the case of C_4 and C_8 spacer arms, γ-aminobutyric acid and ω-aminocaprylic acid were used to coupling reactions, respectively. For anionic MMCD preparation, introduction of a spacer arm to dextran was carried out using 6-bromohexanoic acid (C_6 spacer) followed by conjugation with MMC. All the MMCD were stabler than MMC against acid-catalyzed hydrolysis and metabolic degradation. MMC was liberated from MMCD with a half-life of 24 hr in the case of cationic conjugates (Kato et al., 1982) . For MMCD having different spacer arm

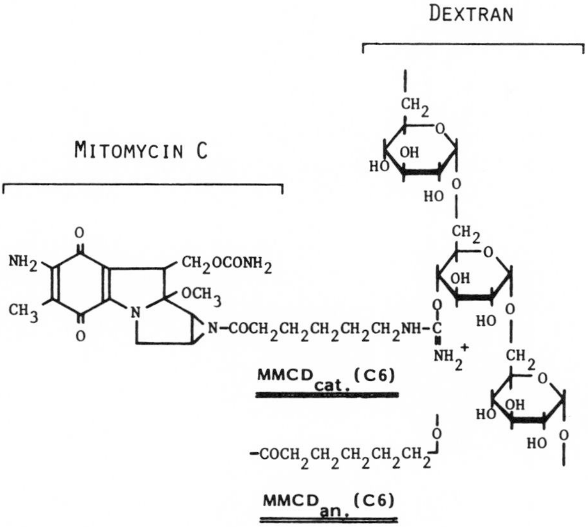

Fig. 2. Representative structure of mitomycin C-dextran

conjugate (MMCD).

lengths but with equal molecular weight dextran moieties, C_8 exhibits the longest *in vitro* release half-life of 42 hr and half-life becomes shorter as the length of the spacer arm shortened. The longest half-life was obtained with dextran T500 (C_6 spacer) bearing anionic charge (TABLE 1).

Cationic MMCD having molecular weight of 70,000 were less active against *E. coli in vitro*. Also they showed about one-tenth of the antitumor activity of MMC *in vitro* in contact with L1210 leukemia cells, but showed almost equal activity in the i.p. - i.p. system *in vivo*, suggesting that they exhibit activity after being regenerated to the parent compound in the body (Hashida et al., 1981).

Several distinct membrane properties are potential targets for a drug molecule. Also, chemotherapeutic agents attached to a carrier complex have been shown to be

TABLE 1 PHYSICO-CHEMICAL CHARACTERISTICS OF MMCD

	$\bar{M}_w$ (Carrier)	Mitomycin C content (weight %)	*in vitro* release* $t_{1/2}(\%)$	Adsorption % at pH 7.2	
				CM-Sephadex	DEAE-Sephadex
T10 (C_6^+)	9,900	10.80	24.4	66.6	0
T70 (C_6^+)	64,400	8.46	23.6	57.3	0
T500 (C_6^+)	487,000	10.10	23.8	70.8	0
T70 (C_4^+)	64,400	3.15	11.0	37.6	0
T70 (C_6^+)	64,400	8.46	23.6	57.3	0
T70 (C_8^+)	64,400	7.20	42.2	61.7	0
T10 (C_6^-)	9,900	9.43	35.0	0	0.3
T70 (C_6^-)	64,400	8.15	35.4	0	38.3
T500 (C_6^-)	487,000	7.80	50.0	0	28.4

* $37°$, pH 7.4

effective in overcoming resistance *in vitro* and to enhance
toxicity to specific tumor cells (Ryser and Shen, 1978).
Therefore, we studied cellular interactions and *in vitro*
antitumor activities of MMCD in a cell culture system. MMCD
having a cationic charge are remarkably adsorbed on tumor
cell surface by an electrostatic force, while MMC, anionic
MMCD, and a negative charge-bearing poly-L-glutamic acid
conjugate of MMC did not (Roos et al., 1984). Also greater
association was observed as the molecular weight of dextran
increased. The association tendency of MMCD with the cells
was unaffected at low temperature, 4°, which suggests a non-
specific character of adsorption. Most of MMCD regenerating
MMC exhibited cytocidal activity almost equivalent to MMC
in the case of continuous contact experiment. In a 1 hr
exposure experiment, however, macromolecular conjugates
with higher interacting tendency with tumor cells showed
higher antitumor activities than MMC. MMCD released MMC by
hydrolysis on the tumor cell surface, which is different
from the behaviour proposed in the case of adriamycin
(Trouet et al., 1972). In the case of anthracyclines and
methotrexate polymeric drugs, which gave the most successful results among numerous attempts to develop polymeric
antineoplastics, the drugs are considered to enter the
tumor cells in combination with the carrier by endocytosis
and to be cleaved to free forms by lysosomal enzymes.
However, MMCD showed different properties. It has slight
toxicity as such, liberate spontaneously MMC not by enzyme-
mediated reaction, and was directly inactivated by tissue
homogenates. Thus, MMCD acts in a free form following
chemical cleavage of MMC from the dextran in the body,
including central circulation, body cavities such as
peritoneal cavity, or at the target cell surface, but not
in the intracellular lysosomes, and is a polymeric drug
different from lysosomotropic agents (De Duve et al.,1974).
Anthracyclines such as adriamycin have previously been
considered to act by intercalation with nuclear DNA, but
recent evidence suggests the possibility that the cell
surface membrane represent an alternative target (Tritton
et al., 1983). Presentation of inactive anthracycline
analog on a solid phase support resulted in the acquisition
of cytotoxic activity (Rogers and Tökes, 1984).Creation of
a new mechanism of cytotoxicity due to covalent attachment
to polymers is a likely interpretation. Regardless, our
results demonstrate that even a simple manipulation of an
electric charge and carrier molecular weight may profoundly
influence the macromolecular drug-cancer cell surface

interaction and cytotoxic demonstration.

Pharmacokinetics and Disposition of MMCD

Although various conjugates of cytotoxic agents with
high molecular weight materials have been synthesized and
evaluated as candidates for tumor specific delivery devices,
surprisingly little is known about the relationship between
the antitumor activities and the physicochemical characteristics of the conjugates. Furtheremore, studies on the role
of the macromolecular carrier moiety on the overall kinetic
behaviour of delivery systems is almost completely unexplored.

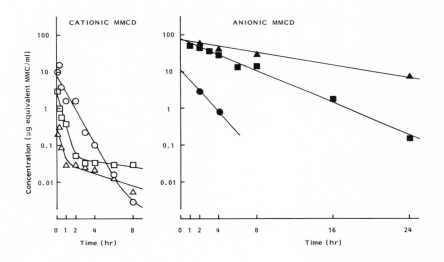

Fig. 3. Plasma concentrations of cationic (open symbol) and
anionic (solid symbol) MMCD in rats following bolus intravenous administration of MMCD with different molecular
weights (○ ●) T10 ; (□ ■) T70 ; (△ ▲) T500.

Disposition of MMCD was investigated following intra-venous bolus administration in rats. Different types of MMCD listed in TABLE 1 were tested and the disposition of MMC, MMCD, and carrier dextran was determined. As shown in Fig. 3, cationic MMCD are more rapidly cleared from the circulation than anionic ones. Tissue distribution studies using ^{14}C-labelled cationic MMCD revealed that they are specifically accumulated in the RES such as the liver, spleen but not in the lung, heart and muscle (Hashida et al., 1984). The polycationic nature of MMCD may play an important role in this large accumulation since much longer retention in plasma was observed in the anionic counterparts as shown in Fig. 3. Electric charges also influence the renal excretory pattern of the conjugates. Unlike free dextrans which tend to readily accumulate in the kidney, charged conjugates are not highly distributed in this vital organ (Takakura et al., 1984) which suggest the possibility for controlling the drug delivery to a specific organ or inversely target an agent by selecting the size and electric charge of the conjugates since the size of carrier dextran also seems to behave as a deter-minant that ordains the disposition pattern of the conjugate.

Plasma concentration data for cationic MMCD and carrier dextran were fitted to a compartment model in which it is assumed that (1) the system is linear; (2) the distribution of conjugates is described by a two-compart-ment body model; (3) the elimination of MMCD by metabolism and urinary excretion occurs in the central compartment; (4) the conversion of MMCD to MMC proceeds at the same rate in both central and peripheral compartments; and (5) the disposition of free MMC is described by a one-compartment body model. Several additional compartment models were derived and tested for describing the sets of data for all cationic MMCD experiments based on general analyses by Notari (Notari, 1981). However, only the one shown in Fig.4 yielded an excellent fit by the evaluation using Akaike's information criteria (Akaike, 1973).

It is noteworthy that the sets of data of three kinds of cationic MMCD of different molecular weight yielded almost identical conversion rate constants of those of *in vitro* hydrolysis, though other pharmacokinetic para-meters varied with the carrier molecular size. These results support our previous observation that MMCD acts in the body

Conjugated MMC   Free MMC

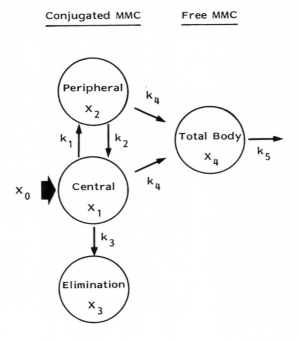

Fig. 4. Pharmacokinetic model describing disposition of MMCD. X_0: initial dose of MMCD ; X_1, X_2, X_3 : amount of conjugated MMC (MMCD); X_4: amount of free MMC; k_1, k_2, k_3, k_4, k_5: first-order rate constant.

as a reservoir which supply MMC at an identical first-order rate constant regardless of their molecular sizes. Many of the cleavage reactions of macromolecule-drug conjugates depend on enzymes. When the enzymatic reaction is at least characteristic of tumor cells as compared with normal ones, such regeneration may be favorable for a site-specific activation of the conjugate. On the other hand, cleavage reaction not mediated by an enzymatic process is generally free from species differences, intersubject variation, and the effect of disease and co-administered drugs. Anionic MMCD is retained in the circulation for a much longer period than cationic ones. If the target is confined in the circulation or readily equilibrated organs or a slow and controlled release of an active agent during circulation is a preferred modality, anionic MMCD seems to suggest a potentially effective method of cancer chemotherapy by sustaining the supply or targeting the cytotoxicity although still dominant accumulation in the RES poses major difficulties in obtaining optimized therapy by a systemic dose of MMCD.

Lymphatic Delivery of MMCD

A sufficient supply of anticancer agents to the lymphatic system seems to offer a promising means of preventing lymph node metastasis. Various kinds of emulsion formulations were adopted as topical delivery systems, and improvement of lymphatic transfer of anticancer agents such as 5-fluorouracil and bleomycin was successfully achieved in our previous studies (Sezaki and Hashida, 1982). In addition to these trials using physical carriers, MMCD was studied as a lymphatic delivery system.

Málek et al.first reported an increased affinity of salts of antibiotics such as streptomycin and neomycin with high-molecular weight anionic substances for the lymphatics (Málek et al., 1958). Concerning conjugates with covalent linkage, Maeda et al. prepared a conjugate of neo-carzinostatin with a poly-(maleic acid) styrene oligomer (Maeda et al., 1979) and observed a selective delivery to lymphatics and to other target tumors, although the role of molecular size remains obscure since the parent drug also has a relatively high molecular weight of 10,700.

Disposition of cationic MMCD following intramuscular administration to rats was different from MMC (Takakura et al., 1984). Polymeric modification remarkably retarded the elimination of MMC from the injection site. The elimination rate was decreased as the molecular weight of carrier dextran increased, suggesting the control of the absorption rate by proper carrier selection. Very high concentrations of MMC in the lymph node continued during the course of the experiments, and the molecular weight of carrier exhibited a significant effect on this. A more remarkable influence of the molecular size was demonstrated

in thoracic lymph transfer, in which MMCD (T10)itself
appeared in the thoracic lymph together with free MMC while
only free MMC was detected following the injection of MMCD
(T500). The former was taken up by the lymphatic vessels,
passed through the lymph node, and appeared in the thoracic
lymph while liberating free MMC. On the other hand, the
latter was accumulated in the regional lymph node and
supplied the active MMC there. MMCD (T70) was an intermediate case. The maximum lymph node concentration of the
drug after injection of MMCD was about 50 times that of the
emulsion formulation containing MMC. MMCD persisted in the
lymph node for longer periods than the parent drug
entrapped in the emulsion formulation.

     The results of chemotherapeutic experiments revealed
the efficacy of local injection of MMCD against lymph node
metastasis. The highest effectiveness was observed in the
group treated with MMCD (T70). On the other hand, MMCD
(T500) showed the most remarkable activity in the prophy-
lactic experiment (Takakura et al., 1984). These results
correspond well to the kinetic characteristics of MMCD as
well as the interaction between MMCD and tumor cells.

                    Intratumor Delivery of MMCD

     Another interesting approach to localized chemotherapy
is the use of macromolecule-drug conjugate for intra-
tumoral administration. Goldberg et al. recently expanded
the idea by introducing affinity ligands (polymeric
affinity drug) which is based on the concept of local chemo-
and immuno-therapy (Goldberg, 1983). In integrated cancer
therapy, surgical resection of the tumor is only a support-
ing mean to reduce the number of the target cells which are
susceptible to chemotherapeutic agents and radiation. There
are many chemotherapeutic modalities for advanced cancers
but the simplest method with high efficiency is the direct
administration of the anticancer drug into the residual
tumor. Obvious difficulties in intratumor application are
rapid diffusion of drug from the injection site into the
circulation and an extensive inflammation and tissue
necrosis at the site of injection which could be avoided by
MMCD.

     MMC and MMCD (0.4 mg eq. MMC/kg) dissolved in isotonic
saline was injected into VX2 tumor, transplanted on the ear

chamber of a rabbit. Following the injection, MMC was
retained at the injection site for about 48 hr in a conjugated form, while it disappeared rapidly when given as a
free form. Free MMC injection resulted in severe necrosis
and penetration in the ear at day 30, while in the case of
MMCD, the tumor regressed without necrosis of the surrounding tissues in 7 days and was replaced by granulatomous
fibrosis. In the recent report on extravascular diffusion
of macromolecules in normal and neoplastic tissue, a graded
series of fluoresceinisothiocyanate dextrans were found to
diffuse more easily into VX2 carcinoma than normal tissues
(Nugent and Jain, 1984). MMCD might diffuse in the interstitial space in tumor from the injection site to outside
of the tumor delivering MMC to the malignant cells.
Preliminary passive cutaneous anaphylactic test was
negative in all cases and no anaphylactic signs appeared in
rabbits that received repeated administration of MMCD.

Experimental therapy using MMCD (T500) has started
from September, 1983 at the Second Surgery Department of
Kyoto University Medical School. MMCD (T500), 5-10 mg
equivalent MMC, was administered to 14 patients with
advanced abdominal cancers including 3 gastric cancers, 8
colon cancers, 1 hepatoma, 1 ovary cancer, and 1 gall-
bladder cancer. The median age was 60 years (range, 42 -
72). In three cases with palatable masses, the conjugate
was injected into the tumor by percutaneous puncture. In
some cases, the tumor responses were evaluated by sono-
graphy and/or computerized tomography of the abdomen. In
other patients, MMCD was given during surgical operation
to the residual malignancies. Two patients received
repeated administration of MMCD without anaphylactic signs.
Eight patients (57 %) had objective tumor responses and
one of them had a complete remission for more than thirty
weeks (Honda et al., 1984). Except for a transient fever,
mild leukopenia, and slight elevation of serum transaminase
level, no serious side effects appeared. Eight patients
had a fever shortly after the administration of MMCD. The
temperature rose as high as $39°$ in two cases but fell to
normal with the use of antipyretic drugs. Repeated administration of MMCD also elevated a fever which was not as high
as that after the first injection.

Conclusion

The examples discussed show the potentials and limitation of the practical use of macromolecule-drug conjugates in directed delivery of drugs. Combination with vectoring devices such as biologically recognizable moieties and with physical carriers and/or sophisticated medical technology certainly hold great promise. Like most rapidly developing fields, polymeric drugs have experienced large swings in mood. It has now reached the stage in which much systematical and yet multidisciplinary information must be accumulated and integrated into quantitative perspectives.

REFERENCES

Akaike, H., A new look at the statistical model identification. IFEE Trans. Aut. Contr., 19 (1973) 716-723.

Alving, C. R., Delivery of liposome-encapsulated drugs to macrophages. Pharmacol. Ther., 22 (1983) 407-424.

Bundgaard, H., Hansen, A. B. and Kofod, H. (Eds) Optimization of drug delivery, Munksgaard, Copenhagen, 1982.

De Duve, C., De Barsy, T., Poole, B., Trouet, A., Tulkens, P. and Van Hoof, F., Lysosomotropic agents. Biochem. Pharmacol., 23 (1974) 2495-2531.

Goldberg, E. P. (Eds) Targeted drugs, John Wiley & Sons, New York, 1983.

Gregoriadis, G. (Eds) Drug carriers in biology and medicine, Academic Press, London, 1979.

Gregoriadis, G., Senior, J. and Trouet, A. (Eds) Targeting of drugs, Plenum Press, New York, London, 1982.

Hashida, M., Kato, A., Kojima, T., Muranishi, S., Sezaki H., Tanigawa, N., Satomura, K. and Hikasa, Y., Antitumor activity of mitomycin C-dextran conjugate against various murine tumors. Gann, 72 (1981) 226-234.

Hashida, M., Kato, A., Takakura, Y. and Sezaki, H., Disposition and pharmacokinetics of a polymeric prodrug of mitomycin C, mitomycin C-dextran conjugate, in the rat. Drug Metab. Dispos. 12 (1984) 492-499.

Honda, K., Matsumoto, S., Takakura, Y., Arimoto, A., Kikuchi, S., Tanaka, K., Hashida, M., Sezaki, H. and Satomura, K., Local administration of mitomycin C conjugated with dextran in the treatment of advanced abdominal cancers. Cancer, submitted.

Juliano, R. L. (Eds) Drug delivery systems, Oxford University Press, New York, Oxford, 1980.

Kato, K., Takakura, Y., Hashida, M., Kimura, T. and Sezaki H., Physico-chemical and antitumor characteristics of

high molecular weight prodrugs of mitomycin C. Chem.
Pharm. Bull., 30 (1982) 2951-2957.

Kato, Y. and Hara, T., Macromolecule-anticancer drug
conjugates. J. Synth. Org. Chem. Jpn., 41 (1983)
1135-1142.

Kojima, T., Hashida, M., Muranishi, S. and Sezaki, H.,
Mitomycin C-dextran conjugate:a novel high molecular
weight pro-drug of mitomycin C. J. Pharm. Pharmacol.
32 (1980) 30-34.

Maeda, H., Takeshita, J., Kanamaru, R., Sato, H., Katoh, J.
and Sato, H., Antimetastatic and antitumor activity
of a derivative of neocarzinostatin:An organic solvent
and water-soluble polymer-conjugated protein. Gann,
70 (1979) 601-606.

Málek, P., Kolc, J., Herold, M. and Hoffman, J., Lymphotropic antibiotics-"Antibiolymphins". In Antibiotics
Annual, Medical Encyclopedia Inc., New York, 1958,
pp. 546-556.

Michels, L. D., Davidman, M. and Keane, W. F., Glomerular
permeability to neutral and anionic dextrans in
experimental diabetes. Kidney Int. 21 (1982) 699-705.

Molteni, L., Dextrans as drug carriers. In Gregoriadis, G.
(Eds) Drug carriers in Biology and Medicine, Academic
Press, London, New York, 1979, pp. 107-125.

Notari, R. E., Prodrug design. Pharmacol. Ther., 14 (1981)
25-53.

Nugent, L. J. and Jain, R. K., Extravascular diffusion in
normal and neoplastic tissues. Cancer Res. 44 (1984)
238-244.

Peterson, T. C. and Renton, K. W., Depression of cytochrome
P-450-dependent drug biotransformation in hepatocytes
after the activation of the reticuloendothelial system
by dextran sulfate. J. Pharmacol. Exp. Ther., 229
(1984) 299-304.

Poznansky, M. J., Shanlding, M., Salkie, M. A., Elliot,
J. and Lau, E., Advantages in the use of L-aspara-
ginase-albumin polymer as an antitumor agent. Cancer
Res. 42 (1982) 1020-1025.

Rogers, K. E. and Tökés, Z. A., Novel mode of cytotoxicity
obtained by coupling inactive anthracycline to a
polymer. Biochem. Pharmacol., 33 (1984) 605-608.

Roos, C. F., Matsumoto, S., Takakura, Y., Hashida, M. and
Sezaki, H., Physico-chemical and antitumor activities
of some polyamino acid prodrugs of mitomycin C.,
Int. J. Pharm., in press.

Ross, A. D. and Angaran, D. M., Colloids vs. crystalloids-

A continuing controversy. Drug. Intell. Clin. Pharm., 18 (1984) 202-212.

Ryser, H. J. P. and Shen, W. C., Conjugation of methotrexate to poly (L-lysine) increaes drug transport and overcome drug resistance in cultured cells. Proc. Natl. Acad. Sci. USA, 75 (1978) 3867-3870.

Senger, D. R., Galli, S. J., Dvorak, A. M., Perruzzi, C.C., Harvey, V. S. and Dvorak, H. F., Tumor cells secrete a vascular permeability factor that promotes accumulation of ascites fluid. Science, 219 (1983) 983-985.

Sezaki, H., Hashida, M. and Muranishi, S., Gelatin microspheres as carriers for antineoplastic agents. In Bundgaard, H., Hansen, A. B. and Kofod, H. (Eds) Optimization of drug delivery, Munksgaard, Copenhagen, 1982, pp. 316-332.

Sezaki, H. and Hashida, M., Macromolecule-drug conjugates in targeted cancer chemotherapy. CRC Crit. Rev. Ther. Drug Carrier System, in press.

Takakura, M., Matsumoto, S., Hashida, M. and Sezaki, H., Enhanced lymphatic delivery of mitomycin C conjugated with dextran. Cancer Res. 44 (1984) 2505-2510.

Tritton, T. R., Yee, G. and Wingard Jr., L. B., Immobilized adriamycin:a tool for separating cell surface from intracellular mechanisms. Fed. Proc., 42 (1983) 284-287.

Trouet, A., Campeneere, D. D. and De Duve, C., Chemotherapy through lysosomes with a DNA-daunorubicin complex. Nature New Biol., 239 (1972) 110-112.

Ventor, J. C., Immobilized and insolubilized drugs, hormones, and neurotransmitters:properties, mechanisms of action and application. Pharmacol. Rev. 34 (1982) 153-187.

Yoshikawa, H., Sezaki, H. and Muranishi, S., Mechanism for selective transfer of bleomycin into lymphatics by a bifunctional delivery system via the lumen of the large intestine. Int.J. Pharm., 13 (1983) 321-332.

Zimmerman, A. L., Sablay, L. B., Aynedjian, H. S. and Bank, N., Increased peritoneal permeability in rats with alloxan-induced diabetes mellitus. J. Lab. Clin. Med., 103 (1984) 720-730.

Zunino, F., Savi, G., Giuliani, F., Gambetta, R., Supino, R., Tinelli, S. and Pezzoni, G., Comparison of antitumor effects of daunorubicin covalently linked to poly-L-amino acid carriers. Eur. J. Cancer Clin. Oncol., 20 (1984) 421-425.

D. BIOLOGICAL-CHEMICAL APPROACHES TO DIRECTED DRUG DELIVERY

MONOCLONAL ANTIBODY MEDIATED DRUG DELIVERY AND ANTIBODY

TOXIN CONJUGATES

David M. Neville, Jr.
Section on Biophysical Chemistry
Laboratory of Molecular Biology
National Institute of Mental Health
Bethesda, Maryland 20205

I. INTRODUCTION

Monoclonal antibody mediated drug delivery systems are relatively new to pharmacology. Early development of monoclonal antibodies and their interaction with unique cell surface determinants was confined largely to immunology groups (Mason and Williams, 1980). As clinical applications appear practical these systems are likely to come increasingly under the purview of pharmacologists. The point of view of this paper is that the questions and tools that are unique to pharmacology will be necessary for the practical development of antibody mediated drug delivery systems.

Monoclonal antibody reagents have many similarities with one class of standard pharmacologic reagents, the class of reagents whose actions are receptor mediated. Just as pharmacokinetic studies have aided our understanding of receptor-mediated drugs, they are particularly important in the study of monoclonal antibody mediated delivery systems. This is because monoclonal antibodies must cross barriers to get to their target sites and during this time period the antibodies or materials conjugated to them are metabolized with a resulting change in pharmacologic specificity. Very small metabolic modifications in antibody structure have profound effects in altering their target specificity. For these reasons pharmacologists should be quite at home with monoclonal antibody systems.

II. STRUCTURAL AND FUNCTIONAL CONSIDERATIONS OF ANTIBODIES

Antibodies are made in a variety of structures that constitute classes and subclasses. However, all antibodies exhibit a basic pattern of domains. These domains are made up of heavy and light chains of variable and constant regions and these domains have different functions (Roitt, 1980). The IgG class has to date proven the most useful for drug delivery systems. This class has a molecular weight of approximately 150,000 and contains two antigen binding sites which arise from a hinge region on the molecule which is flexible and permits bivalent binding over a range of antigen site configurations. Other major domains on IgG bind complement and bind cells of the monocyte-macrophage lineage of the immune system. By activating complement or by activating cellular immune responses antibodies in themselves constitute an endogenous drug delivery system.

When antibodies are used to target radioactive isotopes, toxins or other drugs, the antibody interactions with complement or macrophages may constitute competing side reactions. These reactions can be eliminated by cleaving the molecule just before the hinge region with pepsin producing what is known as a divalent $F(ab')_2$ piece having the same full affinity towards the antigen as the parent antibody. The $F(ab')_2$ piece of approximately 100,000 daltons can be cleaved into two monovalent pieces of equal size by reduction of the disulfide bonds in the hinge region. When divalent antibodies bind to determinants on the external plasma membrane surface, they tend to bind in a divalent fashion, although the fraction of antibody binding divalently versus monovalently varies with the antigen and antibody in question (Mason and Williams, 1980). Generally, all binding is not divalent and binding isotherms are therefore heterogeneous. In general, the apparent affinity of divalent antibodies are 10^2 to 10^3 higher than their monovalent counterparts for cell surface determinants. Monoclonal antibodies obtained by cloning the progeny resulting from the fusion of an immunized lymphocyte and a myeloma cell line exhibit sequence homogeneity providing that the parental myeloma line does not make its own heavy or light chains, which can become randomly mixed with lymphocyte heavy or light chains (Galfrè and Milstein, 1981). When the myeloma does not make heavy or light chains, the antibodies are quite homogeneous, however, dimers and higher aggregates may exist that alter important properties.

Monoclonal antibodies can exhibit enormous specificity and can recognize a single amino acid substitution in a protein. An antibody directed toward such a determinant may have an affinity in the order of $10^{10}M^{-1}$ which corresponds to a dissociation rate constant expressed as a half-life in the range of 10 - 20 hrs, whereas binding to the allotype is undetectable indicating an affinity of 10^4M^{-1} or less (Williams and Gagnon, 1982; Mason and Willians, 1980). High affinity antibodies such as these provide enormous specificity when used at high dilutions. Immunoassays utilizing monoclonal antibodies coupled with colorometric enzyme or radioactive readouts are highly useful diagnostic products which have reached today's market place.

III. ADVANTAGES OF MONOCLONAL ANTIBODIES

The advantages of monoclonal antibodies over polyclonal antibodies are the result of their inherent homogeneity and can be divided into three categories. (1) Data Interpretation: Homogeneity of affinity, class and subclass means that physical chemical concepts can be realistically applied to these systems. Equilibrium constants, rate constants, receptor number and diffusion rates across barriers can be determined and interpreted in meaningful ways. This also applies to interactions with other systems such as complement or binding to macrophages or other cells involved in clearance. In addition the ability to generate monoclonals of varying properties against the same antigenic determinant allows one to dissect out the importance of all of the above mentioned variables in any system of interest. (2) Reproducibility of Effects: A homogeneous reagent can be passed from laboratory to laboratory or clinic to clinic and results compared. This is of particular importance in the development of commercial reagents. With proper care the clone will be immortal providing a continuous supply which can be expanded or contracted on demand. Reproducibility also exists in methods of chemical modification such as conjugations to other drugs. (3) Tailored Specificity: Because a variety of classes and subclasses with different properties can be raised against the same determinant, antibodies can be sought that have unique specificities at each of their functional domains. In addition it is possible to chemically link monoclonals of differing specificities (Nisonoff and Rivers, 1961).

IV. ANTIBODIES AS THEIR OWN DELIVERY SYSTEM.

Exogenous antibodies have been administered to both laboratory animals and humans as anti-cancer agents. The antibodies have been directed against cell surface determinant present on the tumor. Prolongation of animal survival time in experimental models of leukemia have been noted, however, these results were no better than conventional drug therapy in similar leukemia models. The results in humans have generally been disappointing (Levy et al., 1983). In both the human and animal studies the effects of exogenously administered antibody when noted appeared to be due to activating cellular immune systems (Bernstein et al., 1980; Kaproski, 1983) or activating complement (Glennie and Stevenson, 1982). Since most monoclonal antibodies are currently raised in mice, it is worthwhile to note that the only mouse IgG sub-class that can extensively bind to human macrophages is the IgG_{2A} sub-class.

Antibodies can act as their own drug delivery systems in one other important case and that is when they are directed against receptors that are involved in the uptake of an essential component for the cell or when they are directed against receptors that provide signaling events. An example of the latter process is an autoimmune disease in which the organism generates antibodies directed against the the thyroid stimulating hormone receptor. These antibodies themselves are stimulating and cause hyperplasia of the thyroid gland and thyrotoxicosis (Roitt, 1980). Antibodies may also exert profound effects when directed against endogenous trophic factors which must be internalized by specific tissues for maintenance of differentiation (Gurney et al., 1984). An example of antibodies blocking a physiologic uptake process are antibodies that have been raised against the transferrin receptor and thereby block essential iron uptake. Cells exposed to monoclonal antibodies directed against a transferrin receptor become starved for iron and exhibit markedly reduced growth (Trowbridge et al., 1982). None of these types of systems has as yet been used clinically.

V.   ANTIBODIES AS CARRIERS OF TOXIC COMPOUNDS: ANALYSIS
     OF THE VARIABLES

A variety of low molecular weight toxic agents have been
linked to monoclonal antibodies (Arnon and Sela, 1982).
Antibodies conjugated with radioisotopes emitting γ-rays,
x-rays and positrons and have provided the most quantitative
data.   These labeled antibodies have been used for both
imaging purposes and as therapeutic tools in an attempt to
destroy unwanted cell populations, particularly malignant
tumors.   Animal and clinical studies have been done in
parallel by utilizing human carcinomas which can be carried
in a nude mouse system.   The antigen receiving most attention has been the carcinoma embryonic antigen or CEA antigen which is present in high concentration on many gastrointestinal malignant tumors, but not extensively present
in normal adult tissues, although the antigen is actually a
fetal antigen.   This antigen is also shed from tumor cells
and appears in the circulation, a situation that compli-
cates imaging procedures and therapeutic procedures using
monoclonal antibodies directed at this antigen.
Studies reported by Haskel and co-workers (1983) have
utilized antibodies with affinities in the order of $10^9 M^{-1}$.
The results of these studies performed both in nude mice
and in humans prior to surgery revealed that following intravenous administration of ^{125}I-antibody the distribution
ratios between the tumor and the surrounding tissues are
low, ranging between 5/1 to 10/1 tumor/surrounding tissue
at the optimum time period post injection which is generally
one to three days.   In humans, tumors 6 cm in diameter could
be detected, whereas tumors 1 cm in diameter were not detected (Mach et al., 1983).   In mice, distribution ratios
of this size resulted in no measurable therapeutic effect.
These studies were performed in some cases with $F(ab')_2$
pieces and these provided the higher distribution ratio.
The stomach and kidney received 10% of the total time average dose and high doses were also received by the thyroid
gland because the isotope was iodine in this case.
A problem in using radioisotopes coupled to monoclonal
antibodies is that the isotope may be catabolically removed
from the antibody prior to degradation of the antibody.
Once the isotope is removed from the antibody, its uptake
in other tissues is determined by the properties of the
isotope.

A second reason for the failure to achieve a high distribution coefficient between the target and non-target organs is the placement of physiologic barriers between the blood stream and the target organ. Barriers of this sort have been documented in a study by Houston et al. (1980) using a murine leukemia model and a monoclonal antibody directed at the Thy 1.1 antigen present in large numbers on AKR murine T cells. These T cells are present in lymph nodes, spleen and thymus. The spleen is essentially exposed to the blood circulation, whereas the other two organs exhibit endothelial barriers. Using ^{125}I-labeled intact antibody, ratios of sequestered spleen and lymph node CPM to injected CPM were still low in the range of 5%. However, when F(ab')$_2$ pieces were used the lymph node received 50% of the injected isotope at 10 hrs. However, the thymus received virtually no isotope indicating a profound barrier. The brain also contains large amounts of the Thy 1.1 antigen and no uptake was noted to this compartment. The lymph nodes of mice positive for the Thy 1.1 antigen contained 140-fold more isotope at the peak concentration than the lymph nodes of allotypic mice not containing this antigen. However, when the organ dose was integrated over time the stomach and kidney received significant doses. This could have resulted from dehalogenation of the antibody because protein bound radioactivity was not determined.

Monoclonal antibodies used in this murine study and in the studies of human colorectal cancer have affinities in the order of $10^9 M^{-1}$. This corresponds to a half-time of dissociation in the order of 1 hr. Thus, antibodies that become bound to the target cell have ample opportunity to dissociate from the target during the time frame over which the maximum target/non-target distribution ratio is achieved. The rate of receptor-mediated endocytosis for the specific receptor in question is an important variable in these systems. Bound antibodies once internalized in the cell may be returned to the cell membrane again by the process of exocytosis. If the target cells are few in number compared to the non-target cells and if non-target cells have either a low affinity for the antibody or for the ligand that is coupled to the antibody, then a crucial variable becomes the ratio of non-target to target cells. In most therapeutic situations, in terms of cancer therapy, the ratio of non-target to target cells is usually at least 1000 and may be as high as 10^5. Thus, even a small affinity of the therapeutic agent for the non-target cell can result in distribution ratios close to 1 to 1.

There is one example in medicine of a highly effective therapy for eliminating unwanted cells using a radioisotope in a drug delivery system. In this case, the drug delivery system is physiologic and it is the delivery of iodide to the thyroid gland. Because this system is so effective and is used routinely to eradicate benign cells in a hyperthyroid gland and is also used to eradicate malignant cells when they have the iodide uptake system intact, it is useful to examine the features of this system. When one plots the ratio of the total rads delivered by various radioiodine isotopes of varying half-lives to the thyroid gland to the rads delivered to the "total body" (minus the thyroid gland), one sees that with the radioisotope having 8 and 60 day half-lives that the ratio is approximately 1800 to 1 (Wellman and Anger 1971). This means that a dose of 2000 to 10,000 rads can be delivered to the thyroid without imposing a significant radiation burden on the remainder of the body. This achieves complete ablation of the gland. The interesting feature of this system is that the isotopes having shorter half-lives deliver a less favorable therapeutic ratio. The ratio of the isotope having a 2.3 hr half-life is 150 and this number corresponds to the distribution coefficient of iodide between the thyroid gland and the general circulation. The uptake of iodide by the thyroid gland is maximal at about 24 hrs when 27% of the total dose has been taken up. The gland gradually eliminates this dose with a t1/2 of 68 days. The reason for this is that as soon as iodide crosses the cell membrane it is converted into iodine and then into iodotyrosine and incorporated covalently into thyroglobulin which is only slowly broken down to release thyroxine as needed. Thus, uptake of iodide by the thyroid gland is a two step process. The first step is reversible and achieves a distribution coefficient of approximately 150. The second slower step is largely irreversible and provides another factor of 12. Radioactive iodine isotopes of half-lives less than the time over which the irreversible step takes place have therapeutic ratios that reflect only the initial reversible step. Delivery systems employing a second irreversible step are highly advantageous.

VI. MONOCLONAL ANTIBODY TOXIN CONJUGATES

The bacterial and plant protein toxins such as diphtheria toxin and ricin are unique in that these structures
contain their own delivery systems. These two protein
toxins have molecular weights of approximately 60,000 and
consist of two chains that are held together by a single
disulfide bond. These toxins enter cells by receptor-
mediated transport systems. The binding site for the cell
receptor is located on the B chain of the toxin. The A
chain of the toxin is an enzyme that catalytically inhibits protein synthesis. In the case of diphtheria toxin
the A chain is an ADP-ribosyl transferase that catalyzes
the transfer of the ADP moiety from endogenous NAD^+ to
elongation factor 2. ADP-ribosylated EF_2 is inactive in
protein synthesis (Pappenheimer, 1977). The turnover number
is such that one molecule of DT A-chain (DTA) can inactivate all of the EF_2 within a single cell in 24 hrs. Ricin
catalytically inactivates ribosomes. The exact mechanism
is unknown (Neville and Youle, 1982a). The substrate for
both of these toxins is the protein synthesizing machinery
located in the cytosol compartment. The toxins kill cells
by 3 sequential steps: binding to cell surface membrane
receptors; a transport step that transports at least the
A-chain of the toxin to the cytosol compartment; and then
the enzymatic inactivation step. The toxins are believed
to enter the cell via receptor-mediated endocytosis. The
transport step is the least understood step in this process.
However, recent work from our laboratory indicates that
diphtheria toxin gains entrance to the cytosol compartment
by destabilizing the vesicle (or a derivative of this
vesicle) into which the toxin is packed. A bolus of toxin
of sufficient size to rapidly inactivate all of the EF_2
within the cell appears to enter the cell in a concerted
process (Hudson and Neville, 1985).
In 1977 our laboratory posed the question whether binding of toxin A-chain to an alternate cell surface receptor
was sufficient for entry and transport to the cytosol compartment. We synthesized disulfide-linked conjugates of
human placental lactogen and diphtheria toxin A-chain.
These conjugates had no detectable activity when assayed
on mammary gland explants containing lactogenic receptors
(Chang et al., 1977). However, we demonstrated that when
toxin B-chains were included within the toxin conjugates,

target cells could specifically be reduced from mixed cell populations (Youle et al., 1979). The extent of reduction of target/non-target cells was approximately 3 logs. These findings were generalized to the case of monoclonal antibody toxin conjugates (Youle and Neville, 1980). Youle and co-workers (1981) attempted to separate the ricin B chain efficiency enhancing effect from B chain binding activity by site specific o-acetylation of the one or two tyrosine residues involved at the galactose binding site. Both activities were reduced and have yet to be separated. Subsequent work has indicated that conjugates made with toxin A-chains do have limited specific toxicity provided that there are sufficient number of receptors present on the target cells and that the number of occupied receptors is high (Cawley et al. 1980; Blythman et al., 1981; Esworthy and Neville, 1984). The variables present in these types of systems are illustrated in Figs. 1 and 2. In Fig. 1 (redrawn from Youle and Neville (1982) we see a dose response curve of the inhibition of protein synthesis by ricin A-chain (RTA), ricin and conjugates made with an antibody OX-7 and ricin A and ricin. Protein synthesis is measured at 24 hrs after addition of toxin to AKR cells which contain receptors for the Thy-1.1 antigen to which OX-7 is directed. There are about 600,000 of these determinants per cell.

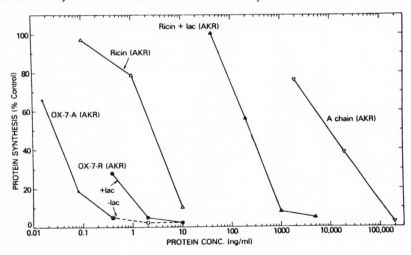

Fig. 1. The inhibition of protein synthesis of AKR cells by ricin A chain, ricin, and conjugates of ricin. + lac indicates the presence of 50 mM lactose during the 24 hr incubation.

Figure 1 shows a 10^5 difference in toxicity between the A-chain of ricin representing the non-target cell toxicity and the antibody A-chain conjugate OX-7-A. The enormous difference between the conjugate dose response curve and that of the A-chain alone is due to several features of the system. The OX-7 monoclonal antibody has an affinity of $10^{10} M^{-1}$. The t1/2 of dissociation of this antibody is in the neighborhood of 20 hrs, so that the antibody is essentially irreversibly bound for the conditions of this experiment. The cell density has been reduced in this experiment to 10^4 cell/ml. Under these conditions at 0.17 ng/ml of conjugate virtually all of the conjugate is bound to the cells, and on the average more than 90% of all the receptors are occupied. The medium is essentially depleted of conjugate. Thus the protein concentration axis represents an input concentration rather than a free ligand concentration. Occupancy of more than 90% of all the receptors present in the system is the requirement for the decreasing protein synthesis to 10% of control value in this system. Therefore, if the cell density is increased, larger amounts of conjugates must be added and the dose response curve will be shifted to the right.

Conjugates such as these have very little therapeutic effect when used in in vivo situations, in spite of the 10^5-fold separation between the non-target cell toxicity and the target cell toxicity shown in Fig. 1. However, in vertebrates the vascular systems allows cells to be bathed in a very low volume of extra-cellular fluid compared to our usual tissue culture systems. The corresponding cell density of vertebrates is in the order of 10^{10} cell/cc, six logs different from the experiment shown in Fig. 1. Therefore, when using a high affinity conjugate in vivo, the differential dose response curves (target vs non-target cell populations) are likely to be compressed compared to their tissue culture counterparts. The amount of compression will be determined by the total load of conjugates put into the system. The total load of conjugates required will be related to the number of target cells which one wishes to eliminate (Neville and Youle, 1982a). Obviously the rate of delivery of a conjugate and its removal by target cells will affect its concentration. This illustrates some of the complexities which arise when these reagents are used in vivo.

Data in Fig. 1 were acquired at the time of maximal action of the conjugates which is 24 hrs. In Fig. 2 the kinetics of intoxication over a 24 hr period of time when all receptors in the system are saturated is shown. One notes that after 24 hrs, cells exposed to OX-7-RTA begin to recover as cell growth continues. The A-chain conjugate of ricin is more effective than the A-chain conjugate of diphtheria toxin OX-7-DTA. When the B-chain of ricin is included in the conjugate along with lactose to block its toxicity towards non-target cells, the killing efficiency increases, and we estimate that a 3 log kill is easily achievable with this system at 24 hrs. However, these efficiencies are much less than the parent toxins (Esworthy and Neville, 1984).

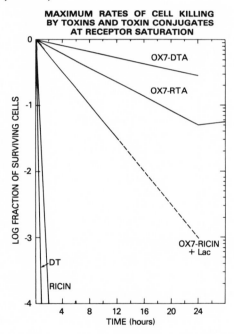

Fig. 2. The kinetics of toxin and conjugate action following the lag period at $\geq$ 90% receptor saturation. All data except diphtheria toxin, DT, is from AKR cells. DTA, conjugate with diphtheria toxin A chain. RTA, conjugate with ricin A chain. Dashed line is an extrapolation. Redrawn from Youle and Neville (1982a); Esworthy and Nevile (1984).

If one is attempting to eradicate a tumor load in an animal or human using antibody toxin conjugates, the log kill in 24 hrs must be equal to the log of the tumor burden (Neville and Youle, 1982a). The log kill of A-chain conjugates can be improved by adding agents to the media which either prevent the degradation of the conjugate or in some manner alter the routing of conjugates within intracellular vesicles, thus, ammonia and chloroquine have been found to double and triple the log kill of certain monoclonal antibody ricin A-chain conjugates (Casellas et al. 1984).

TABLE I

CONJUGATE OR TOXIN	CELL TYPE	K_I logs/hr	n	$\frac{K_I 5 \times 10^5}{n}$	CONC. 91% SAT $10 \times Kd$ (M)
hPL-DTA	mam. gland	<.005 [1]	~2x10⁴ [2]	<.1	10^{-8}
EGF-DTA	3T3	<.005 [1]	6x10⁴	<.04	10^{-8}
EGF-RTA	3T3	.04 [1]	6x10⁴	.3	10^{-8}
OX7-DTA	AKR	.02	6x10⁵	.02	10^{-9}
OX7-RTA	AKR	.07	6x10⁵	.06	10^{-9}
OX7-RTA+B	AKR	.3	6x10⁵	.25	10^{-9}
OX7-RICIN+lac	AKR	.3	6x10⁵	.25	5×10^{-9} [3]
OX7-DT	AKR	.1	6x10⁵	.08	10^{-9} [3]
RTA	L	.08	—	—	3×10^{-6} [3]
DTA	L	.05	—	—	2×10^{-5}
DT	L	.2	— [4]	—	5×10^{-5}
DT	CV-1	4.0	2x10⁵ [5]	10.	10^{-8} [5]
RICIN	AKR	6.7	7.5x 10⁵	4.5	10^{-6}

K_I = 1st order inactivation rate constant of protein synthesis
n = number of receptors per cell for conjugate or toxin

The type of data shown in Fig. 2 is summarized in Table I (reprinted from Esworthy and Neville, 1984) where the entry efficiency of various toxin conjugate toxins and toxin A chains are compared. The slopes K_I are the slopes taken at 90% or greater of receptor saturation and are first order rate constants of protein synthesis   inactivation and are listed in units of hr^{-1}. Since the number of occupied receptors is an important variable we have normalized these rate constants per 10^5 occupied receptors in the next to furthest right-hand column. Again one sees that the efficiencies of the parent toxins, ricin and diphtheria toxin, are approximately 30-fold higher than our best conjugates and these differences translate into exponential differences when computing log survivors.

Currently our most effective conjugates are ricin conjugates linked to monoclonal antibodies via a thioether bond. A maleimide residue is added to ricin via an N-hydroxysuccinimide ester reactive towards the amino groups of ricin. Sulfhydryl groups are exposed on the antibody by a brief reduction with DTT. The two are mixed together and the thioether conjugate is formed within 30 min (Youle and Neville, 1980; Neville and Youle, 1980). This structure then has two binding specificities, one directed at all cells which contain ricin receptors which consist of branched galactose and N-acetylgalactosamine residues present on all vertabrate cells.

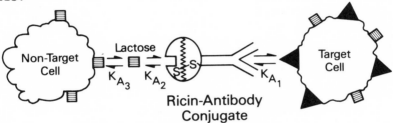

Fig. 3. Schematic representation of a monoclonal antibody thioether conjugate made with intact ricin and utilizing lactose to reduce non-target cell toxicity due to the affinity, KA_3 of ricin for its galactose containing receptors present on all vertebrate cells.

The affinity of ricin for these receptors is about $10^7 M^{-1}$. The sugar lactose will bind to ricin with affinity of approximately $10^3 M^{-1}$ and 100 mM lactose produces approximately 100-fold shift in the dose response curve of ricin as shown in Fig. 1. We therefore use ricin conjugates in the presence of 100 mM lactose to reduce the non-target cell toxicity. This scheme is illustrated in Fig. 3. This methodology is not tenable in <u>in vivo</u> situations where it is very difficult to raise lactose concentrations much higher than 20 mM for brief periods of time. Moreover, the ratio of non-target cells to target cells <u>in vivo</u> is likely to range between 10^3 to 10^6 and even a very small degree of binding of the conjugate to non-target cells will be increased by the above factors when the entire non-target cell population is considered.

Conjugates or immunotoxins patterned after the illustration in Fig. 3 are useful reagents in in vitro systems for eliminating unwanted cell populations from a mixture of cells. Currently, conjugates of this type synthesized in our laboratory (Neville and Youle, 1982b) are being evaluated at the University of Minnesota, as an adjunct to human bone marrow transplantation (Filipovich et al., 1984a). Bone marrow transplantation is a therapeutic regimen used to treat leukemia, aplastic anemia or other immunodefficiency syndromes. It also has potential as a treatment for morbid autoimmune diseases. Bone marrow transplantation is performed by ablating the host's diseased marrow with a combination of radiation and cytotoxic drugs, and injecting a new donor marrow which can reconstitute a near normal hemeapoetic and immune system. The major problem in bone marrow transplantation is that the new bone marrow graft reacts against the host if it considers the host to be non-self. This disease known as graft-versus-host disease, GVHD, is severely debilitating and has a high mortality rate. It occurs because the marrow transplant from the donor contains T cells which contain the memory of self and non-self (Storb and Thomas, 1983; Korngold and Sprent, 1983).

Using a cocktail of an equal mixture of three different immunotoxins directed at three different human T cell surface membrane determinants, the reduction of T cell responses are shown in Fig. 4 on the left-hand verticle axis as a function of dose (redrawn from Vallera et al., 1983). The inhibition of T cell response is also compared to the inhibition of the stem cell growth by clonogenic assays and the stem cell inhibition is seen to be minimal. Stem cells are the cells which will repopulate the bone marrow in the host. Between 600 and 1000 ng/ml of immunotoxins, a three log inhibition of T cell response is achieved without significant inhibition of stem cells. When one of the immunotoxins is substituted for the mixture at the same total concentration the inhibition of T cell responses is approximately 1 log less (Vallera et al., 1983). This probably occurs because in the range of 100 to 300 ng/ml of each of the conjugates receptor saturation is occurring. Therefore, with an equal part mixture of 100 ng/ml there are more total receptors occupied than at 300 ng/ml of the single component. In addition, it is possible that there are T cell subsets which contain only one of the three determinants (Vallera et al., 1983).

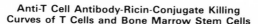

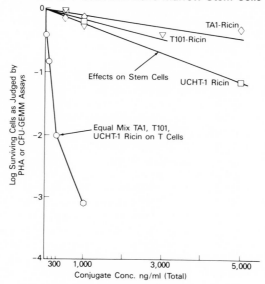

Fig. 4. The effect of a 2 hr exposure at 37° of anti–human T cell monoclonal antibody–ricin conjugates in the presence of 100 mM lactose on human T cell survival and human bone marrow stem cell survival (Vallera et al., 1983).

At the University of Minnesota, to date, sixteen patients with leukemia receiving transplants from HLA matched siblings have been treated using immunotoxin therapy. The donor marrow following isolation has been treated with the immunotoxin cocktail shown in Fig. 4, in doses between 300 and 900 ng/ml before washing and infusing into the recipient (Filipovich et al., 1984a and b). Engraftment has been prompt in all cases and the procedure appears quite safe. In the preliminary data a trend is seen in that no severe cases of GVHD have been observed in a group where 4 to 6 such cases might have been expected. Mild GVHD has been observed so that all T cells have not been eliminated as one would expect from analyzing Fig. 4 data. (About 10^8 nucleated cells per kg, patient weight are administrated during bone marrow transplantation and about 25% of these are T cells unless T cell depletion methodology is performed [Filipovich et al., 1984a]).

The type of study cited above is in its infancy. Only recently has it been possible to perform bone marrow transplants with elimination of specific subsets of donor cells. The biology of this system is not well understood. Radiation resistant cells in the recipient can cause graft rejection in animals (Von Melchner and Bartlett, 1983). Certain donor T cells subsets may be required for engraftment when radiation is less than totally ablative (Vallera et al., 1982). Other or the same donor T cell subsets may participate in a useful graft-versus-leukemia reaction eliminating leukemic cells surviving the ablative procedure (Storb and Thomas, 1983). Many T cell antigens residing on various subsets can be utilized for immunotoxins. As we develop more efficient immunotoxins, receptors common to subsets occurring at low density, i.e., less than 10^4 per cell could be effectively utilized. Immunotoxins are now and will continue to be an important tool for exploring the biology of bone marrow transplant systems.

Monoclonal antibodies toxin conjugates or immunotoxins are a new class of pharmacologic reagents with unique potential. Currently they have in vitro utility. More research is required to achieve reagents which will also function effectively in vivo. These reagents have been dubbed "magic bullets" by some but they are not. They are reagents which combine the physical and chemical attributes of both monoclonal antibodies and their parent toxins. They operate according to physical chemical principles and we have a fair degree of understanding of their actions in these terms especially in the in vitro system. In vivo systems require more basic knowledge of toxin transport processes and detailed pharmacokinetic studies which consider all of the various compartments involved.

REFERENCES

Arnon, R. and Sela, M., In vitro and in vivo efficacy of conjugates of daunomycin with anti-tumor antibodies. Immunol. Rev., 62 (1982) 5-27.

Bernstein, I. D., Tam, M. R., and Nowinski, R. C., Mouse leukemia: Therapy with monoclonal antibodies against a thymus differentiation antigen. Science, 207 (1980) 68-71.

Blythman, H. E., Casellas, P., Gros, O., Gros, P., Jansen, F. K., Paolucci, F., Pau, B., and Vidal, H., Immunotoxins: Hybrid molecules of monoclonal antibodies and a toxin subunit specifically kill tumour cells. Nature, 290 (1981) 145–146.

Casellas, P., Bourrie, B. J. P., Gros, P., and Jansen, F. K., Kinetics of cytotoxicity induced by immunotoxins. J. Biol. Chem., 259 (1984) 9359–9364.

Cawley, D. B., Hershman, H. R., Gilliland, D. G., and Collier, R. J., Epidermal growth factor-toxin A chain conjugates: EGF-ricin A is a potent toxin while EGF-diphtheria fragment A is nontoxic. Cell, 22 (1980) 563–570.

Chang, T. M., Dazord, A., and Neville, D. M., Jr., Artificial hybrid protein containing a toxic protein fragment and a cell membrane receptor-binding moiety in a disulfide conjugate. II. Biochemical and biological properties of diphtheria toxin fragment A-S-S-human placental lactogen. J. Biol. Chem., 252 (1977) 1515–1522.

Esworthy, R. S. and Neville, D. M., Jr., A comparative study of ricin and diphtheria toxin-antibody-conjugate kinetics of protein synthesis inactivation. J. Biol. Chem., 259 (1984) 11496–11504.

Filipovich, A. H., Vallera, D. A., Youle, R. J., Quinonas, R. R., Neville, D. M., Jr., and Kersey, J. H., Ex-vivo treatment of donor bone marrow with anti-T cell immunotoxins for the prevention of graft-versus-host disease. The Lancet (1984a) 469–472.

Filipovich, A. H., Vallera, D. A., Youle, R. J., Neville, D. M., Jr., and Kersey, J. H., Ex vivo T cell depletion with immunotoxins in allogeneic bone marrow transplantation: The pilot clinical study for prevention of graft-versus-host disease. Transplantation Proc., (1984b) (in press).

Galfrè, G. and Milstein, C., Preparation of monoclonal antibodies: Strategies and procedures. Meth. Enz., 73 (1981) 1–46.

Glennie, M. J. and Stevenson, G. T., Univalent antibodies kill tumor cells in vitro and in vivo. Nature, 295 (1982) 712–714.

Gurney, M. E., Belton, A. C., Cashman, N., and Antel, J. P., Inhibition of terminal axonal sprouting by serum from patients with amyotrophic lateral sclerosis. New Eng. J. Med., 311 (1984) 933–939.

Haskell, C. M., Buchegger, F., Schreyer, M., Carrel, S.,
    and Mach, J.-P., In vitro screening of new monoclonal
    anti-carcinoembryonic antigen antibodies for radio-
    imaging human colorectal carcinomas. In Boss, B. D.,
    Langman, R., Trowbridge, I., and Dulbecco, R. (Eds)
    Monoclonal Antibodies and Cancer, Academic Press,
    1983, pp. 275-283.
Houston, L. L., Nowinski, R. C., and Bernstein, I. D.,
    Specific in vivo localization of monoclonal antibodies
    directed against the Thy 1.1 antigen. J. Immunol. 125
    (1980) 837-843.
Hudson, T. H. and Neville, D. M., Jr., Quantal entry of
    diphtheria toxin to the cytosol. J. Biol. Chem., 260
    (1985) in press.
Koprowski, H., Mouse monoclonal antibodies in vivo. In
    Boss, B. D., Langman, R., Trowbridge, I., and Dulbecco,
    R. (Eds) Monoclonal Antibodies and Cancer, Academic
    Press, 1983, pp. 17-38.
Korngold, R. and Sprent, J., Lethal GVHD across minor histo-
    compatibility barriers: Nature of the effector cells
    and role of the H-2 complex, Immunol. Rev. 71 (1983)
    5-29.
Levy, R., Miller, R. A., Stratte, P. T., Maloney, D. G.,
    Link, M. P., Meeker, T. C., Oseroff, A., Thielemans,
    K., and Warnke, R., Therapeutic trials of monoclonal
    antibody in leukemia and lymphoma: Biologic considera-
    tions. In Boss, B. D., Langman, R., Trowbridge, I.,
    and Dulbecco, R. (Eds) Monoclonal Antibodies and
    Cancer, Academic Press, 1983, pp. 5-16.
Mach, J. P., Chatal, J. F., Lumbroso, J. D., Buchegger, F.,
    Forni, M., Ritschard, J., Berche, C., Douillard, J. Y.,
    Carrel, S., and Herlyn, M., Tumor localization in
    patients by radiolabeled monoclonal antibodies against
    colon carcinoma. Cancer Res., 43 (1983) 5593-5600.
Mason, D. W. and Williams, A. F., The kinetics of antibody
    binding to membrane antigens in solution and at the
    cell surface. Biochem. J., 187 (1980) 1-20.
Neville, D. M., Jr. and Youle, R. J., Monoclonal antibody-
    ricin or ricin A chain hybrids. Kinetic analysis of
    cell killing for tumor therapy. Immunol. Rev., 62
    (1982a) 75-91.
Neville, D. M., Jr. and Youle, R. J., Monoclonal antibody-
    ricin hybrids as a treatment of animal graft-versus-
    host disease. U. S. Patent 4,440,747. (Related U. S.
    patents pending SN 399,257, SN 456,401) (1982b)

Neville, D. M., Jr., and Youle, R. J., Anti-Thy 1.2 monoclonal antibody hybrid utilized as a tumor suppressant. U.S. Patent 4,359,457 (1980)

Nisonoff, A. and Rivers, M. M., Recombination of a mixture of univalent antibody fragments of different specificity. Arch. Biochem. Biophys., 93 (1961) 460-467.

Pappenheimer, A. M., Jr., Diphtheria toxin. Ann. Rev. Biochem., 46 (1977) 69-94.

Roitt, I., Essential Immunology, 4th Ed., Blackwell Scientific Publications, Oxford, 1980.

Storb, R. and Thomas, E. D., Allogeneic bone-marrow transplantation. Immunol. Rev. 71 (1983) 77-102.

Trowbridge, I. S., Lesley, J., and Schulte, R., Murine cell surface transferrin receptor: Studies with an anti-receptor monoclonal antibody. J. Cell Physiol., 112 (1982) 403-410.

Vallera, D. A., Ash, R. C., Zanjani, E. D., Kersey, J. H., LeBien, T. W., Beverly, P. C. L., Neville, D. M., Jr., and Youle, R. J., Anti-T-cell reagents for human bone marrow transplantation: Ricin linked to three monoclonal antibodies. Science, 222 (1983) 512-515.

Vallera, D. A., Soderling, C. C., Carlson, G. J., and Kersey, J. H., Bone marrow transplantation across major histocompatibility barriers in mice. II. T cell requirement for engraftment in total lymphoid irradiation-conditioned recipients. Transplantation 33 (1982) 243-248.

Von Melchner, H. and Bartlett, P. F., Mechanisms of early allogeneic marrow graft rejection, Immunol. Rev. 71 (1983) 31-56.

Wellman, H. N. and Anger, R. T., Jr., Radioiodine dosimetry and the use of radioiodines other than ^{131}I in thyroid diagnosis. Sem. in Nuc. Med., 1 (1971) 356-378.

Williams, A. F. and Gagnon, J., Neuronal cell Thy-1 glycoproteins and homology with immunoglobulin. Science, 216 (1982) 696-703.

Youle, R. J., Murray, G. J., and Neville, D. M., Jr., Studies on the galactose-binding site of ricin and the hybrid toxin Man6P-ricin. Cell, 23 (1981) 551-559.

Youle, R. J., Murray, G. J., and Neville, D. M., Jr., Ricin linked to phosphomannan binds to fibroblast lysosomal hydrolase receptors resulting in a cell type specific toxin. Proc. Natl. Acad. Sci. USA, 76 (1979) 5559-5562.

Youle, R. J. and Neville, D. M., Jr., Kinetic of protein
    synthesis inactivation by ricin-anti Thy 1.1 monoclonal
    antibody hybrids: Role of the ricin B subunit demon-
    strated by reconstitution. J. Biol. Chem., 257 (1982)
    1598-1601.
Youle, R. J. and Neville, D. M., Jr., Anti-Thy 1.2 mono-
    clonal antibody linked to ricin is a potent cell-type-
    specific toxin. Proc. Natl. Acad. Sci. USA, 77 (1980)
    5483-5486.

DRUG DELIVERY VIA CELL-SURFACE RECEPTORS

T. Y. Shen

Merck Sharp & Dohme Research Laboratories

Rahway, New Jersey   07065

Cell-surface receptors are noted for their high degree of specificity in their interactions with appropriate ligands. In receptor mediated drug delivery the drug is attached to or associated with a ligand which recognizes a specific receptor on the surface of a target cell. The ligand can be a component of a phospholipid vesicle, e.g. liposome, a lipoprotein particle or a chemical derivative of a macromolecule, small peptide or oligosaccharide (Fig. 1). After ingestion the active free drug is liberated by intracellular enzymes to exert its pharmacological effect.

For example the well defined cell surface lipoprotein receptors may be used as a potential target-specific entrance. The interaction of low density lipoprotein (LDL) with its membrane receptor and its subsequent metabolism have been well characterized (Goldstein & Brown, 1977, Mahley & Innerarity, 1983). On the surface of many cell types there are approximately 50-100,000 LDL receptors per cell with molecular weight in the range of 100-160,000. The receptor recognizes two lipoproteins, Apoprotein B and Apoprotein E, each composed of approximately 300 amino acids. Apparently several lysine and arginine residues are critical for receptor binding. LDL has an inner lipid core containing cholesterol and esters, triglycerides and phospholipids with Apoprotein B on the outside for recognition by the receptor (Table 1). The cholesterol esters can be removed by solvent extraction and replaced by other lipophilic molecules or

Receptor Specific Ligands

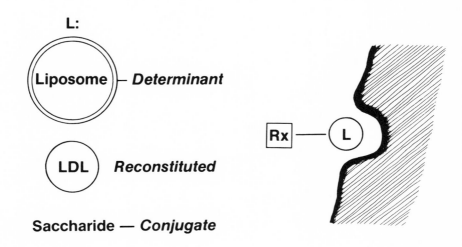

FIG. 1. A schematic representation of targeted drug delivery via cell surface receptors. L, carrier with receptor-specific ligands, R_x, drug or biologically active substance, e.g., enzyme, DNA or biochemical markers.

drug derivatives to form a reconstituted LDL (r-LDL) which can still be recognized by the LDL receptor and internalized into lysosomes (Krieger, et al., 1978a).

The effectiveness of such a Trojan horse approach was demonstrated by the selective cytotoxicity of r-LDL containing 25-hydroxy cholesterol (Krieger, et al., 1978b), which is a cholesterol synthesis inhibitor, or the photosensitizer pyrene (Mosley, et al., 1981). In the latter case, only cells having LDL-receptors to take in r-LDL are killed upon irradiation. A recent study further demonstrated that oleoyl cholesterol is a good anchor for

LOW DENSITY LIPOPROTEINS (LDL)

DIAMETER	215 $\overset{\circ}{A}$
MOL. WT.	2.5 $\times$ 10^6

COMPOSITION (moles)

APOPROTEIN B	60
CHOLESTEROL	540
CHOLESTEROL ESTERS	1400
TRIGLYCERIDES	200
PHOSPHOLIPIDS	750

TABLE 1. The composition of low density lipoproteins (LDL).

keeping nitrogen mustards inside reconstituted LDL with minimal leakage in the serum. After cellular uptake, the nitrogen mustard is efficiently released to exert cytotoxicity with good selectivity against SV-589 cells versus normal human fibroblasts. The involvement of LDL receptor was confirmed by the lack of cytotoxicity when the conjugates were incorporated into methylated LDL which is not accepted by the LDL receptor (Firestone, et al., 1984).

It should be pointed out that the therapeutic advantage of this approach depends much upon a quantitative difference in the density of LDL receptor in different tissues. Abnormal cells like some leukemic cells may contain highly elevated numbers of LDL receptors. On the other hand, the adrenal gland, with its high density of LDL receptor, is of special concern. It is also of interest to note that the intracellular pathway of LDL is, with minor variations, a mechanism for the receptor mediated endocytosis of many polypeptide hormones, growth factors and plasma proteins (Mahley & Innerarity, 1983). The peptide region involved in their receptor interactions might also be receptor specific ligands.

Another approach is to use cell-surface saccharide receptors as a means of drug delivery. It is well known that membrane polysaccharides or glycoproteins on the surface of many cells, such as macrophages, play important roles in cellular functions. They also serve as cell surface determinants involved in cellular interactions. Furthermore, in the coated-pit region of the cell surface, there are receptors which recognize and internalize glycoproteins with specific carbohydrates determinants. The specificity of these saccharide receptors is illustrated by the D-galactose binding site on the surface of hepatocytes and by the receptor on Kupffer cells and macrophages which recognize D-mannose or L-fucose and, to a lesser extent, N-acetyl-D-glucosamine. As with many other receptors, the saccharide receptors are multivalent. For example, the well known hepatic receptor has higher affinity for a cluster of galactose terminals. Using a group of synthetic lactosyl peptides which have very high affinity for the hepatic lectin, the probable geometry of the binding site was delineated recently (Lee, et al., 1984). A triangular cluster of galactose terminals attached to flexible backbones with interdistances of 15, 22 and 25Å appears to be optimal for binding. The minimal structural requirement for receptor binding and endocytosis by the mannose receptor of macrophages and Kupffer cells was also defined as an oligosaccharide unit (Fig. 2).

Both the galactose and mannose determinants have been investigated in several drug delivery experiments, either with liposomes or with chemical conjugates. We have used a group of synthetic glycolipids, consisting of saccharides attached through a C6 spacer arm to the 3-hydroxy group in cholesterol, to prepare liposomes with

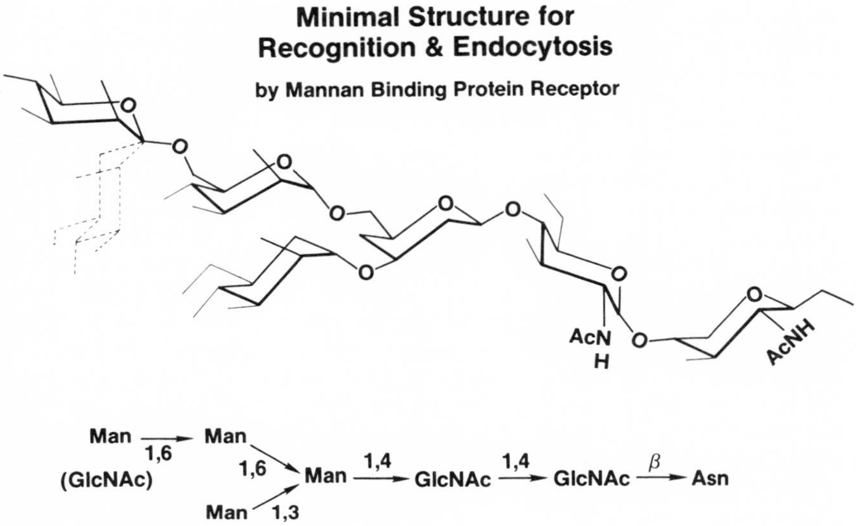

Minimal Structure for
Recognition & Endocytosis

by Mannan Binding Protein Receptor

FIG. 2. Proposed minimal structure of oligosaccharide for the recognition and endocytosis by the mannan receptor of macrophages.

specific saccharide determinants on the surface (Ponpipom, et al., 1980). A variety of mono- and disaccharide determinants can be introduced this way. Instead of cholesterol, other lipophilic groups, e.g. diglycerides or ceramide, have also been used to anchor the carbohydrate groups in the liposome bilayer. But liposomes prepared from cholesterol glycoconjugates appear to be more stable than ceramide liposomes in vivo (Wu, et al., 1982).

The head group interactions and membrane properties of liposomes containing the naturally occurring glyceroglycolipids with glucose or galactose terminals were investigated in detail (Iwamoto, et al., 1982). The interaction between neighboring disaccharide head groups is structure specific, much influenced by the stereo configuration of the hydroxyl groups, and may be stronger than the interaction among phosphatidyl choline head groups As a result, the phase transition temperatures of the glycolipid liposomes are increased by 11-15°.

The selective delivery of liposomal contents to different cell types in the liver, as directed by the surface carbohydrates, was clearly demonstrated in an improved delivery of plasmid DNA (Soriano, et al., 1983, Nicolau, et al., 1984). Hepatocytes are secretory cells which contain enzymes required for the expression of liposome transported preproinsulin gene I. After i.v. injection of the genetic material incorporated in ordinary liposomes, plasmid DNA was mainly taken up by the phagocytic Kupffer cells in the liver. When lactosylceramide was incorporated into the liposome membrane to provide surface galactose terminals, very significant increases of plasmid DNA in hepatocytes and endothelial cells, which possess galactose receptors, were observed. Because of their relative tissue abundance, nearly 20% of total plasmid were delivered to hepatocytes (Table 2). In a similar manner, using α-globulin as a marker, the uptake of liposomes by liver cells was shown to be influenced by the surface carbohydrates of the liposome (Ghosh, et al., 1982, Latif & Bachhawat, 1984). Asialoganglioside or galactose determinants favor the uptake by hepatocytes, whereas α-mannose determinants enhance the uptake by non-parenchymal cells.

For pharmaceutical applications, certain practical limitations of liposomes remain to be resolved. Seeking an alternative to liposomes, we have also explored the feasibility of using chemical conjugates of carbohydrate ligands for drug targeting (Robbins, et al., 1981). A group of synthetic ligands consisting of mannose thioglycoside attached through a propionyl group to the ε-amino groups in lysine, lysyl-lysine and trilysine were synthesized by a general procedure (Fig. 3). These conjugates competitively block the binding and uptake of labeled mannosyl-BSA by macrophages. The inhibitory potency increases with increasing number of mannose terminals. The trivalent ligand, Man_3Lys_2, with $K_i = 4$ μM, is approximately 200 times more potent than simple mannosides. The chirality of the lysine peptide backbone is not important. The K_i values of both L and

Uptake of Liposome Plasmid DNA

Cell Type	PL Liposome Plasmid/cell	Lac Cer Liposome Plasmid/cell	Lac Cer Liposome Plasmid %
Kupffer	12	16	31
Hepatocyte	<0.2	1	19
Endothelial	<0.2	8	50

Soriano et al, '83

TABLE 2. The influence of liposome surface determinants on the distribution of plasmid DNA in different hepatic cells.

D isomers are about the same but the binding is decreased by the presence of a basic amidine group in the spacer arm. The carbohydrate specificity of the macrophage receptor is clearly demonstrated by its low affinity for the corresponding D–galactose analog, Gal_3Lys_2. The L–fucose analog, Fuc_3Lys_2, is only moderately active. These observations are in accordance with the specific binding of glycoproteins to alveolar macrophages.

The affinity of the synthetic ligand for the macrophage receptor is, fortunately, not much reduced by the attachment of other groups such as an aminohexyl side–chain, the trisaccharide raffinose, and the Bolton–Hunter reagent (p–hydroxy–phenylpropionyl group) which is suitable for iodination. With an iodine[125] labeled Bolton–Hunter derivative, we obtained a

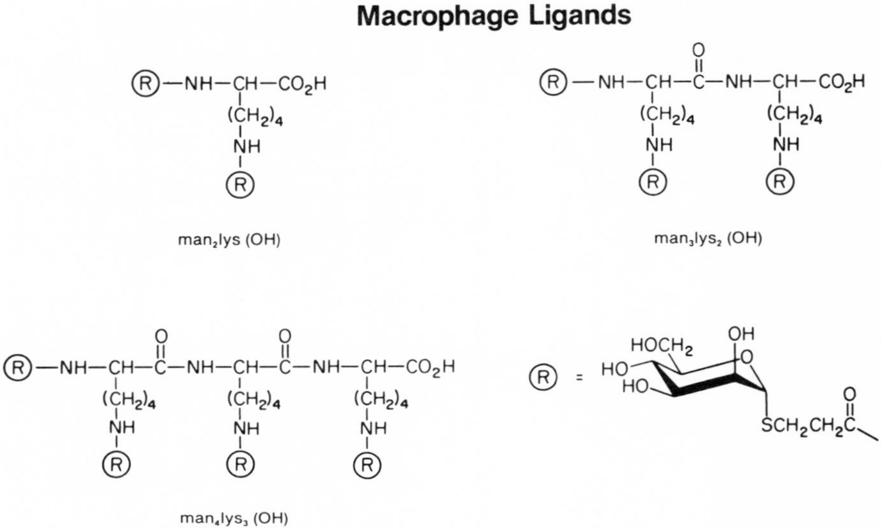

Macrophage Ligands

man$_2$lys (OH)

man$_3$lys$_2$ (OH)

man$_4$lys$_3$ (OH)

FIG. 3. Chemical structures of synthetic macrophage ligands with 2–4 mannose determinants.

dissociation constant K_D of 2.7 µM for this ligand and estimated a maximal binding of 5.2×10^5 molecules per cell at $0°C$. This number of receptors per cell is very similar to that for LDL receptors. All of the labeled ligand bound specifically at $0°$ could be removed by EDTA, thus indicating its surface location. At room temperature, receptor binding is followed by internalization and no longer releasable. By carrying out the uptake experiment at $21°$ we could estimate the Michaelis-Menten constant K_m of uptake to be 5.6 µM and a maximum velocity (V_{max}) of 1.7×10^5 molecules per minute per cell. That means the rate of entry of the ligand conjugate into macrophage is roughly one molecule per receptor every three minutes, again very similar to the estimated $t_{1/2}$ of 5 minutes for the uptake of LDL (Table 3).

Mannose Receptor Mediated Endocytosis by Macrophages

Recognition: multiple non - reducing (Man - R)$_n$

Binding: 6×10^5 mol / cell, $0°C$

   Kd $2 \mu M$

Internalization: 1.7×10^5 mol / min / cell

   Km $6 \mu M$

TABLE   3.   Characteristics   of   the   macrophage   ligand Man$_3$Lys$_2$.

The Man$_3$Lys$_2$ ligand was also labeled by reductive amination with ^{3}H–raffinose to give a conjugate which does not readily diffuse from lysosomes and whose label should remain in lysosomes after hydrolysis to sucrose. Activated mouse peritoneal macrophage in culture took up this ligand much faster and to a much greater extent than they took up ^{3}H–raffinose itself. The blockade of this uptake by mannan again confirmed that it is a receptor–mediated process. The in vivo targeting of this ligand was demonstrated by the uptake of ^{125}I–labeled Man$_3$Lys$_2$–Bolton Hunter derivative by the liver in rats. The uptake is inhibited by coinjection with unlabeled Man$_3$Lys$_2$ but not by Gal$_3$Lys$_2$.

To explore the possibility of using the mannan receptor for targeted delivery of biologically active substances, the Man$_3$Lys$_2$ ligand was first coupled to

corticosteroids and other drugs. The affinity of several
dexamethasone derivatives (Fig. 4) for the mannan-receptor
are nearly identical, but the rate of release of free
dexamethasone in vitro and in vivo varies according to the
linkage. As expected, the stability of linkage increases
from ester to carbonate and carbamate. The Man$_3$Lys$_2$
ligand was also attached to the polysaccharide antigen of
the meningococcus group C bacteria in an attempt to
increase its uptake by macrophage for antigen processing.
It is remarkable that the macromolecular polysaccharide
conjugate, but not the antigen itself, is still readily
recognized by the macrophage receptor.

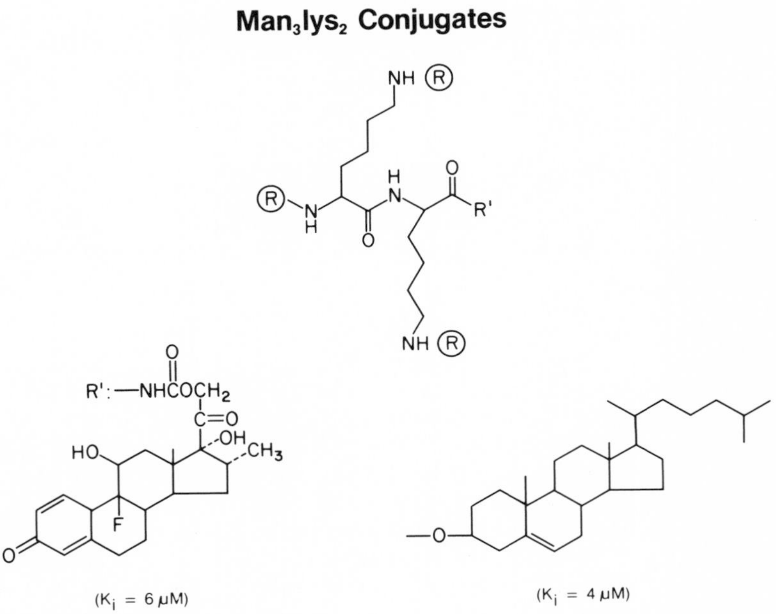

Man$_3$lys$_2$ Conjugates

FIG. 4. Chemical structures of dexamethasone and
cholesterol conjugates of the macrophage ligand
Man$_3$Lys$_2$.

Furthermore, we have explored the possible application of Man_3Lys_2 in enzyme replacement therapy. Gaucher's disease is a genetic disorder due to a deficiency of β-gluco-cerebrosidase in the Kupffer cells of the patient. The polysaccharide portion of this enzyme carries galactose terminals. As a consequence, intravenous administration of exogenous native enzyme to the patient resulted in the delivery of the enzyme mainly to the hepatocytes and less to the Kupffer cells. It would seem that attachment of our mannose ligand should in theory increase the distribution to the Kupffer cells which have mannose receptors (Fig. 5). For this purpose a partially purified human placental enzyme supplied by Dr. Brady's group at NIH was coupled with the Man_3Lys_2 ligand (Doebber, et al., 1982). The modified enzyme contains approximately 8 to 9 molecules of ligand per enzyme subunit and retains its enzymatic characteristics

ENZYME REPLACEMENT THERAPY
(GAUCHER'S)

Delivery of Glucocerebrosidase

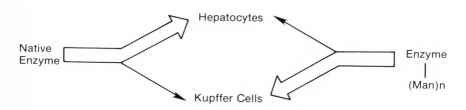

FIG. 5. A scheme to divert the delivery of glucocerebrosidase from hepatocytes to Kupffer cells in the liver by the attachment of mannose ligands.

(Fig. 6). In the macrophage culture the uptake of the enzyme is indeed faster and to a greater extent than the native enzyme. At an enzyme concentration of 0.7 µM, alveolar macrophages in vitro endocytose an amount of Man₃Lys₂-β -glucocerebrosidase equal to more than 11 times their endogenous β-glucosidase level after one hour. The modified enzyme also appears to be reasonably stable inside the macrophage to maintain activity for several hours in vitro. In the rat it is cleared more rapidly than the native enzyme from circulation. The clearance of the modified enzyme, but not the native enzyme, can be dramatically inhibited by coinfusion with mannan. An analysis of enzyme distribution in isolated liver cells indicates an 18-fold increase in enzyme specific activity in non-parenchymal cells and only 1.5 fold for hepatocytes compared to uninjected control animals. This again showed that the mannan receptors are mainly responsible for the enzyme uptake. Such an

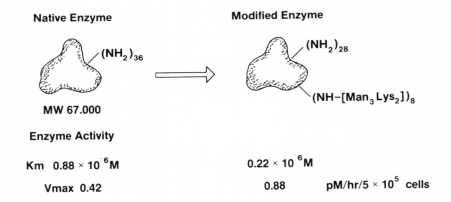

FIG. 6. Properties of chemically modified gluco-cerebrosidase.

increase in non-parenchymal cells is more than 1/3 of the increase obtainable after injection of partially deglycosylated glucocerebrosidase. Further optimization of enzyme-modification may result in a higher uptake form for therapeutic trials (Murray, et al., in press).

In conclusion, preliminary biochemical results have demonstrated the methodology and feasibility of receptor mediated selective drug delivery. The selective delivery of cytotoxic agents by reconstituted low density lipoproteins, plasmid DNA by saccharide-liposomes and glucocerebrosidase by mannose-conjugates are encouraging examples. Conceptually, other receptor ligands, e.g., peptides and hormones etc. may also be used in a similar manner to deliver drugs to different target cells. For practical applications, this approach to drug-targeting is still at its infancy. Critical in vivo parameters such as pharmacodynamics of each preparation, the rate of release of the active drug from the ligand, and efficacy in appropriate animal models must be optimized in specific cases. The full potential of such receptor-mediated drug-targeting remains to be explored.

ACKNOWLEDGEMENT

The author wishes to thank Mrs. Marita J. Herman for her valuable assistance in the preparation of this manuscript.

REFERENCES

Doebber, T.W., Wu, M.S., Bugianesi, R.L., Ponpipom, M.M., Furbish, F.S., Barranger, J.A., Brady, R.O. and Shen, T.Y., Enhanced macrophage uptake of synthetically glycosylated human placental β-glucocerebrosidase. J. Biol. Chem., 257, (1982) 2193-2199.

Firestone, R.A., Pisano, J.M., Falck, J.R., McPhaul, M.M. & Krieger, M., Delivery of cyto-toxic compounds to cells by the LDL pathway. J Med. Chem., 27 (1984) 1037-1043.

Ghosh, P., Das, P.K., and Bachhawat, G.K., Targeting of liposomes towards different cell types of rat liver through the involvement of liposomal surface glycosides. Arch. of Biochem. and Biophysics, 213 (1982) 266-270.

Goldstein, J.L. and Brown, M.S., The low density lipo-protein pathway and its relation to atherosclerosis. Annu. Rev. Biochem., 46 (1977) 897-930.

Iwamoto, K., Sunamoto, J., Inoue, K., Endo, T. and Nojima, S., Importance of surface structure in liposomal membranes of glyceroglycolipids. Biochimica et Biophysica Acta, 691 (1982) 44-51.

Krieger, M., Goldstein, J.L. & Brown, M.S., Receptor-mediated uptake of low-density lipoprotein reconsitituted with 25-hydroxycholesteryl oleate suppresses 3-hydroxy-3-methylglutaryl-coenzyme-a reductase and inhibits growth of human fibroblasts. Proc. Natl. Acad. Sci. USA, 75 (1978) 5052-5056.

Krieger, M., Brown, M.S., Faust, J.R. & Goldstein, J.L., Replacement of endogenous cholesteryl esters of low densitylipoprotein with exogenous cholesteryl linoleate - reconsitution of a biologically active lipoprotein particle. J. Bio. Chem., 253 (1978) 4093-4101.

Latif, N. & Bachhawat, B.K., The effect of surface sugars on liposomes in immunopotentiation. Immuno. Letters, 8 (1984) 75-78.

Lee, R.T., Lin, P., and Lee, Y.C., New synthetic cluster ligands for galactose/N-acetylgalactosamine specific lectin of Mammalian liver. Biochem., 23, (1984) 4255-4261.

Mahley, R.W. and Innerarity, T.L., Lipoprotein receptors and cholesterol homeostasis. Biochimica et Biophysica, Acta., 737 (1983) 197-222.

Mosley, S.T., Goldstein, J.L., Brown, M.S., Falck, J.R. & Anderson, R.G., Targeted killing of cultured cells by receptor dependent photosensitization. Proc. Natl. Acad. Sci. USA, 78 (1981) 5717–5721.

Murray, G.J., Doebber, T.W., Wu, M.S., Bugianesi, R.L., Ponpipom, M.M., Shen, T.Y., Brady, R.O., & Barranger, J.A., Targeting of synthetically glycosylated human placental glucocerebrosidase. (In press)

Nicolau, C., Legrand, A., & Soriano, P., Liposomes for gene transfer and expression in vivo. Ctr. Biophys. Molec., CNRS, Ciba Foundation Symposia, No. 103, (1984) 254–264.

Pompipom, M.M., Bugianesi, R.L., and Shen, T.Y., Cell surface carbohydrates for targeting studies. Canadian J of Chem., 58, (1980) 214–220.

Robbins, J.C., Lam, M.H., Tripp, C.S., Bugianesi, R.L., Ponpipom, M.M. and Shen, T.Y., Synthetic glycopeptide substrates for receptor mediated endocytosis by macrophages. Proc. Natl. Acad. Sci. USA, 78 (1981) 7294–7298.

Soriano, P., Dijkstra, J., Legrand, A., Spanjer, H., Londos-Gagliardi, D., Roerdink, F., Scherphos, G. and Nicolau, C., Targeted and nontargeted liposomes for in vivo transfer to rat liver cells of plasmid containing the preproinsulin I gene. Proc. Natl. Acad. Sci. USA, 80 (1983) 7128–7131

Wu, P.S., Wu, H.M., Tin, G.W., Schuh, J.R., Croasmun, W.R., Baldeschwieler, J.D., Shen, T.Y., and Ponpipom, M.M., Stability of carbohydrate modified vesicles in vivo: Comparative effects of ceramide and cholesterol glycoconjugates. Proc. Natl. Acad. Sci. USA, 79, (1982) 5490–5493.

PRODRUGS: A CHEMICAL APPROACH TO TARGETED DRUG DELIVERY

Valentino J. Stella and Kenneth J. Himmelstein

University of Kansas and Interx Research Corp.

Lawrence, Kansas 66045

The term Prodrug is used to describe compounds which must undergo chemical transformation prior to exhibiting their pharmacologic or therapeutic action. The concept is not new since compounds such as acetylsalicylic acid (aspirin), as a prodrug of salicylic acid, and methenamine, as a prodrug of formaldehyde, were discovered in the late 19th century. The term "pro-drug or "pro-agent" was first used by Albert (1958) who suggested that this approach could be used to alter the properties of drugs, in a temporary manner, to increase their usefulness, and/or decrease associated toxicity.

The idea of preparing these bioreversible derivatives was applied by various investigators in both a foresighted as well as a serendipitious manner to solve a number of pharmaceutical problems. This chemical approach to the solving of various formulation and transport problems gained renewed interest soon after the publication of a review by Sinkula and Yalkowsky (1975) and a book edited by Higuchi and Stella (1975). Numerous research reports and and reviews (see Table 1) have been published on the subject. The reader is directed to these reviews for a comprehensive general discussion of the subject.

Before the question of prodrugs and drug targeting is discussed in detail, it is worthwhile to mention two points about prodrugs in relation to their traditional uses. First, since medicinal chemists are becoming more sensitive to the fact that optimal drug design must take into account

247

Table 1. A list of comprehensive review articles on
          prodrugs

Albert, 1973	Notari, 1981
Ariens, 1966	Roche, 1977
Ariens, 1971	Sinkula and Yalkowsky, 1975
Bodor, 1982	Sinkula, 1975
Bundgaard, 1982	Stella, 1973
Digenis and Swintosky, 1975	Stella, 1977
Harper, 1959	Stella and Himmelstein, 1980
Harper, 1962	Yalkowsky and Morozowich, 1980
Higuchi and Stella, 1975	

the physical/chemical form of the drug as it pertains to
stability, solubility, and other formulation factors, as
well as pharmacokinetic factors, such as the transport
properties of the drug, it is quite likely that the prodrug
approach to optimizing those properties will become an
integral part of basic drug design. As such, there is
likely to be fewer examples where prodrugs will have to be
used in a hindsighted manner to solve problems. Two recent
examples of the foresighted use of prodrugs are enalapril,
as a better orally absorbed prodrug of MK-422 (Ulm, 1983),
and sulindac as a more soluble, better absorbed and less GI
irritating prodrug of sulindac sulfide (Duggan, 1981;
Duggan et al., 1977; Shen and Winter, 1977). In the future
"drugs need to be designed with delivery components in
mind" (Higuchi, 1984). Prodrugs will be one tool available
for achieving this goal. Second, in this book various
means of achieving directed drug delivery, other than prodrugs, have been discussed. Many of these techniques can
only be effectively used with drugs with certain physical/
chemical properties. For example, the entrapment of a drug
in a microparticulate may require the drug to have one set
of properties whereas the optimal dermal delivery of that
same drug may require it to have completely different
properties. If the properties of a drug can be optimized,
either intrinsically or via prodrugs, then more drugs can
be accommodated into these newer delivery systems.

Future research in prodrugs will continue to provide
better examples of the traditional use of prodrugs, to show
it as a powerful tool to compliment the newer approaches to
optimal drug delivery, and finally to demonstrate the
technique as a relatively new approach to chemically based
targeted drug delivery. This last topic will be the
subject of the balance of this paper.

DRUG TARGETING VIA PRODRUGS

Even though the idea of targeting of drugs for specific organs, cell lines etc., was proposed as early as the turn of the century by Ehrlich when he suggested his "magic bullet" concept, and targeting is the goal of rational, basic drug design, it has rarely been success- fully achieved in a true foresighted manner. The use of prodrugs as a means of achieving targeting has also met with only marginal success. The lack of "break-through" progress in the area of prodrug based drug targeting can probably be traced to the flawed nature of many of the hypotheses proposed to achieve such targeting. If it is possible to identify the basis for those few successes and critically evaluate the causes of the many failures, it may be possible to be more rational and realistic, in the future, in the design of prodrugs for targeting.

Drug targeting has been defined as the selective delivery, relative to the rest of the body, of a therapeutic agent to its site of action. Note that this definition emphasizes the term <u>delivery</u>. During mathematical model testing of various hypotheses for achieving targeting via prodrugs, Stella and Himmelstein (1980, 1982) showed that at least three factors are necessary for targeting to be successful via prodrugs.

1. The prodrug must be readily transported to the target site and uptake must be reasonably rapid.

2. Once at the site, the prodrug must be selectively cleaved to the active drug relative to its conversion at other sites in the body.

3. The active drug, once selectively generated at the site must be somewhat retained by the tissue.

Perhaps, therefore, a better definition of targeting is the selective delivery and retention of a therapeutic agent to its site of action resulting in high target site, cell line, organ, etc. concentration of the therapeutic agent and a lowered drug burden to the rest of the body.

We have recently expanded our earlier mathematical model for testing various hypotheses for achieving drug targeting via prodrugs. This was necessary because the old model could not be used to test some of the hypotheses that had been proposed for macromolecular-drug conjugates acting as prodrugs, where targeting was proposed to occur via the selective binding of the prodrugs to particular cell surface determinants. The expanded model is illustrated in Fig. 1. This hybrid pharmacokinetic model is used here to assess some of the previously tested hypotheses as well as some of the newer ones.

Basically this model describes a system where a prodrug or a drug is inputed into a body volume (50L). In the case of drug input, the drug is carried to the target organ extracellular fluid (50 ml) at a perfusion rate of 10 ml/min (Q), and once in this fluid, it can partition into the intracellular volume (50 ml) via a clearance term, $Cl_{in, out}^{D}$. The drug is eliminated from the body with a clearance of 250 ml/min. This corresponds to a drug with a biological half-life of about 2 hr, and a distribution half-life to the target organ extracellular fluid of less than 5 min. $Cl_{in, out}^{D}$ was varied from 10 ml/min, to represent a drug that readily permeated from the

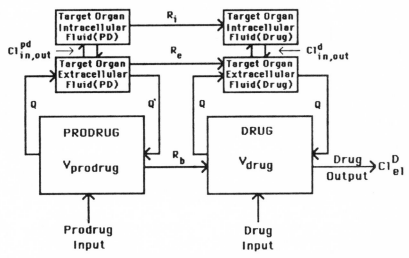

Fig. 1.   A hybrid pharmacokinetic model used for testing various hypotheses as to whether targeting can be achieved via prodrugs

extracellular fluid into the intracellular fluid, to 0.1
ml/min for a drug that had slow access to the intracellular
fluid. Even though we have assigned the two target organ
volumes as extra- and intracellular spaces, these spaces
could just as easy represent pharmacodynamically productive
versus non-productive volumes, or other subcellular units
or subdivisions of the overall target organ.

Prodrug input (350 mg, parent drug equivalent) is the
same as for the drug, except that the prodrug can undergo
biotransformation, via a Michaelis-Menten mechanism, in the
body (R_b), extracellular fluid (R_e), and/or the
intracellular fluid (R_i). Kms for these three possible
sites of metabolism were arbitrarily set at 10 mcg/ml and
the Vmaxs (Vmax, Vmax', Vmax" respectively) were varied so
that selective metabolism in either the target organ extra-
or intracellular space could be modelled. Vmax was fixed
at 10^4 mcg/min which gives a pseudo first order half-life
for prodrug conversion to drug in the body of about 35 min.
In this paper we will only be presenting simulations where
the prodrug is selectively cleaved in either the target
organ extra- or intracellular space 100 times faster than
in the body proper. Also varied for the prodrug was Q'.
Q' was generally set equal to Q except for an illustration
of the effect of extracellular binding on drug disposition
and targeting. This was mathematically effected by setting
Q' equal to 0.1 ml/min. All the simulations were performed
by setting up the appropriate mass balance equations and
solving them numerically by computer.

As stated earlier, various hypotheses have been
proposed for achieving targeting via prodrugs. One such
hypothesis is "I WILL ACHIEVE TARGETING BY DESIGNING A
PRODRUG THAT HAS BETTER ACCESSIBILITY TO THE TARGET SITE
THAN THE PARENT DRUG". This better accessibility may be
due to altered passive permeability to the site, or the
utilization of a carrier mediated transport mechanism to
gain better site delivery. This hypothesis is severely
flawed if the researcher does not take into account the
fact that the prodrug reaching the site must then be
capable of releasing the drug at the site for any advantage
to be achieved. For example, Shashoua et al. (1984)
recently studied the brain uptake of γ-aminobutyric acid
(GABA) in the form of various aliphatic and steroidal
esters of GABA. All the esters were taken up into the
brain substantially faster than GABA but only the

cholesteryl ester depressed the general motor activity of
mice and rats, presumably due to GABA release. The authors
concluded that the activity of the esters "was dependent on
their capacity to release GABA by enzymatic activity and
their lipid solubility". The higher lipid solubility of
the esters, compared to GABA itself, resulted in better
blood brain barrier permeability by the esters but only
those esters capable of undergoing brain cleavage to GABA
showed any activity. To illustrate this point quantitatively, Fig. 2 shows two plots, extra- and intracellular
target organ drug concentration versus time after input of
prodrug and drug to the body. The simulation is one where
the prodrug has a 100 fold faster access to the
intracellular space compared to the parent drug. Also in
this case, the prodrug was 100 fold more selectively
cleaved in the extracellular space compared to the rest of
the body i.e., Vmax' = 100 Vmax and no intracellular
cleavage occured (Vmax" = 0). The two plots show that
under these conditions the prodrug input resulted in only a
minimal improvement in drug delivery to either the intra-
or extracellular space relative to just drug input.

An alternative hypothesis for achieving targeting is
"SINCE THE LEVEL OF ENZYME X IN ORGAN Y IS HIGHLY ELEVATED
RELATIVE TO OTHER ORGANS IN THE BODY, WE WILL ACHIEVE
TARGETING BY DESIGNING PRODRUGS THAT UTILIZE THIS ENZYME X
FOR BIOREVERSION SO RESULTING IN THE SELECTIVE RELEASE OF
THE ACTIVE DRUG IN ORGAN Y". Again this appears to be an
attractive hypothesis. For example, Table 2 contains some
data from Double and Workman (1977) on the relative
distribution of acid and alkaline phosphatase levels in
tumors and livers of mice. It has been postulated that the
approximate 100 fold greater alkaline phosphatase activity
in the tumor cells could be used to effect targeting.
However, a prodrug that would be a substrate for alkaline
phosphatase i.e., a phosphate ester, is likely to have
difficulty penetrating into the target organ because of its
high polarity. Transport to the target organ or cell line
can be limited not only by permeability considerations but
also by perfusion limitations. For example in the above
case of tumor versus liver conversion of a phosphate
prodrug, the liver is a highly perfused tissue whereas
cells in a tumor are quite poorly perfused (Workman and
Double, 1978). Rapid conversion in the body of a prodrug
competing with target organ conversion can be seen in the
data of Orlowski et al. (1980) on the relative cleavability

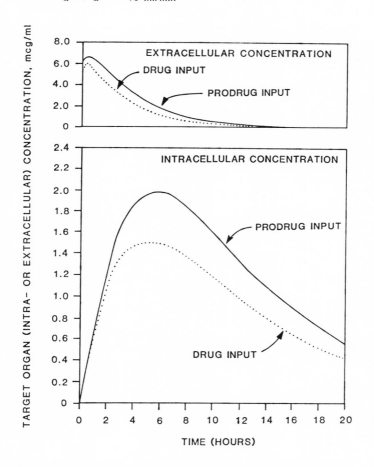

GOOD PRODRUG TRANSPORT (Cl $^{PD}_{IN,OUT}$ = 10 ml/min)

SELECTIVE EXTRACELLULAR CONVERSION

POOR PARENT DRUG TRANSPORT (Cl $^{D}_{IN, OUT}$ = 0.1 ml/min)

Q = Q' = 10 ml/min

Fig. 2.   A simulation demonstrating the need for
selective target site metabolism for
targeting to be achieved via prodrugs.

of L-γ-glutamyl-sulfamethoxazole and N-acetyl-L-γ-glutamyl-sulfamethoxazole shown in Table 3. As can be seen, both of these potential prodrugs of sulfamethoxazole, designed for the selective delivery of sulfamethoxazole to the kidney, are more susceptible to bioreversion in the mice kidney by L-γ-glutamyl-transpeptidase relative to other organs. However, only the N-acetyl prodrug resulted in better

Table 2. Enzyme-Specific Activities of Tumors and Corresponding Liver (Double and Workman, 1977)

	Specific Activity micromol/min/g protein	
	Acid Phosphatase	Alkaline Phosphatase
HT67 Tumor	41.3	207
CBA Liver	152	3.27
ADJ-PC6A Tumor	41	230
BALB/c Liver	125	1.86

Table 3. Rates of Release of Sulfamethoxazole from L-γ-Glutamyl-Sulfamethoxazole and N-Acetyl-L-γ-Glutamyl-Sulfamethoxazole by Homogenates of Various Mice Organs (Orlowski et al. 1980)

Organ	Sulfamethoxazole Release Rate nmol/mg protein/min	
	L-γ-Glutamyl-Sulfamethoxazole	N-Acetyl-L-γ-Glutamyl-Sulfamethoxazole
Kidney	71.5	0.46
Pancreas	10.4	0.001
S. Intestine	1.25	0.001
Liver	0.02	0.002
Spleen	0.126	0.001
Lung	0.094	0.001
Heart	0.005	0.001
Brain	0.25	0.05

kidney delivery of sulfamethoxazole when compared to the
administration of sulfamethoxazole itself. It was argued
that the L-γ-glutamyl prodrug was too rapidly cleaved
systemically to compete with kidney uptake and cleavage,
whereas the N-acetyl prodrug had better access to the
kidney tissue and deacetylation was required before the
L-γ-glutamyl transpeptidase could act on the prodrug.

If the drug has difficulty reaching the target organ
due to poor permeability characteristics and a prodrug can
be designed that has greater permeability to the site while
also being capable of undergoing non-selective cleavage to
the drug at the target site, significant impovement in drug
delivery can be achieved. For example Bodor et al. (1975,
1976, 1983), and Shek et al. (1976a, 1976b) have shown that
the delivery of the quarternary aromatic ammonium drugs,
2-PAM and berberine to the brain is very significantly
improved when they are administered as their dihydro
prodrugs. These prodrugs, being uncharged at physiological
pH, are able to passively permeate the blood brain barrier,
pass into the brain, where they are oxidized to their
parent drugs. Similarly, dopamine is incapable of passing
across gastrointestinal (GI) mucosal cells and through the
blood brain barrier. Transport of dopamine into systemic
circulation and into the CNS was improved by the
administration of L-DOPA as a prodrug of dopamine. L-DOPA
is actually more polar than dopamine but it is capable of
being actively transported from the GI tract and across the
blood brain barrier by the carrier mechanism responsible
for the transport of aromatic L-amino acids (Shindo et al.,
1977). L-DOPA is metabolized in the CNS by L-DOPA
decarboxylase to release dopamine. Since the decarboxylase
enzyme is not only found in the CNS but also in the rest of
the body, considerable systemic dopamine is also produced,
resulting in some systemic side effects. These side
effects could be reduced by the co-administration of a
L-DOPA decarboxylase inhibitor incapable of entering the
CNS. By selectively inhibiting systemic L-DOPA metabolism
to dopamine a significant degree of targeting for the CNS
can be achieved.

Increasing the polarity of an agent can be used to
help direct delivery to a specific site by limiting uptake
to other sites that require the drug to be non-polar. Two
specific examples of this possibility are prodrugs of
5-aminosalicylic acid (Goldman, 1982), sulphasalazine and

azodisal sodium (Jewel and Truelove, 1981), and some glycosidic prodrugs of two steroidal anti-inflammatory agents (Friend and Chang, 1984). These prodrugs are poorly absorbed from the GI tract after oral dosing because of their polarity but are metabolized to their active components in the colon by anaerobic bacteria. The released drugs are useful in the treatment of inflammatory bowel disease. If the active drugs themselves were administered orally, they undergo GI absorption such that little of the drug reaches the colon membrane where they can exert their maximal effect. Also their systemic absorption exposes the rest of the body to the drugs with their unwanted systemic side effects.

Researchers have focused on the importance of target site accessibility and the target site selective metabolism of prodrugs as important criteria for targeting. However there are numerous literature examples of where, even when these two factors were optimized, targeting was not achieved. Stella and Himmelstein (1980), as a result of some computer simulations, showed that a third factor was required before selective delivery could be achieved. The property of the parent drug had to be considered. Figure 3 is a plot of intracellular target organ drug concentration versus time for prodrug input compared to drug input for a prodrug that is rapidly transported to the target site, and is 100 fold more selectively metabolized at the target site relative to the rest of the body. The parent drug itself, however, has good accessibility to the target site (identical to the prodrug). As can be seen, prodrug input only marginally improves delivery relative to drug input. The problem here is that the drug liberated from the prodrug rapidly equilibrates with the rest of the body tissues after its enzymatic release. This result tends to suggest that the targeting of most currently useful therapeutic agents will not be successful via prodrugs. Since most researchers have tended to choose already known active drugs as model compounds for targeting studies this fact can probably account for a large number of failures seen in this field.

Figure 4 is a similar plot to that shown in Fig. 3, however, in this simulation the drug being targeted has poor target organ accessibility to begin with, whereas its prodrug has all the same characteristics as the prodrug shown in Fig. 3. Note the significant, both absolute and

GOOD PRODRUG TRANSPORT ($Cl^{PD}_{IN, OUT}$ = 10 ml/min)

SELECTIVE INTRACELLULAR CONVERSION

GOOD PARENT DRUG TRANSPORT ($Cl^{D}_{IN, OUT}$ = 10 ml/min)

$Q = Q' = 10$ ml/min

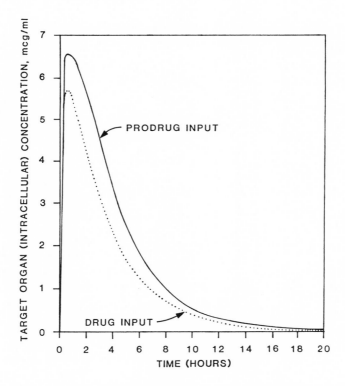

Fig. 3. A simulation demonstrating the importance
of target site retention of the parent
drug for targeting to be effected via
prodrugs. In this case the drug rapidly
equilibrates with the extracellular fluid
resulting in no targeting even when other
factors have been optimized. See Fig. 4
for a simulation where the drug is retained
by the site.

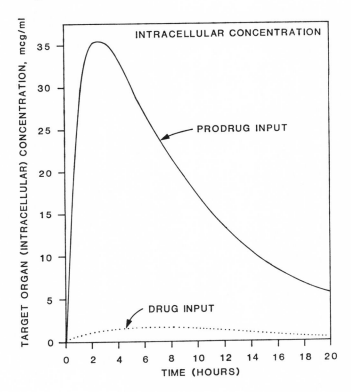

GOOD PRODRUG TRANSPORT (CI $^{PD}_{IN,\ OUT}$ = 10 ml/min)

SELECTIVE INTRACELLULAR CONVERSION

POOR PARENT DRUG TRANSPORT (CI $^{D}_{IN,OUT}$ = 0.1 ml/min)

Q = Q' = 10 ml/min

Fig. 4. A simulation demonstrating the importance of target site retention of the parent drug for targeting to be effected via prodrugs. See Fig. 3 for comparison.

relative, increase in target site delivery of drug brought about by not only optimizing prodrug transport to its selective metabolism at the site, but also by SITE RETENTION of the drug. It is interesting to note that such a drug i.e., one with poor site accessibility, probably would have shown up as an inactive drug in traditional in vivo drug screening procedures. The drug, however, may have shown considerable potential as a possible therapeutic agent if it was screened in an in vitro assay such as in a receptor binding screen or an enzyme inhibition based screen.

There are a few good examples of targeting or improved delivery to target sites where the importance of site retention has been confirmed. The previously discussed examples of prodrugs of 2-PAM, berberine, and dopamine all produced parent drugs with poor site accessibility and loss. These prodrugs, however, did not have the advantage of site selective metabolism. Wilk et al. (1978) and others (Kyncl et al., 1979) developed L-γ-glutamyl derivatives of L-DOPA and dopamine as kidney specific prodrugs for the delivery of the renal vasodilator, dopamine. In the case of L-γ-glutamyl-dopamine, the prodrug is only slowly cleaved on passage through the kidney. The released polar dopamine is then rapidly metabolized and excreted into the urine without re-entering the systemic circulation where it would produce adrenergic stimulation of the heart and other side effects. In the case of the L-DOPA derivative, Wilk et al. (1978) showed that L-γ-glutamyl-L-DOPA is selectively accumulated in the kidney and that the L-DOPA released from the L-γ-glutamyl prodrug by the action of L-γ-glutamyl transpeptidase is decarboxylated to dopamine by L-DOPA decarboxylase, which is also abundant in the kidney (Louenberg et al., 1962).

Pipkin and Stella (1978) and Stella (1977) demonstrated that thiamine was inadvertently selectively delivered (76% of an I.V. dose) to the red blood cell fraction of whole blood after I.V. administration to rats of thiamine as its prodrug, thiamine tetrahydrofurfural disulphide (TTFD). It was shown that the lipid soluble TTFD rapidly entered the red blood cells, reacted with red blood cell glutathione to generate thiamine, which was then only slowly released from the red blood cells because of thiamine's very polar nature. On the other hand, thiamine itself given I.V. remained in the plasma fraction of blood

from which it was rapidly excreted. Negligable red blood
cells uptake occured.

Viruses are less selective in their phosphorylation of
potential nucleotide precursors. This fact has been
utilized in the development of some of the newer antiviral
agents such as acyclovir (Fyfe et al., 1978). These
putative prodrugs are not phosphorylated by mammalian cells
but are phosphorylated by the less selective viral enzyme.
The active agent is actually the phosphorylated prodrug
which is incorporated into viral DNA, disrupting the
virus's replication cycle. The selectivity in this case
comes primarily from the activation process, prodrug
accessibility to the phosphorylating enzyme, and possibly
drug retention by the virus. Even if there is release of
the phosphorylated prodrug to systemic circulation, it may
not be a problem in that the polar phosphate may not be
readily taken up by mammalian cells.

Other examples of site directed delivery are
methenamine as a prodrug of formaldehyde for the treatment
of bladder infections, the earlier examples of azodisal
sodium as a prodrug of 5-aminosalicylic acid, and the
glycosidic derivatives of various steroidal
anti-inflammatory drugs. These examples really represent
illustrations of local drug delivery, in that the treatment
site is not systemic tissue. In the case of methenamine,
acidification of the urine of patients causes the renally
excreted methenamine to release formaldehyde. The
selectivity here comes from the fact that methenamine is
renally excreted and does not breakdown rapidly at
physiological pH. Once formaldehyde is released in the
bladder as a result of urine acidification, the formaldehye
is able to act locally. Site retention is not really a
problem in this case. Similarly, when 5-aminosalicylic
acid and the steroids are released from their prodrugs in
the colon, the treatment of the bowel tissue is effected.

Another hypothesis often heard for achieving targeting
is "A PRODRUG WILL BE SYNTHESIZED BY COUPLING A SMALL DRUG
MOLECULE TO A MACROMOLECULAR PROMOIETY THAT WILL HAVE AN
AFFINITY FOR A SURFACE DETERMINANT OF A PARTICULAR CELL
LINE. THIS PRODRUG, ONCE BOUND TO THIS CELL SURFACE WILL
BE INTERNALIZED VIA AN ENDOCYTIC MECHANISM AND WILL BE
METABOLIZED IN A LYSOSOME, THEREBY SELECTIVELY DELIVERING
THE ACTIVE AGENT TO THAT SPECIFIC CELL LINE". Overall this

hypothesis seems well grounded and would seem to show
promise as a targeting technique. However the idea does
have some weaknesses. If the target site is in the extravascular bed, can the macromolecular–drug conjugate diffuse
from the capillary vessels to its binding site or will the
conjugate be taken up by the phagocytic cells of the
reticular endothelial systems, especially those of highly
perfused organs like the liver (Poste and Kirsch, 1983).
How quickly will the conjugate be metabolized systemically
relative to the uptake? If bound at the desired site and
internalized, will lysosomal cleavage of the conjugate to
release the active drug, present the drug to the target
site, or will the drug be trapped or rapidly inactivated in
the lysosome? If the drug can rapidly leave the lysosome,
it can probably also rapidly leave the cell. Site
retention of the drug, then becomes a problem. Many
examples of site specific antibody–drug, monoclonal
antibody–drug, and glycopeptide–drug conjugates have been
proposed as drug targeting techniques. In an attempt to
see if these techniques hold any promise, we did attempt to
simulate their pharmacokinetics using our model system.
Figure 5 is a plot of intracellular target organ drug
concentration against time after I.V. administration of a
drug, with poor target site (assumed to be the intracelluar
fluid) accessibility ($Cl_{in, \ out}$ = 0.1 ml/min) but to a
reasonably well perfused tissue (Q = 10 ml/min). The
prodrug was one that also had slow intracelluar fluid
uptake from the extracelluar space, to simulate a
relatively slow endocytotic process (more correctly, this
process should be simulated as a unidirectional process).
The prodrug, however, is strongly bound in the extracellular space. This is mathematically effected by making
Q' = 0.1 ml/min. The prodrug was also programmed to
breakdown intracellularly at a rate of 100 fold faster than
in the rest of the body. As can be seen from Fig. 5,
targeting is achieved via input from such a prodrug. Note,
however, that the metabolism of the conjugate to release
the drug must occur in such a way that the drug has
accessibility to the receptor phase. What this simulation
suggests is that the concept of cell line specific binding
may be useful as a prodrug targeting technique provided
other factors, such as site accessibility by the conjugate
(prodrug), availability of an internalization mechanism,
site/s or conjugate breakdown and site retainability of the
active drug are all carefully considered.

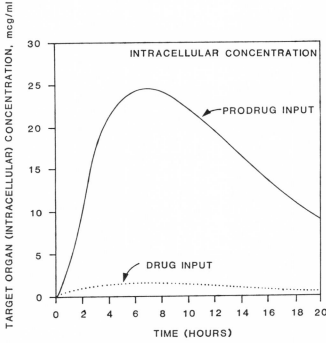

POOR PRODRUG TRANSPORT (CI $^{PD}_{IN,OUT}$ = 0.1 ml/min)

SELECTIVE INTRACELLULAR CONVERSION

POOR PARENT DRUG TRANSPORT (CI $^{D}_{IN, OUT}$ = 0.1 ml/min)

Q = 10 ml/min   Q' = 0.1 ml/min

(STRONG BINDING OF PRODRUG IN EXTRACELLULAR SPACE)

Fig. 5.   A simulation showing how cell surface binding
          or strong extracellular affinity can be used
          to effect targeting via prodrugs even when
          intracellular uptake is slow. Note that
          selective intracellular metabolism of the
          prodrug and site retention of the parent drug
          are still required for targeting. This
          simulation is used to demonstrate the possible
          utility of prodrugs prepared by coupling a
          small drug to a macromolecular promoiety which
          has an affinity for a surface determinant of
          a particular cell line.

In conclusion, TARGETING based on the prodrug approach, could be successful if a proper strategy is applied. This would involve;

1) The identification of diseased states with well delineated etiologies such as aberrant receptors or biochemical pathways.

2) The site of the aberration is well defined and isolated to a single organ or cell line with clearly defined anatomical boundaries e.g. the blood brain barrier for the brain or red blood cell membranes for red blood cells.

3) This site should be studied to identify any unique cell surface properties, membrane transporting properties, or metabolic activity properties, that could be utilized to help effect targeting.

4) The candidate drug chosen as a targeting possibility must have been shown to be very effective at the receptor level (receptor here is broadly defined) but based on physical/chemical properties, and not other shortcomings, is poorly able to reach the receptor after in vivo administration. It is unlikely that most currently useful therapeutic agents would fit this description unless it had been established that the performance of the agent is less than ideal because it is unable to efficiently reach its site of action.

5) The drug proposed as a targeting candidate must have a "handle in its structure that will permit the synthesis of a derivative (prodrug) with the physical/chemical/biochemical characteristics that will allow the prodrug to reach its targeting site and there, very efficiently release the active drug.

The interplay, therefore, between the properties of the TARGET SITE, the proposed PRODRUG, the DRUG and the disease state to be treated will determine whether a TARGETING STRATEGY based on the prodrug approach is scientifically feasible and economically worthwhile.

REFERENCES

Albert, A., Chemical aspects of selective toxicity. Nature, 182 (1958) 421–423.

Albert, A., Selective Toxicity, 3rd Edn., John Wiley and Sons Inc., New York, N.Y., 1965, p. 63.

Albert, A., Selective Toxicity, 5th ed., John Wiley, New York, 1973, pp. 21–26.

Ariens, E.J., Molecular pharmacology, a basis for drug design. In Jucker (Ed) Progress in Drug Research, Vol. 10, Birkhauser Verlag, Basel, 1966, pp. 429–529.

Ariens, E.J., Modulation of pharmacokinetics by molecular manipulation. In Ariens (Ed) Drug Design Volume II, Academic Press, New York, 1971, pp. 1–127.

Bodor, N., Shek, E. and Higuchi, T., Delivery of a quaternary pyridinium salt across the blood-brain barrier by its dihydropyridine derivative. Sci., 190 (1975) 155–156.

Bodor, N., Shek, E. and Higuchi, T., Improved delivery through biological membranes. 1. Synthesis and properties of 1-methyl-1,6-dihydropyridine, a prodrug of N-methylpyridinium-2-carbaldoxime chloride. J. Med. Chem., 19 (1976) 102–107.

Bodor, N., Novel approaches in prodrug design. In Bundgaard, Hansen and Kofod (Eds) Optimization of Drug Delivery, Munksgaard, Copenhagen, 1982, pp. 156–177.

Bodor, N. and Brewster, M.E., Improved delivery through biological membranes XV - Sustained brain delivery of berberine. Europ. Med. Chem., 18 (1983), 235–240.

Bundgaard, H., Novel bioreversible derivatives of amides, ureides, amines and other chemical entities not readily derivatizable, In Bundgaard, Hausen and Kofod (Eds) Optimization of Drug Delivery, Munksgaard, Copenhagen, (1982), pp. 178–198.

Digenis, G.A. and Swintosky, J.V., Drug latentiation, In Gillette and Mitchell (Eds) Handbook of Experimental Pharmacology, Vol. 28 (part 3), Springer-Verlag Berlin (1975) pp. 86–112.

Double, J.A. and Workman, P., A new high-glucuronidase mouse tumor curable by aniline mustard therapy, Canc. Treat. Rept., 61 (1977) 909–911.

Duggan, D.E., Sulindac: Therapeutic implications of the prodrug/pharmacophore equilibrium. Drug Met. Rev., 12 (1981) 325–337.

Duggan, D.E., Hare, L.E., Ditzler, C.A., Lei, B.W. and
    Kwan, K.C., The disposition of sulindac. Clin,
    Pharmacol. Therap., 21 (1977) 326–335.
Friend, D.R. and Chang, G.W., A colon-specific drug
    delivery system based on drug glycosides and
    glycosidases of colonic bacteria. J. Med. Chem., 27
    (1984) 261–266.
Fyfe, J.A., Keller, P.M., Furman, P.A., Miller, R.L. and
    Elion, G.B., Thymidine kinase from herpes simplex
    virus phosphorylates the new antiviral compound,
    9-(2-hydroxyethoxymethyl)guanine. J. Biol. Chem. 253
    (1978) 8721–8727.
Goldman, P., Will there be a next generation of
    sulfasalazine? Gastroenterol., 83 (1982) 1138–1141.
Harper, N.J., Drug latentiation. J. Med. Pharm. Chem. 1
    (1959) 467–500.
Harper, N.J., Drug latentiation. Prog. Drug Res. 4 (1962)
    221–294.
Higuchi, T. and Stella, V. (Eds) Pro-drugs as Novel Drug
    Delivery Systems, American Chemical Society,
    Washington, D.C. 1975.
Higuchi, T. (1984) personal communications.
Jewell, D.P. and Truelove, S.C., Disodium azodisalicylate
    in ulcerative. Lancet ii (1981) 1168.
Kyncl, J.J., Minard, R.N. and Jones, P.H., L-γ-glutamyl
    dopamine, an oral dopamine prodrug with renal
    selectivity. In Impsand and Schwartz (Eds) Peripheral
    Dopaminergic Receptors, Pergamon Press, New York,
    (1979) pp. 369–380.
Louenberg, W., Weissbach, H. and Udenfriend, S., Aromatic
    L-amino acid decarboxylase. J. Biol. Chem. 237 (1962)
    89–93.
Notari, R.E., Prodrug design. Pharmacol. Therap. 14 (1981)
    25–53.
Orlowski, M., Mizoguchi, H. and Wilk, S., N-Acyl-γ-glutamyl
    derivatives of sulfamethoxazole as models of
    kidney-selective prodrugs. J. Pharmacol. Exp. Therap.,
    212 (1980) 167–172.
Pipkin, J.D. and Stella, V.J., Thiamine whole blood
    pharmacokinetics in rats using both a specific
    [3]5S-thiamine liquid scintillation assay and the
    thiochrome fluorescence assay. J. Pharm. Sci. 67
    (1978) 818–821.

Poste, G. and Kirsch, R., Site specific drug delivery in
    cancer therapy. Biotechnology 1 (1983) 869–878.
Roche, E.B. (ED) Design of Biopharmaceutical Properties
    Through Prodrugs and Analogs. American Pharmaceutical
    Association, Washington, D.C., 1977.
Shashoua, V.V. Jacob, J.N., Ridge, R., Campbell, A. and
    Baldessarini, R.J., γ-Aminobutyric acid esters.
    1. Synthesis, brain uptake, and pharmacological
    studies of aliphatic and steroidal esters of
    γ-aminobutyric acid. J. Med. Chem. 27 (1984) 659–664.
Shek, E., Higuchi, T. and Bodor, N. Improved delivery
    through biological membranes. 2. Distribution,
    excretion and metabolism of N-methyl-1,6-dihydro-
    pyridine-2-carbaldoxime hydrochloride, a prodrug of
    N-methylpyridinium-2-carbaldoxime chloride. J. Med.
    Chem. 19 (1976a) 108–112.
Shek, E., Higuchi, T. and Bodor, N., Improved delivery
    through biological membranes. 3. Delivery of
    N-methylpyridinium-2-carbaldoxime chloride through the
    blood brain barrier in its dihydropyridine pro-drug
    form. J. Med. Chem. 19 (1976b) 113–117.
Shen, T-S., and Winter, C.A., Chemical and biological
    studies on indomethacin, sulindac and their analogs.
    In Harper and Simmonds (Eds) Advances in Drug Research
    Vol. 12, Academic Press, New York, 1977, pp. 89–246.
Shindo, H., Komai, T. and Kawai, K., Mechanism of
    intestinal absorption and brain uptake of
    L-5-hydroxytryptophan in rats, as compared to those of
    L-3,4-dihydroxyphenyl-alanine. Chem. Pharm. Bull. 25
    (1977) 1417–1425.
Sinkula, A., Prodrug approach in drug design. Ann. Rep.
    Med. Chem. 10 (1975) 306–316.
Sinkula, A. and Yalkowsky, S. Rationale for design of
    biologically reversible drug derivatives: Prodrugs.
    J. Pharm. Sci. 64 (1975) 181–210.
Stella, V.J., Drug substances in particular prodrugs:
    Problems and methods of approach. In Polderman (Ed)
    Formulation and Preparation of Dosage Forms,
    Elsevier/North-Holland, Amsterdam, 1977, pp. 91–111.
Stella, V.J. and Himmelstein, K.J., Prodrugs and site
    specific delivery. J. Med. Chem. 23 (1980) 1275–1282
    (1980).

Stella, V.J. and Himmelstein, K.J., Critique of prodrugs and site specific delivery. In Bundgaard, Hansen and Koford (Eds) Optimization of Drug Delivery-Alfred Benzon Symposium 17, Munksgaard, Copenhagen, 1982, pp. 134-155.

Ulm, E.H., Enalapril maleate (MK 421), a potent nonsulfhydryl angiotension-converting enzyme inhibitor: Absorption, disposition and metabolism in man. Drug Metab. Rev. 14 (1983) 99-110.

Wilk, S., Mizoguchi, H. and Orlowski, M., γ-Glutamyl dopa: A kidney specific dopamine precursor. J. Pharmacol. Exp. Therap. 206 (1978) 227-232.

Workman, P. and Double, J.A., Drug latentiation in cancer chemotherapy, Biomed. 28 (1978) 255-262.

Yalkowsky, S.H. and Morozowich, W., A physical chemical basis for the design of orally active prodrugs, In Ariens (Ed) Drug Design Vol. IX, Academic Press, New York, 1980, pp. 121-185.

NEW DRUG DELIVERY SYSTEMS: PHYSICO-CHEMICAL CONSIDERATIONS

Ian H Pitman DSc

Victorian College of Pharmacy Ltd

381 Royal Parade Parkville, 3052   Australia

INTRODUCTION

As illustrated by the preceding papers in this symposium, contemporary technology provides clinicians with an exciting array of drug delivery systems. However, the selection of the most appropriate delivery system for any particular drug continues to be based on:

1   the pharmacodynamic demands of the disease or pathological condition being treated, and

2   the physico-chemical properties of the drug which is to be delivered.

This presentation is concerned with the influence that the physico-chemical properties of the drug have on the selection of the delivery system and on the steps that can be taken to optimize drug delivery.   The aim of the presentation is to direct interested readers to pertinent reviews rather than to attempt to comprehensively cover the field.

In an attempt to give the presentation cohesion I will concentrate on a scenario that currently recurs in hospital pharmacy departments around the world.   Imagine that the decision has been taken to employ constant infusion therapy for an ambulatory patient.   This is an advanced drug delivery option which has been reported to be beneficial in the delivery of insulin (Rupp et al., 1982, Brownlee et al., 1984) and cancer chemotherapeutic agents (Lokich and Ensminger, 1983; Gyves et al., 1984).

The initial step that the pharmacist is likely to take to fulfil this request is to select from the shelf one of a number of skilfully engineered constant infusion pumps. He may select one that is worn externally (e.g. Cormed®, Cormed, Medina, NY; Auto Syringe®, Travenol Laboratories, Chicago, Ill; Ar-Med®, Alza Corporation, Palo Alto, Ca) or an implantable pump (e.g. Infusaid®, Infusaid Corporation, Mass). The next step for the pharmacist is to charge the pump with a formulation of the drug that will enable it to infuse the drug at the specified rate. To achieve this goal it will be necessary to:

> solubilize the drug: i.e. get a sufficient amount of
>   drug into solution so that the pump can deliver
>   drug at the required rate;

> stabilise the drug and the formulation against
>   chemical and physical degradation;

> ensure that the drug is bioavailable.

SOLUBILIZATION OF DRUGS FOR PARENTERAL INFUSION

Whenever possible parenteral dosage forms should consist of the drug dissolved in an aqueous solution. Thus, the first question that the pharmacist must address "is the water solubility of the drug sufficiently high to produce the desired concentration of drug in the formulation?" If the answer is no the pharmacist will have to decide which, if any, of a number of solubilization options is most likely to result in an appropriate formulation. Useful leads towards the solution of this problem are likely to be found in the monograph "Techniques of Solubilization of Drugs" (Yalkowsky 1981a).

A strategy for increasing the water solubility of drugs, which are nonelectrolytes, has been suggested by Yalkowsky (1981b) on the basis of the following semi-empirical equation which relates aqueous solubility of a wide variety of compounds S_W to their octanol/water partition coefficient (PC), the entropy of fusion of their crystal (ΔS_f), and their melting point (MP) (Yalkowsky and Valvani, 1980):

$$\log S_W = -1.00 \log PC - 1.11 \Delta S_f (MP-25)/1364 + 0.54 \quad ..(1)$$

The strategy is:

1   if MP>300°, forces within the crystal are a major factor in reducing aqueous solubility (methods E and F in Table 1 are likely to be useful for increasing solubility);

2   if MP=200-300,° forces between molecules within the crystal are probably a major factor in reducing aqueous solubility (methods E and F in Table 1 are likely to be useful for increasing water solubility although methods A,B,C, and D should be considered);

3   if MP<100° or the compound is a liquid, the most fruitful way of increasing aqueous solubility is to minimize the difference between the sum of solute: solute (D:D) and solvent:solvent (W':W') interactions and the solute:solvent interactions (D:W') i.e. minimize the value of the activity coefficient of the drug ($\gamma_{w'}$) as defined in equation 2:

$$\log \gamma_{w'} = (D:D) + (W':W') - 2(D:W') \quad ....(2)$$

The value of ($\gamma_{w'}$) is reflected by the octanol/water partition coefficient of the drug in equation (1). The most fruitful ways of solubilizing such compounds are likely to be those designated as A,B,C, and D in Table 1.

The above considerations apply to drugs that are non-electrolytes.

Strong electrolytes, which dissociate completely into ions in water, normally have high water solubility because of strong solute:solvent (ion-dipole) interactions in water. On the other hand, a high percentage of drugs are weak electrolytes (weak acids and bases) and exist as both neutral molecules and ions in water.

Table 1
Methods of Solubilizing Drugs

Drug Type	Solubilization Code	Solubilization Method
Non-electrolyte	A	Use of surfactants
Non-electrolyte	B	Use of fat emulsions
Non-electrolyte	C	Use of cosolvents
Non-electrolyte	D	Use of complexation
Non-electrolyte	E	Drug derivatization
Non-electrolyte	F	Solid state manipulation
Electrolyte	G	pH adjustment

The generally low water solubility of the neutral molecules can be understood and manipulated on the basis of the above considerations concerning non-electrolytes. However, water solubility of weak electrolytes can normally be increased by adjusting the pH of the solution to a value where the molecules exist significantly as ions (i.e. to pH values above the pKa values of acids or below the pKa values of bases) - method G in Table 1.

Solubilization Code A : Use of Surfactants

Recent Review : Florence (1981).

The dissolution of surface active agents in water at concentrations above their critical micelle concentration (cmc) produces micellar solutions which are characterised by a lipophilic region (the core) and a hydrophilic region. Such solutions are usually good solvents for molecules of low polarity that have low water solubility.

Although a large number of surfactants with a range of solubilizing potential have been identified, the majority of them have such high intrinsic toxicity that they cannot be used for solubilizing drugs in parenteral dosage forms. The intrinsic toxicity of surfactants arises because they have a high affinity for biological membranes and they frequently adsorb to and penetrate the membranes and thereby change their fluidity and barrier properties.

Additional problems frequently arise because of:

interactions between surfactants and polymers;

solubilization of other formulation constituents by surfactants;

surfactant molecules catalysing the degradation of drugs or of other formulation constituents.

The most widely used surface active agent as a solubilizer in parenteral formulations is polyoxyethylated castor oil (Cremophor EL). However, a recent World Health Organisation Bulletin (1984) noted that the Italian Ministry of Health has suspended the marketing authorisation of two products (Alfathesin®, Glaxo, and Epontol®; Bayer) that contain Cremophor EL. This action was taken in the belief that there was a high probability that Cremophor EL was associated with:

allergic/analphylactic reactions,

hyperlipidaemia and abnormal electrophoretic distribution of lipoproteins which develops after long treatment.

Information on these reactions has been published by Moneret-Vautrin et al., (1983), Clarke (1981), Huttle et al., (1980), Doenicke et al., (1973).

In man, the incidence of adverse reactions remains low and they appear to be idiosyncratic. Reactions seen include hypotension (with concomitant tachycardia), sometimes with anaphylactoid signs. In some subjects, serum histamine was elevated but of these, only some experienced anaphylactoid reactions, which responded to antihistamine therapy.

It is possible that the adverse reactions may be

caused by impurities in the Cremophor EL or by specific effects involving Cremophor EL and the drugs alphaxalone or alphadolone in (Alfathesin®) and propanidid (in Epontol®). Cremophor EL certainly appears to be less toxic in parenteral solutions than anionic surfactants (e.g. sodium lauryl sulfate), cationic detergents (e.g. dodecyltrimethylammonium bromide) and many non-ionic surfactants.

One of the potential problems with using parenteral dosage forms in which the solubility of the drug has been elevated by solubilization techniques, is that the drug is likely to precipitate in the biological medium into which it is introduced. This is less likely to occur when the drug has been solubilized by the use of surfactants than when pH adjustment, the use of cosolvents, or complexation is the solubilization technique, because precipitation will not occur until dilution has proceeded to a point where the concentration of surfactant is below its cmc.

Solubilization Code B : Use of Fat Emulsions

An alternative method of solubilization, that is related to the use of surfactant solutions, involves the use of oil in water emulsions as solvents for lipophilic drugs. The oil phase in the emulsions, which corresponds to the core in micellar solutions, is the site of solubilization of lipophilic drugs. Commercial fat emulsions (e.g. Liposyn®, Abbott Laboratories; Intralipid®, Cutter-Vitrum Laboratories) are readily available solvents. This technique has been used to solubilize antineoplastic agents (El-Sayed and Repta 1983), diazepam (Jeppsson and Ljunberg 1975) cyclandelate (Jeppsson and Ljunberg 1973) barbiturates (Jeppsson 1972), and valinomycin (Repta 1981a).

Solubilization Code C : Use of Cosolvents

Recent reviews: Yalkowsky and Roseman (1981), Spiegel and Noseworthy (1963).

The addition to water of miscible solvents (cosolvents) such as ethanol, propylene glycol, polyethylene glycol, and glycerol is probably the most widely used technique for solubilizing drugs for parenteral dosage forms. However, while cosolvents increase solubility of many drugs (mainly non-polar drugs), they decrease the solubility of some drugs (mainly polar drugs) and they have little effect on the solubility of other drugs (mainly semi-polar drugs). Examples of these three effects are given in Fig. 1, 2, and 3.

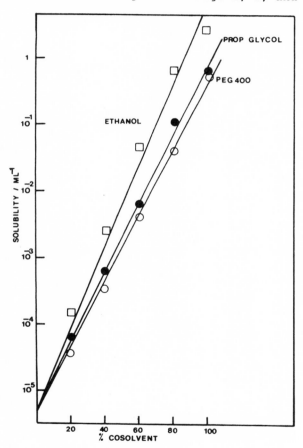

Fig. 1. Solubility vs cosolvent fraction relationship for non-polar case, ticonazole. (Reproduced from Gould et al., 1984 with permission of the copyright owners).

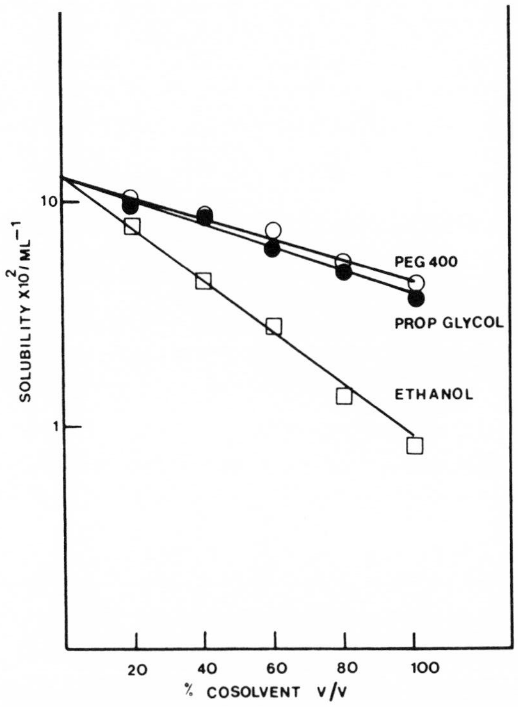

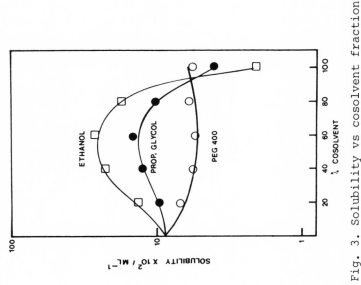

Fig. 3. Solubility vs cosolvent fraction relationship for semi-polar case, caffeine. (Reproduced from Gould et al., 1984 with permission of the copyright owners).

Fig. 2. Solubility vs cosolvent fraction relationship for polar case, oxfenicine. (Reproduced from Gould et al., 1984 with permission of the copyright owners).

The effect of cosolvents depends on the polarities of both the drug and the cosolvents and a number of empirical relationships have been developed which assist in the development of cosolvent systems for particular purposes. (Yalkowsky and Roseman 1981, Gould et al., 1984).

For example, Gould et al., (1984) report that the solubility of a non polar drug, ticonazole, S_M in a mixture of ethanol (E) propylene glycol (PG) and polyethylene glycol 400 (PEG 400) can be accounted for by using equation 3

$$\log S_M = (0.059 \pm 0.003)\%E + (0.047 \pm 0.003)\%PG +$$

$$(0.050 \pm 0.003) \%PEG\ 400 - 5.136 \qquad \ldots\ldots(3)$$

Yalkowsky and Roseman (1981) draw attention to the fact that dilution of a solution prepared by dissolving a drug in a cosolvent mixture (e.g. following parenteral administration) can lead to precipitation of the drug. Ways of predicting whether precipitation is likely to occur, which are based on knowledge of the solubilities of the drug in water and in pure cosolvents and on the octanol/water partition coefficient of the drug, are suggested.

Solubilization Code D : Use of Complexation

Recent Review: Repta (1981b).

The formation of one or more molecular complexes by a drug and a ligand in water has been suggested as a way of increasing the aqueous solubility of a number of drugs. The principles involved and the rules for selecting appropriate ligands are well presented by Repta (1981b). An example of the type of solubilization that can be achieved by complexation is illustrated in Fig. 4. which shows solubilization of an antineoplastic adenine derivative (NSC 263164) using nicotinamide.

Repta (1981b) has pointed out the following potential limitations on the use of complexation as a means of solubilizing drugs:

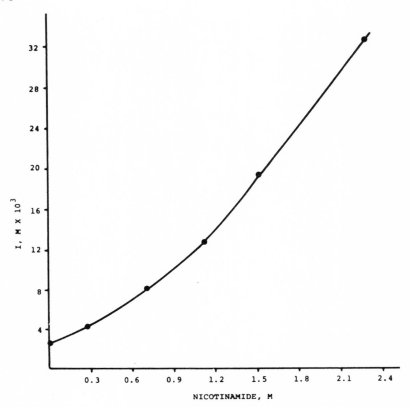

Fig. 4. The influence of nicotinamide concentration on the solubility of NSC 263164(I) in 0.1 M phosphate buffer at pH 3 and 25°C. (Reproduced from Truelove et al., 1984 with permission of the copyright owners).

1   the rapid and total reversibility of the complexation reaction may result in an unacceptably high rate of release and precipitation of drug upon dilution of the dosage form.

2   the fact that the ligand will be present in equimolar or higher concentrations relative to the drug places stringent requirements on its toxicity and aesthetic properties.

3   the degree of solubilization that can be expected following complexation is normally less than an order of magnitude.

Solubilization Code E : Drug Derivatization

Recent Review: Amidon (1981), Higuchi and Stella (1975).

An important option that exists for the formulator of solution dosage forms is to present the drug as a transient derivative (a pro-drug) that possesses the desired properties of solubility, stability, and bio-availability, but which will be transformed to active drug within the body. The topic of pro-drugs has been adequately reviewed in the above-mentioned papers and is the subject of the previous presentation.

Solubilization Code F : Solid State Manipulation

Recent Review: Shefter (1981).

As discussed in the introduction to this paper, intermolecular forces have a profound effect on the solubility of non-electrolytes with melting points above 200°. The above-mentioned review considers ways in which forces within the crystal can be modified to increase aqueous solubility. However, many of these methods (e.g. selection of polymorphs or solvates) have little effect on equilibrium solubility and have only minor relevance to the formulation of solution dosage forms for parenteral administration.

Solubilization Code G : pH Adjustment

A large number of drugs are weak organic acids or weak organic bases and exist as both neutral molecules and ions in aqueous solution. Water is a good solvent for ions because of its high dielectric constant and because of the possibilities it offers for ion-dipole interactions. It is generally a poor solvent for neutral molecules because they break up the water structure without providing the opportunity for compensation interactions. Consequently, drugs that are acids can be solubilized in water by increasing the pH value (up to and above the pKa value) whereas drugs that are bases can be solubilized in water by lowering the pH value (down-to and below the pKa value).

However, such changes in pH value may adversely effect the stability of the drugs or of the formulation or may result in formulations with unacceptably high or low pH values from a physiological point of view.

Thus, the pharmacist will frequently be called on to make a compromise between solubility and stability.

STABILIZATION OF DRUGS AND FORMULATIONS AGAINST
CHEMICAL AND PHYSICAL DEGRADATION

Because the desirable solvents for parenteral dosage forms contain a high percentage of water, the drugs which they contain will be exposed to a wide variety of hydrolytic reactions including:

> hydrolysis (e.g. esters and amides)
> hydration (e.g. hydrochlorothiazide)
> deamination (e.g. cytosine)
> dehydration (e.g. tetracycline)
> isomerization (e.g. penicillin)
> epimerization (e.g. pilocarpine)
> transesterification (e.g. aspirin and
>   polyethylene glycol)
> transamination (e.g. thiamine and aromatic
>   amines).

The magnitude of the problems presented by these reactions will frequently be exacerbated by substances that were added to the formulation to solubilize the drug. For example:

> hydrolysis reactions are catalysed by hydrogen
>   and hydroxide ions
>
> hydrolysis reactions are influenced by
>   surfactants (Florence, 1981)
>
> hydrolysis reactions are catalysed by polyhydric
>   alcohols (Wyatt and Pitman, 1979; Bundgaard
>   and Larsen, 1983).

Furthermore, because many constant infusion pumps are fabricated from plastics, there is the possibility that oxygen will diffuse into the formulation and participate in auto-oxidation reactions.

Several excellent reviews are available to assist the pharmacist in taking steps to protect parenteral formulations against chemical degradation. These include:

Handbook of Injectable Drugs (Trissel, 1983)

Chemical Stability of Pharmaceuticals (Connors et al., 1979).

Stability of Pharmaceuticals (Mollica et al., 1978).

The pharmacist who is preparing a formulation for use in a constant infusion pump will also have to consider the possibilities of:

loss of drug due to sorption to components of the infusion system,

problems caused by the flow of formulation from the pump.

Sorption of Drugs to Container Materials

Constant infusion pumps and their associated catheters are fabricated from a variety of materials including polymers. Consequently, the formulator of drug solutions for such delivery systems must consider the possible losses of drug caused by sorption to the materials of the pumping system.

The adsorption of proteins and peptides onto glass and plastic surfaces has been reported by a number of workers (Petty and Cunningham, 1974; Mizutani and Mizutani, 1978; Bitar et al., 1978; Christensen et al., 1978; Ogino et al., 1979). The most common methods of minimizing loss of drug by this means include the addition to the formulation of proteins such as gelatin and albumin (Petty and Cunningham, 1974; Kraegan et al., 1975). A recent report (Anik and Hwang, 1983) shows that adsorption of a decapeptide onto glass could be reduced by the presence of 0.1 M phosphate ion and 0.16 M acetate ion at pH 5.

Drug loss from solutions into plastic containers can also occur by absorption into the plastic (e.g. the unionised forms of various drugs (Illum et al., 1983; Illum and Bundgaard, 1982), or by penetration through the plastic (e.g. nitroglycerine Roberts et al., 1979, 1980). Illum et al., (1983) suggest that the octanol/water partition coefficient of the drug is a useful parameter for predicting its sorption behaviour by plastic containers.

Problems Caused by Flow of Formulations

Up to this point, it has been assumed that all the formulations employed in constant infusion pumps are solutions. However, this mode of delivery is commonly used for suspensions of insulin in water. A recent report in the Lancet (Brownlee et al., 1984) drew attention to the fact that serum concentrations of serum amyloid A protein were nearly twice as high in patients receiving insulin by continuous subcutaneous infusion using an infusion pump as in patients receiving subcutaneous injections. The probable cause of this effect was the greater tendency of insulin to aggregate during the infusion pump treatment than when it was administered by subcutaneous injection. The authors suggested that "the use of high-potency non-aggregating insulins in the pump treatment of type I diabetic patients may be necessary for optimum therapy".

The shear forces that accompany flow from constant infusion pumps may cause problems with other heterogenous formulations.

BIOAVAILABILITY FROM MODIFIED-RELEASE DELIVERY SYSTEMS

Very few, if any, bioavailability problems are likely to be involved with the use of a well designed constant infusion pump that is charged with a stable drug solution. However, this is not the case with the majority of modified release systems that are currently appearing in the market place.

The major problems in the assessment of bio-availability of modified-release dosage forms arise because of our ignorance of the environment within the body where the dosage form will be releasing its drug.

Theeuwes (1984) has prepared a useful review of the steps that will have to be taken to establish in vitro vs in vivo correlations of bioavailability of such dosage forms. However, much research remains to be done before confident validations can be performed. In the meantime, the USP (Leeson et al., 1984) has taken a useful step in describing a dissolution test, which is aimed at establishing that a modified-release system:

does not "dose dump",

is likely to prolong tissue drug levels.

CONCLUSION

The foregoing pages describe the steps that a pharmacist can take in an attempt to fulfil a request to charge a constant infusion pump with a drug so that the pump will deliver the drug in a programmed fashion. The constraints placed upon the pharmacist arise because of the physico-chemical properties of the drug and the methods available to him to:

solubilize the drug;

stabilize the formulation;

ensure bioavailability of the drug.

Approximately 3000 constant infusion pumps are currently being used in Australia and world usage must be substantial. However, little information is available in a convenient form to guide pharmacists in formulating appropriate drug solutions.

Although the formulator will be called on to solve different problems when faced with other modified-release dosage forms, he will be constantly restrained by the physico-chemical properties of the drug. It is suggested that he will be assisted in overcoming these constraints by an application of the general principles outlined in this presentation.

REFERENCES

Amidon, G.L., Drug derivatization as a means of solubilization: Physicochemical and biochemical strategies. In Yalkowsky, S.H., (Ed) Techniques of Solubilization of Drugs, Marcel Dekker, Inc; New York, 1981, pp. 183-211.

Anik, S.T. and Hwang, J-Y. Adsorption of D-Nal (2) ^{6}LHRH, a decapeptide, onto glass and other surfaces. Int. J. Pharm., 16 (1983) 181-190.

Bitar, K.N., Zfass, A.M. and Makhlorf, G.M., Binding of secretin to plastic surfaces. Gastroenterology, 75 (1978) 1080-1082.

Brownlee, M., Cerami, A., Li, J.J., Vlassara, H., Martin, T.R. and McAdam, K.P.W.J., Association of insulin pump therapy with raised serum amyloid A in Type 1 diabetes mellitus. Lancet 1 (1984) 411-413.

Bundgaard, H. and Larsen, C., The influence of carbohydrates and polyhydricalcohols on the stability of cephalosporins in aqueous solution. Int. J. Pharm., 16 (1983) 319-325.

Clarke, R.S.J., Adverse effects of intravenously administered drugs used in anaesthetic practice. 22 (1981) 26-41.

Christensen, P., Johansson, A. and Nielsen, V., Quantification of protein adsorbance to glass and plastics: investigations of a new tube with low adherence. J. Immunol. Meth., 23 (1978) 23-28.

Connors, K.A., Amidon, G.L. and Kennon, L., Chemical Stability of Pharmaceuticals. John Wiley and Sons, New York, 1979, pp. 1-367.

Doenicke, A., Lorenz, W., Beigl, R., Bezecny, H., Unlig, G., Kalmar, L. Praetorius, B. and Mawn, G., Histamine release after intravenous application of short-acting hypnotics. Br. J. Anaesthesia, 45 (1973) 1007-1104.

El-Sayed, A-A, A. and Repta, A.J., Solubilization and stabilization of an investigational antineoplastic drug (NSC no. 278214) in an intravenous formulation using an emulsion vehicle. Int. J. Pharm. 13 (1983) 303-312.

Florence, A.T., Drug solubilization in surfactant systems. In Yalkowsky, S.H., (Ed.) Techniques of Solubilization of Drugs, Marcel Dekker, Inc., New York, 1981, pp. 15-89.

Gould, P.L., Goodman, M. and Hanson, P.A., Investigation of the solubility relationships of polar, semi-polar and non-polar drugs in mixed co-solvent systems. Int. J. Pharm. 19 (1984) 149-159.

Gyves, J.W., Ensminger, W.D., Stetson, P., Niederhuber, J.E., Meyer, M., Walker, S., Janis, M.A. and Gilbertson, S., Constant intraperitoneal 5-fluorouracil infusion through a totally implanted system. Clin. Pharmacol. Ther., 35 (1984) 83-89.

Higuchi, T. and Stella, V., Pro-drugs as novel drug delivery systems. American Chemical Society, Washington D.C., 1975.

Huttle, M.S., Olesen, A.S. and Soffersen, E., Complement-mediated reactions to diazepam with Cremophor as solvent (STESOLID MR). Br. J. Anaesthesia, 52 (1980) 72-79.

Illum, L., Budgaard, H. and Davis, S.S., A constant partition model for examining the sorption of drugs by plastic infusion bags. Int. J. Pharm., 17 (1983) 183-192.

Illum, L. and Bundgaard, H., Soprtion of drugs by plastic infusion bags. Int. J. Pharm., 10 (1982) 339-351.

Jeppsson, R. and Ljungberg, S., Anticonvulsant activity in mice of diazepam in an emulsion formulation for intravenous administration. Acta Pharmacol. Toxicol., 36 (1975) 312-320.

Jeppsson, R. and Ljungberg, S., Intraarterial administration of emulsion formulations containing cyclandelate and nitroglycerin. Acta Pharm. Suec., 10 (1973) 129-140.

Jeppsson, R., Effects of barbituric acids using an emulsion form intravenously. Acta Pharm. Suec., 9 (1972) 81-90.

Kraegen, E.W., Lazarus, L., Meler, H., Campbell, L. and Chia, Y.O., Carrier solutions for low-level intravenous insulin infusion. Br. Med. J., 23 Aug (1975) 464-466.

Leeson, L.J., Petersen, R.V. and Robinson, J.R., Pharmacopeial Forum, March-April 1984 pp. 4103-5.

Lokich, J. and Ensminger, W., Ambulatory pump infusion devices for hepatic artery infusion. Seminars in Oncology, 10 (1983) 183-190.

Mollica, J.A., Ahuja, S. and Cohen, J., Stability of pharmaceuticals. J. Pharm. Sci., 67 (1978) 443-465.

Moneret-Vautrin, D.A., Laxenaire, M.C. and Viry-Babel, F., Anaphylaxis caused by anti-Cremophor EL lgG STS antibodies in a case reaction to Althesin. Br. J. Anaesthesia, 55 (1983) 469-471.

Mizutani, T. and Mizutani, A., Estimation of adsorption of drugs and proteins on glass surfaces with controlled pore glass as a reference. J. Pharm. Sci., 67 (1978) 1102-1105.

Ogino, J., Noguchi, K. and Terato, K., Adsorption of secretin on glass surfaces. Chem. Pharm. Bull., 27 (1979) 3160-3163.

Petty, C. and Cunningham, N.L., Insulin adsorption by glass infusion bottles, polyvinyl chloride infusion containers and intravenous tubing. Anaesthesiology, 40 (1974) 400-404.

Repta, A.J., In Breimer, D.D. and Speiser, P. (Eds.) Topics in Pharmaceutical Sciences, Elsevier/North-Holland Biomedical Press, 1981a, pp. 131-151.

Repta, A.J., Alteration of apparent solubility through complexation. In Yalkowsky, S.H. (Ed.), Techniques of Solubilization of Drugs, Marcel Dekker, Inc., New York, 1981b, pp. 135-157.

Roberts, M.S., Cossum, P.A., Galbraith, A.J. and Boyd, G.W., The availability of nitroglycerin from parenteral solutions. J. Pharm. Pharmacol., 32 (1980) 237-244.

Roberts, M.S., Polack, A.E., Martin, G. and Blackburn, H.D., The storage of selected substances in aqueous solution in polethylene containers: the effect of some physicochemical factors on the disappearance kinetics of the substances. Int. J. Pharm., 2 (1979) 295-306.

Rupp, W.M., Barbosa, J.J., Perry, M.D., Blackshear, P.J., McCarthy, H.B., Thomas, M.D., Rhode, T.D., Goldenberg, F.J., Rublein, T.G., Dorman, F.D., and Buchwald, H., The use of an implantable pump in the treatment of Type 11 diabetes. N. Engl. J. Med., 307 (1982) 265-270.

Shefter, E., Solubilization by solid-state manipulation. In Yalkowsky, S.H., (Ed.), Techniques of Solubilization of Drugs, Marcel Dekker, Inc., New York, 1981, pp. 159-182.

Spiegel, A.J. and Noseworthy, M.M., Use of non-aqueous solvents in parenteral products. J. Pharm. Sci., 52 (1963) 917-927.

Theeuwes, F., Validation of rate-controlled dosage forms. To be published in the proceedings of the Second International Conference on Drug Absorption, Edinburgh, 1982.

Trissel, L.A., (Ed.), Handbook on injectable drugs. Third. Ed., American Society of Hospital Pharmacists Inc., 1983 pp. 1-538.

Truelove, J., Bawarshi-Nassar, R., Chen, N.R. and Hussain, A., Solubility enhancement of some developmental anti-cancer nucleoside analogs by complexation with nicotinamide. Int. J. Pharm., 19 (1984) 17-25.

World Health Organization Bulletin, January 6 (1984)

Wyatt, K.A. and Pitman, I.H., Some effects of polyhydric alcohols on the degradation of esters. Aust. J. Pharm. Sci., 8 (1979) 77-85.

Yalkowsky, S.H. (Ed.), Techniques of Solubilization of Drugs, Marcel Dekker, Inc., New York, 1981a, pp. 1-224.

Yalkowsky, S.H., Solubility and solubilization of nonelectrolytes. In Yalkowsky, S.H., (Ed.), Techniques of Solubilization of Drugs, Marcel Dekker, Inc., New York, 1981b, pp. 1-14.

Yalkowsky, S.H. and Roseman, T.J., Solubilization of drugs by cosolvents. In Yalkowsky, S.H. (Ed.), Techniques of Solubilization of Drugs, Marcel Dekker, Inc., New York, 1981, pp. 91-134.

Yalkowsky, S.H. and Valvani, S.C., Solubility and Partitioning I: Solubility of nonelectrolytes in water, J. Pharm. Sci., 69 (1980) 912-922.

E. ANALYTICAL ASPECTS OF DRUG DELIVERY

ANALYTICAL ASPECTS OF DRUG DELIVERY: AN IMPORTANT AND OFTEN OVERLOOKED PROBLEM

Larry A. Sternson and Thomas Malefyt

Dept. of Pharmaceutical Chemistry
University of Kansas
Lawrence, KS   66045

A flurry of activity has recently taken place aimed at developing improved delivery systems for drugs. Such systems are being designed to release drugs at controlled rates, to selectively direct the agent to appropriate "target sites" (located either within or on the surfaces of particular cell types) while reducing drug exposure to "non-target" areas and to control the absorption, transport, distribution and cellular uptake of pharmacologically active agents. The motivation for these efforts include: (1) the realization that many candidate drugs that have been found clinically unsuitable would be therapeutically and commerically valuable if properly delivered, (2) interest in developing products derived from genetic engineering (and other compounds) as drugs whose potency, short biological and/or chemical half lives or peculiar disposition profiles necessitate controlled, regiospecific release from a formulation, (3) potential exploitation of cytotoxic agents (or other materials) with narrow therapeutic indices requiring precise temporal and spacial control of drug release, (4) therapeutic advantage gained by less fluctuation in drug levels, better patient compliance and ultimately "personalized" systems whose release program is responsive to physiological/ pharmacological events and (5) marketing considerations.

Sophisticated analytical support in the form of improved technology and methodology is necessary to evaluate these delivery systems. Furthermore, advances in

analytical chemistry will also be required to give
pharmaceutical scientists a mechanistic understanding at
the cellular/molecular level of luminal movement of
solutes and their transepithelial transport as will be
required for rational design of improved delivery systems.
The necessary analytical methodology must offer sufficient
specificity to monitor the drug and key degradation
products in the presence of matrix components. In certain
situations, ability to monitor the intact delivery device
or specific products of its bio-erosion may be avantageous
to optimize overall performance. Evaluation of such
therapeutic systems will also require analytical support
offering exquisitely high sensitivity. The sensitivity
requirement is based on (1) the low levels of drug
anticipated to be found following this type of delivery
due both to the therapeutic advantage gained by delivering
certain drugs slowly and the tendency to deliver potent
drugs with short biological half lives with such systems
and (2) the need to access drug localization at organ,
cellular and even subcellular levels to design and
evaluate sophisticated formulations. A final area
requiring the development of improved analytical
technology is the evolution of closed-loop delivery
systems, in which physiological processes occurring
systemically feed signals back to the delivery system
resulting in appropriate alteration in the drug release
profile. Such devices require the incorporation of a
highly sensitive sensor which is in contact with the
biological environment and capable of sending a control
signal to the delivery system to alter its therapeutic
program appropriately.

SPECIFICITY CONSIDERATIONS

Monitoring any drug in a biological system is
complicated by the heterogeneity of the matrix in which
the analyte(s) reside(s). Matrix composition is unknown
and variable, not only differing from patient to patient,
but also showing intrapatient variability influenced by
diet, emotional and physical status, and secondary agents
administered with the drug of interest. The drug must be
separated from these matrix components, which are often
present at concentrations order of magnitudes greater than
the analyte itself.

Many drugs are of limited stability in biological systems. Some undergo facile chemical degradation; others require enzymatic transformation to produce the active species; and still others undergo extensive metabolic degradation. Thus, methodology must not only offer specificity adequate to separate the drug from matrix components, but it must also be capable of differentiating among drug-derived species (e.g., metabolities, degradation products) which differ only subtly from one another. More recently with interest in polypeptide and protein delivery, concerns of accessing physical stability (e.g., fibril formation, folding) have been raised. Consequently, a great deal of concern exists and a significant effort is often expended in order to introduce adequate specificity in the design of bioanalytical methodology.

Generally, a bioanalytical procedure can be separated into four stages: (a) gross separation of analytes from the biological matrix, (b) high efficiency separation of compound(s) of interest from their (bio)degradation products and from endogenous contaminants, (c) detection and, (d) signal processing and data manipulation. Specificity can be introduced into the methodology at any of these stages.

Immunochemical techniques can be used to provide selectivity where specificity is determined by the magnitude of the binding constant between antigen and antibody and the cross-reactivity of the latter with other haptens. Immunoassays are generally based on the principle of competition between analyte and a tracer form of the analyte (i.e., tagged radiochemically, with an enzyme or with a fluorescent probe) for specific sites on an antibody (which views the analyte as an antigen). The specificity and reproducibility of these techniques have been vastly improved by the availability of monoclonal (from hybridomae technology) antibodies. Furthermore, adaptations of this methodology, no longer require physical separation of "free" and "bound" pools of the tracer as part of the analysis sequence.

Enzyme-based methods of analysis also offer a high level of specificity which not only provide for structural recognition but chiral discrimination as well. Both direct and indirect enzyme assays have been described.

Specificity in drug analysis has most commonly been introduced in a chromatographic step. HPLC has emerged as a powerful tool for achieving the selectivity required for informative clinical analysis. For some applications, however, the specificity provided by common HPLC systems is insufficient. For example, in situations where discrimination among enantiomeric mixtures is required, modifications of stationary phase or mobile phase have been made to provide chiral recognition. Chiral stationary phases have been prepared and then covalently or ionically bonded to γ-mercapto- (Pirkle & House, 1979) or γ-aminopropyl (Pirkle & Finn, 1981) silanized silica microparticles. Such materials have been successfully used to resolve racemates without the need for converting them into diastereomeric mixtures prior to chromatography. Most notable have been the efforts of Pirkle, who, using a chiral fluoro alcohol phase (Pirkle & House, 1979), was able to separate enantiomeric sulfoxides, amines, amino acids, alcohols, hydroxy acids, lactones and mercaptans, and on a chiral N-(3,5-dinitrobenzoyl) phenyl glycine phase (Pirkle & Finn, 1981) could resolve enantiomeric arylalkylcarbinols.

A second approach to resolve optical isomers is to add chiral reagents to the mobile phase that interact with asymmetric analytes via metal ion-based complexation, as demonstrated by Nakazawa and Yoneda (1978). Hare and Gil-Av (1979) have separated some underivatized D,L-amino acids on an ion-exchange column through the direct addition of the L- (or D-) proline-Cu(II) complex to the mobile phase. More recently, amino acid racemates have been resolved (as their dansyl derivatives; Lindler et al, 1979) on reverse phase columns by the addition of the chiral chelate L-2-isopropyl-4-octyl-diethylenetriamine-Zn(II) to the mobile phase. A possible structure of the resulting "diastereomeric" mixed complex is shown below (1). Thus, manipulation of stationary phases and more often mobile phases can be utilized to achieve dramatic specificity advances in bioanalysis of drugs, not only in optical isomer separation, but for a wide variety of separation problems.

SENSITIVITY CONSIDERATIONS

One of the greatest therapeutic benefits to be derived

1

from controlled release systems will be in the delivery of potent, short-lived drugs, where exquisitely low ($\leq$ pg/ml) analyte levels will be achieved. Accordingly, an increased demand on improved detectability (without compromising precision and accuracy) is being placed on analytical technology. Several approaches have been taken to achieve the necessary sensitivity. Instrumental techniques are preferred from a time- and cost-effective perspective; due to specificity considerations, the detection device must usually be interfaced with a module that separates the components in the mixture. Techniques such as spectrofluorimetry, amperometry and mass spectrometry provide the potential for low level detectability, but only for a limited population of molecules that incorporate specific structural features that yield maximal response from the transducer. Very few drugs possess the physical properties that allow their direct detection at levels much below micromolar. Thus, methodology capable of monitoring the majority of drug molecules at subnanomolar levels requires an indirect approach, where something other than the actual analyte is detected and is then related to drug concentration. Examples of this approach include (1) chemical derivatization of analyte, (2) immunochemical methods and (3) enzyme-based techniques.

CHEMICAL DERIVATIZATION

Derivatization may be introduced into an analytical scheme (a) to enhance the stability of the analyte, (b) to

improve the separation of the analyte from the sample
matrix, (c) to refine the subsequent chromatographic
separation (by improving band shape and/or increasing
resolution of adjacent bands), and (d) to improve
detectability by increasing response to the detector or
by introducing an additional element of specificity into
the determination due to the limited reaction
possibilites of the reagent.

The HPLC analysis of the antineoplastic agent dianhy-
drogalactitol (DAG,2) (Munger, et al, 1977) includes a
prechromatographic derivatization step that incorporates
many of the features delineated below. The hydrophilicity
of the drug prevents its efficient extraction into water-
immiscible solvents, even from salt saturated solutions.
Furthmore, DAG is unstable, binding irreversibly to red
blood cells (in the sample containers) through attack by
endogenous nucleophiles at the epoxide, and also
undergoing intramolecular rearrangement to the thermodynamically more stable 2,3-epoxy isomer, 3. The lack of
chromophoric groups in 2 provides detection limits (> 10
µg ml^{-1} of plasma) that are above that necessary for
clinical monitoring of the drug. These difficulties were
overcome by derivatizing DAG with diethyldithiocarbamate.
Reaction was carried out directly in the blood sample (at
room temperature) and conversion to the bis-dithiocarba-
mate, 4, was quantitative and complete in less than 5 min.
Elimination of the epoxides by conversion of 2 to 4
stabilized the analyte from subsequent nucleophilic
attack. The derivative is more hydrophobic that the
parent drug and can be quantitatively extracted into
chloroform. The derivative chromatographs efficiently and

$$\underline{2} \quad + \quad \begin{array}{c} Et \\ \diagdown \\ N\text{--}C \\ \diagup \quad \diagdown \\ Et \qquad S^{\ominus} \\ \overset{Et \quad S}{} \overset{\parallel}{} \end{array} \longrightarrow \begin{array}{c} \overset{S \quad Et}{\underset{\parallel \quad \diagup}{CH_2\text{--}S\text{--}C\text{--}N}} \\ | \qquad\qquad \diagdown Et \\ H\text{--}C\text{--}OH \\ | \\ H\text{--}C\text{--}OH \\ | \\ H\text{--}C\text{--}OH \\ | \\ H\text{--}C\text{--}OH \qquad Et \\ | \qquad\qquad \diagup \\ CH_2\text{--}S\text{--}C\text{--}N \\ \underset{S \quad Et}{\overset{\parallel}{}} \end{array}$$

$\underline{4}$

strongly absorbs uv light, thus providing a route to its clinical monitoring in blood.

Although this application illustrates the multipurpose nature of derivatization, the approach has been primarily used to extend the utility of sensitive HPLC detectors to compounds that are relatively insensitive to them, by chemically transforming the molecule of interest into a more readily detectable species.

For example, tamoxifen (5a) (used in treatment of metastatic breast cancer) and its two major and potentially therapeutically-active metabolites (5b, 5c) have been analyzed in whole blood by HPLC with fluorescence detection after photochemically-induced oxidation of the drug species to the corresponding phenanthrene, 6 (Mendenhall et al, 1978; Golander & Sternson, 1980). Similarily, trace analyses of amino acids and peptides has often relied on their derivatization by reagents that yield fluorescent or electroactive products (Sternson et al, 1984).

IMMUNOCHEMICAL METHODS

Immunoassays (involving an appropriately "tagged" antigen (Kostenbauder et al, 1974) and immunoradiometric ("tagged" antibody) methods (Secher, 1981) also offer a

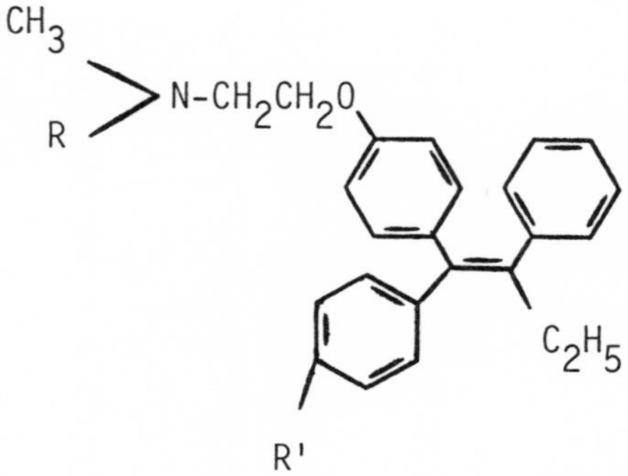

5a R = CH₃; R' = H
5b R = CH₃; R' = OH
5c R = H; R' = H

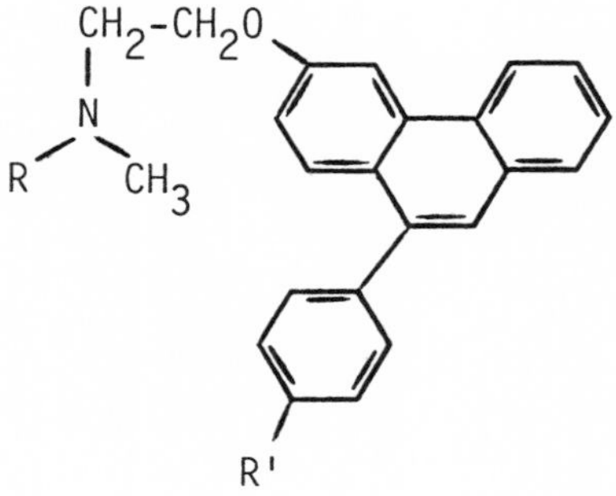

6 (a-c)

high level of sensitivity. These techniques owe their
sensitivity to the remarkably high binding constants (ca
10^{13} M^{-1}) for antibody-ligand interactions and the
nature of the tag. Homogenous assays (not requiring
separation of bound and free fractions) have been
developed and employ enzymes or fluorescent moieties as
tags; they also eliminate the need for radioactive tracers
(Bleka, 1983; Rubenstein et al, 1972).

ENZYMATIC ASSAYS

The specificity of enzymes offers the advantage of
being able to assay appropriate substrates within a
complex mixture with minimal need for their prior
isolation, but this reagent selectivity also limits the

generality of such enzyme-based methods. Most assays
involving enzymes are kinetic methods and often involve
measuring cofactors required of the enzymatic reaction
being exploited. Redox cosubstrates such as the
nicotinamides, allow the site specific oxidation-reduction
of substrates. More importantly to the analyst,
nicotinamides offer a spectroscopic handle on the
reaction. Reduced nicotinamides have a molar absorptivity
of 6220 $M^{-1}cm^{-1}$ at 340 nm (Horecker & Kornberg, 1948).
This allows their detection to about 16 nanomoles (1 ml
16 μM, A_{340} = 0.1, 1 cm pathlength). An increase in
sensitivity of about 50 fold is possible using
fluorescence detection of the reduced nicotinamides.
Chemical alteration of the oxidized nicotinamide using
acetone (Huff & Perlzwerg, 1947; Kaplan et al, 1951) or
strong alkali (Kaplan et al, 1951; Lowry et al, 1957)
produces a highly fluorescent species enabling still
greater sensitivity. Just two of many examples where
optically silent molecules were assayed at very low
concentrations within a complex mixture using enzymes and
fluorometric analysis of the nicotinamide coproduct are
1) the detection of glutamine and asparagine in biological
samples (Nohorski, 1971) and 2) the determination of
aspartate, glutamate and γ-amino butyrate in nerve tissue
(Graham & Aprison, 1966). Therapeutically important
drugs, such as methotrexate (Mtx), can also be monitored
in patient plasma with minimal purification. The strong
competition between the drug and tetrahydrofolate for
sites on the enzyme tetrahydrofolate reductase has been
exploited to determine Mtx concentrations (Seegopaul &
Rechnitz, 1964).

A new dimension in sensitive enzyme-based analysis has
been established, primarily through the creative efforts
of O.H. Lowry with the introduction of enzyme cycling
(Lowry & Passonneau, 1972).

Enzyme cycling is a method of chemical amplification.
Scheme I shows Lowry's nicotinamide cycle in its simplest
form. Any molecule that can be made to enzymatically
oxidize or reduce a nicotinamide cosubstrate can be
measured by this technique. The molecule is first allowed
to enzymatically react (Step A) producing a stoichiometric
equivalent of nicotinamide coproduct. The excess
nicotinamide cosubstrate is then selectively destroyed
(Lowry et al, 1961). The cycling reagent (step B, Scheme I)

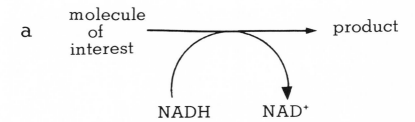

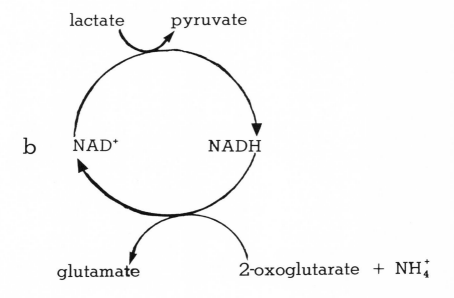

c   pyruvate + NADH ⟶ lactate + NAD⁺

d   NAD⁺ + 6N NaOH ⟶ fluorophore

SCHEME I: Nicotinamide Enzyme Cycling System

is then added, and the remaining nicotinamide coproduct from (A) is cycled between its oxidized and reduced forms. On every complete turn of the cycle, a molecule of glutamate and pyruvate is formed. If cycling is allowed to continue for an hour (at 37°C), an 8000 fold amplification of pyruvate and glutamate results, which can then be measured in a detection step (C & D, Scheme I). Double cycling techniques, taking the nicotinamide product formed in step C and recycling through B have enabled the measurement of 10^{-18} moles of certain cellular metabolites. This represents an amplification factor of about 400,000,000!

We have recently attempted to employ enzyme cycling in peptide analysis (Malefyt & Sternson, 1984). Since enzymes do not exist that are specific for peptides, analysis of these molecules might best be made selective by analyzing one of the constituent amino acids liberated by enzymatic or non-enzymatic hydrolysis of the parent peptide. Glutamate was a logical choice, since it is a terminal residue on a number of hormone peptides, a central product of amino acid and α-keto acid metabolism, and is a neurotransmitter in mammalian brain tissue.

In an attempt to develop a sensitive method based on enzyme-cycling for determination of glutamate, the reactions shown in Scheme II were exploited. Unlike previously described methods, this procedure introduces the principle of geometric amplification, i.e. with every revolution of the cycle, the amount of material within the cycle (i.e. glutamate and glutamine) and the rate of cycling should double. Thus, every 3.2 turns of the cycle will produce a ten-fold increase in the concentration of the coproducts. A geometric scheme should then amplify at a much faster rate. The enzymatic reactions chosen for this cycle are thermodynamically favorable; the reactions catalyzed by glutamine synthetase and glutamate synthase having equilibrium constants[1] of 1200 and 1×10^7,

---

[1] Keq, g. synthetase $= \dfrac{[NH_4^+]\ [ATP]\ [Glutamate]}{[ADP]\ [Pi]\ [Glutamine]}$;

   Keq, g. synthase $= \dfrac{[Glutamate]^2\ [NADP]}{[Glutamine]\ [2\text{-}Oxoglutarate]\ [NADPH]}$

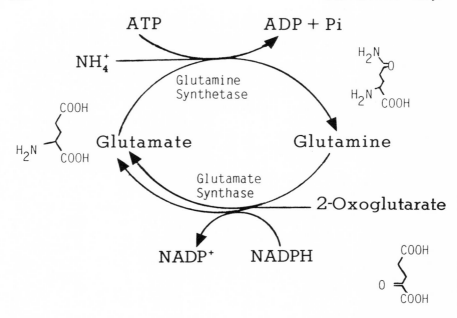

SCHEME II: Glutamine-Glutamate Geometric
             Enzyme Amplification System

respectively. Although a viable approach in theory, this
cycle proved unacceptable for glutamate trace analysis due
to inherent NH3-dependent activity associated with
glutamate synthase (which is induced during enzyme
purification).

     Although we were successful in getting the system to
cycle as predicted, the NH3- activity produces a
background signal that masks the enzyme cycling product at
picomolar levels. Higher levels are detectable by
limiting the amount of glutamate synthase used. Although
Miller et al (1972), Sakamoto (1975) and Schmidt & Jervis
(1980) suggest that the enzyme is glutamine specific and
any ammonia activity arises from glutamate dehydrogenase
contamination, our results support the reports of Mantsala
et al (1976), Bower et al (1983) and Trotta et al (1974)
who claim that glutamate synthase, like all other known
glutamine amidotransferases, has ammonia activity. In

principal, however, the development of cycles involving geometric amplification offer distinct advantage both from the perspective of sensitivity and analysis time. The clever use of enzymes as specific reagents for drug and clinical analysis is an area which offers tremendous potential for achieving additional sensitivity advantages over presently achievable limits.

IMPLANTABLE SENSORS TO CONTROL CLOSED-LOOP DELIVERY SYSTEMS

The development of delivery systems that can vary their release program in response to physiologic or pharmacokinetic events is dependent on the availability of sensitive sensors, in contact with the biological environment that can (1) monitor levels of drug or key endogenous chemicals, (2) process and feed back this information to the delivery device with (3) subsequent appropriate alteration in the release profile. To date, development of the "artificial pancreas" with its associated glucose sensor is the prime example of a closed loop system.

Several versions of sensors to measure blood glucose have been developed. In the first of these devices, a continuous stream of blood drawn from the patient through a special double-lumen catheter was diluted and anticoagulated and then dialyzed against alkaline potassium ferricyanide. Glucose was determined colorimetrically. The more recently developed units use enzyme electrode-based sensors. Glucose oxidase is immobilized in a semipermeable polymer matrix and attached to an oxygen electrode (Clark, 1956). The enzyme catalyzes the reaction between glucose and O_2 to form gluconic acid and hydrogen peroxide. Glucose concentration is measured potentiometrically or amperometrically (Updike & Hicks, 1967) as a function of O_2 depletion. A modification of this sensor was developed by Layne et al (1976) who used two polarographic oxygen probes. The working electrode was covered with the covalently bonded glucose oxidase matrix; a reference electrode was covered with a matrix containing no enzyme. A final version of the enzyme electrode measures hydrogen peroxide polarographically rather than O_2 depletion (Clarke & Santiago, 1977). Protective membranes with differential pore sizes protect

the electrode from substances that could interfere with
the measurement.

While this type of sensor works well in an extracor-
poreal device, it has several drawbacks when considered
for implantation uses. First, the length of time during
which an enzyme electrode sensor retains its sensitivity
and stability is short. Second, it becomes encapsulated
by fibrotic tissue and communication with surrounding
body fluid is disrupted shortly after implantation.

One way to avoid the problem of rapid degradation of
enzyme electrodes is to design a sensor that can operate
without enzymes. Noble metals such as platinum can be
substituted for glucose oxidase to catalyze the oxidation
of glucose. Chang et al (1973) used a fuel cell sensor to
avoid oxide formation on the electrode resulting from the
polarizing potential, and signal drift due to degradation
of the reference electrode. The fuel cell consists of
nonconsumable catalytic anode and cathode, an electrolyte,
and a system of membranes to separate anodic and cathodic
environments. Since the fuel cell measures the electrical
energy generated by the electrochemical oxidation of
glucose, the system needs no applied current nor reference
electrode. This sensor was designed to provide short-term
cycles of negative and positive potential pulses to limit
"poisoning" of the electrode surface. In vivo tests were
conducted with these units for up to 117 days. Sensor
derived values were not compared with standard methods of
blood glucose determination although responses following
meals and during glucose tolerance tests appeared to be
within anticipated ranges. One major difficulty with the
electrochemical sensor is that it is relatively
nonspecific, responding to a variety of endogenous
substances such as ethanol, urea, monosaccharides other
than glucose, and amino acids.

From the examples described in this paper, it is clear
that advances in analytical methodology and technology
will be essential prerequisites in the design, development
and evaluation of sophisticated drug delivery systems -
both in terms of the necessary analytical support to
design improved delivery systems, answer fundamental
questions relating to drug transport as well as for
actual incorporation into delivery devices offering
"personalized" released profiles.

REFERENCES

Blecka, L.J. (1983) Amer. Assoc. Clin. Chem., March issue 1-6. "Fluorescence Polarization Immunoassay: A Review of Methodology and Applications".

Bower, S. and Zalkin, H. (1983) Biochem., 22, 1613-1620. "Chemical Modification and Ligand Binding Studies with Escherichia coli Glutamate Synthase".

Chang, K.W., Aisenberg, S., Soeldner, J.S. and Heibert, J.M. Trans. Am. Soc. Artif. Intern. Organs, 19, 352-360. "Validation and Bioengineering Aspects of an Implantable Glucose Sensor".

Clark, L.C. (1956) Trans. Am. Soc. Artif. Inter. Organs, 2, 41-43. "Monitor and Control of Blood Tissue Oxygen Tension".

Clarke, W.L. and Santiago, J.V. (1977) Artif. Organs, 1, 78-82. "The Characteristics of a New Glucose Sensor for Use in an Artificial Pancreatic Beta Cell".

Golander, Y. and Sternson, L.A. (1980) J. Chromatogr., 181, 41-49. "Paired-ion Chromatographic Analysis of Tamoxifen and Two Major Metabolites in Plasma".

Graham, L.T., Jr. and Aprison, M.H. (1966) Anal. Biochem., 15, 487-497. "Fluorometric Determination of Aspartate, Glutamate, and gamma-Aminobutyrate in Nerve Tissue Using Enzymatic Methods".

Hare, P.E. and Gil-Av, E. (1979) Science, 204, 1226-1228. "Separation of D and L Amino Acids by Liquid Chromatography: Use of Chiral Eluents".

Horecker, B.L. and Kornberg, A. (1948) J. Biol. Chem., 175, 385-390. "The Extinction Coefficients of the Reduced Band of Pyridine Nucleotides".

Huff, J.W. and Perlzwerg, W.A. (1947) J. Biol. Chem., 167, 157-167. "The Fluorescent Condensation Product of N^1-Methyl Nicotinamide and Acetone II: a Sensitive Method for the Determination of N^1-methyl Nicotinamide in Urine".

Kaplan, N.O., Colowick, S.P. and Barnes, C. (1951) J. Biol. Chem., 191, 461-472. "Effect of Alkali on Diphosphopyridine Nucleotide".

Kingdon, H.S. and Stadtman, E.R. (1967) J. Bacteriol., 94, 949-957. "Regulation of Glutamine Synthetase X: Effect of Growth Conditions on the Susceptibility of Escherichia coli Glutamine Synthetase to Feedback Inhibition".

Kostenbauder, H.B., Foster, T.S. and McGovren, J.P. (1974)
    Amer. J. Hosp. Pharm., 31, 763-770. "Radioimmunoassay
    in Pharmacy Practice".
Layne, E.C., Shultz, R.D., Thomas, L.J., Slama, G., Sayler,
    D.F. and Bessman, S.P. (1976) Diabetes, 25, 81-89.
    "Continuous Extracorporeal Monitoring of Animal Blood
    Using the Glucose Electrode".
Lindner, W., LePage, J.N., Davies, G., Seitz, D.E. and
    Karger, B.L. (1979) J. Chromatogr., 185, 323-343.
    "Reversed-phase Separation of Optical Isomers of
    DNS-Amino Acids and Peptides Using Chiral Metal
    Chelate Additives".
Lowry, O.H., Roberts, N.R. and Kapphahn, J.I. (1957) J.
    Biol. Chem., 224, 1047-1064. "The Fluorometric
    Determination of Pyridinium Nucleotides".
Lowry, O.H., Passonneau, J.V. and Rock, M.K. (1961) J.
    Biol. Chem., 236, 2756-2759. "The Stability of
    Pyridine Nucleotides".
Malefyt, T.R. and Sternson, L.A. (1985) Manuscript in
    preparation.
Mantsala, P. and Zalkin, H. (1976) J. Biol. Chem., 251,
    3294-3299. "Glutamate Synthase: Properties of the
    Glutamine Dependent Activity".
Mendenhall, D.W., Kobayashi, H., Shih, F.M. and Sternson,
    L.A. (1978) Clin. Chem., 24, 1518-1524. "Clinical
    Analysis of Tamoxifen, An Anti-neoplastic Agent in
    Plasma".
Miller, R.E. and Stadtman, E.R. (1972) J. Biol. Chem., 247,
    7407-7419. "Glutamate Synthase from Escherichia coli:
    An Iron Sulfur Protein".
Munger, D., Sternson, L.A., Repta, A.J. and Higuchi, T.
    (1977) J. Chromatogr., 143, 375-382. "High Performance
    Chromatographic Analysis of Dianhydrogalacticol in
    Plasma by Derivatization with Sodium
    Diethyldithiocarbamate".
Nahorski, S.R. (1971) Anal. Biochem., 42, 136-142.
    "Fluorometric Measurement of Glutamine and Asparagine
    Using Enzymatic Methods".
Nakazawa, H. and Yoneda, H. (1978) J. Chromatogr., 160,
    89-99. "Chromatographic Study of Optical Resolution.
    II: Separation of Optically Active Cobalt(III)
    Complexes Using Antimony D-tartrate as Eluent".

Pirkle, W.H. and House, D.W. (1979) J. Org. Chem., 44, 1957-1960. "Chiral High-Performance Liquid Chromatographic Stationery Phases. 1: Separation of Enantiomers of Sulfoxides, Amines, Amino Acids, Alcohols, Hydroxy Acids, Lactones and Mercaptans".

Pirkle, W.H. and Finn, M.J. (1981) J. Org. Chem., 46, 2935-2938. "Chiral High-Pressure Chromatographic Stationary Phases. 3: General Resolution of Aryl-alkylcarbinols".

Rubenstein, K.E., Schneider, R.S. and Ullman, E.F. (1972). Biochem. Biophys. Acta, 47, 846-851. "Homogeneous Enzyme Immunoassay: A New Immunochemical Technique".

Sakamoto, N., Kotre, A.M. and Savageau, M.A. (1975) J. Bacteriol., 124, 775-783. "Glutamate Dehydrogenase from Escherichia coli: Purification and Properties".

Schmidt, C.N.G. and Jervis, L. (1980) Anal. Biochem., 104, 127-129. "Affinity Purifiaction of Glutamate Synthase from Escherichia coli".

Secher, D.S. (1981) Nature (London), 290, 501-503. "Immunoradiometric Assay of Human Leucocyte Interferon Using Monoclonal Antibody".

Seegopaul, P. and Rechnitz, G.A. (1984) Anal. Biochem., 56, 852-854. "Enzyme Amplified Determination of Methotrexate with a pCO_2 Membrane Electrode".

Sternson, L.A., Stobaugh, J.F. and Repta, A.J. (1985) Anal. Biochem., in press.

Trotta, P.P., Platzer, K.E.B., Haschemeyer, R.H. and Meister, A. (1974) Proc. Natl. Acad. Sci. USA, 71, 4607-4611. "Glutamine Binding Subunit of Glutamate Synthase and Partial Reactions Catalyzed by this Glutamine Amidotransferase".

Updike, S.J. and Hicks, G.P. (1967) Nature (London), 214, 986-988. "The Enzyme Electrode".

Woolfolk, C.A., Shapiro, B. and Stadtman, E.R. (1966) Arch. Biochem. Biophys., 116, 177-192. "I. Purification and Properties of Glutamine Synthetase from Escherichia coli".

APPLICATIONS OF MINIATURE ELECTRODES TO BIOMEDICAL STUDIES

RALPH N. ADAMS

DEPARTMENT OF CHEMISTRY, UNIVERSITY OF KANSAS

LAWRENCE, KANSAS 66045

Beginning in the 1970s our laboratory began applying modern electroanalytical techniques to problem-solving in neurochemistry and neurobiology--particularly the determination of biogenic amines and related substances both in vitro and in vivo. The in vivo approach utilizes very small graphite electrodes implanted in brain tissue to directly detect catecholamines in the brain extracellular fluid (ECF) space. Several aspects of the in vivo electrochemistry remain exploratory. The techniques have not, in general, been applied to monitoring drug delivery. However, one of their main applications has been to study the effect of drugs on brain biogenic amines. This kind of secondary detection can be utilized as a measure of drug delivery. Furthermore, many electroactive drugs, if present in concentrations greater than those of the endogenous species, could be directly monitored. Thorough treatments of the experimental details have recently appeared (Adams and Marsden, 1982; Marsden, 1984) and the following is a general overview which attempts to summarize some of the applications involving peripherally applied drugs.

BASIC IN VIVO ELECTROCHEMICAL EXPERIMENT

The in vivo electrochemical measurements are, in a sense, quite restricted. They measure only easily electrooxidized components in ECF. Compounds which are reducible cannot generally be studied because of the ubiquitous presence of oxygen in tissue fluid. Oxygen is easily reduced

309

and this signal swamps the detection of other species.

The ease of oxidation of any catecholamine is well known and its initial state proceeds as:

$$\text{(catechol)}\ \longrightarrow\ \text{(quinone)} + 2H^+ + 2e$$

Similarly, although the exact electro-oxidation mechanism is unknown, indoleamines such as 5-hydroxytryptamine (5-HT) and its analogs react as:

$$\text{(5-hydroxyindole)}\ \xrightarrow{\ ?\ }\ P + ne$$

where the questioned arrow indicates oxidation to products, P, and the overall number of electrons liberated, n, is probably 2 to 4. The detailed electrochemistry of these and similar species has been studied and the experimental approaches, applicable to a variety of pharmaceutical systems, have been reviewed (Adams, 1969).

The above reactions involve basic voltammetry experiments. The potential which needs to be applied, E_{App}, is a qualitative indication of the species undergoing oxidation. The current is a quantitative measure of the concentration of electroactive species which react at the electrode surface.

Unfortunately, the catecholamines [dopamine (DA), norepinephrine (NE), etc.] and the indoleamines such as 5-HT and its principal metabolite, 5-hydroxyindoleacetic acid (5-HIAA), are not the only electro-oxidizable species in the ECF. About 200 µM ascorbic acid (AA) and 20-30 µM uric acid (UA) are also present, and these compounds oxidize at potentials very similar to DA, NE and 5-HT. Also it can be noted that the catecholamine structures written above are generic--the side-chain -R indicates any catecholamine or its (non-methoxylated) metabolite. The effect of -R on the ease of oxidation is minimal. Almost all the parent amines and their non-methoxylated metabolites are oxidized at about the same potential. Thus, the major problem, recognized from the beginning of these in vivo electrochemical studies, is one of obtaining selectivity. Although this problem is

still under investigation, several practical solutions have
been found. Electrochemical modification of electrode surfaces has allowed separation of several components (Falat
and Cheng, 1982; Cespuglio et al., 1984; Gonon et al.,
1984). The use of extremely small electrodes provides differentiation (Ewing et al., 1982). Selective ion-exchange
films on the electrode or incorporation of stearic acid in
the electrode matrix work to eliminate interferences
(Blaha and Lane, 1983; Gerhardt et al., 1984). For example,
with a thin film of the anionic polymer Nafion, a graphite
electrode becomes very responsive to the primary neuro-
transmitters DA^+, NE^+ and $5-HT^+$, which are cationic at
physiological pH, but virtually does not "see" the acidic
metabolites and AA or UA (Gerhardt et al., 1984). Although
one still cannot differentiate, for example, DA from NE,
separation of primary transmitters from acidic metabolites
and AA is no longer a problem.

The electrodes themselves are glass capillaries packed
with a mixture of graphite and epoxy resin, or may be carbon fibers suitably sealed in glass capillaries. Sizes
range from 50-250 µm for the graphite epoxy capillary (GEC)
type electrodes to 40 µm or even 8-10 µm for fiber types.
All can be coated with Nafion films or chemically modified
as mentioned above. These working electrochemical (EChem)
electrodes are stereotaxically implanted in the tissue
region desired. They may be used in acute or chronic implants (Adams and Marsden, 1982; Cespuglio et al., 1984;
Gonon et al., 1984; Marsden, 1984). They may also be coupled into multi-electrode arrays with neurophysiological
probes for measuring brain electrical activity. Most recently, we have combined them with ion-selective micro-
pipets (ISMs) to monitor both neurotransmitter and ECF ion
fluxes (Nagy et al., submitted for publication). Further
details of all of the experimental approaches, etc. are
given in the references cited up to this point.

SELECTED EXAMPLES OF IN VIVO ECHEM MEASUREMENTS

The in vivo electrochemistry literature contains numerous examples of measurements of catecholamine release or
increase in turnover, etc. which was induced by various
i.p. drug manipulations. One which is particularly pertinent to the delivery of drugs to target areas and selective
interactions at these sites is discussed below. This work
compared the electrochemical response of two neuroleptic

drugs, chlorpromazine (CPZ) and clozapine (CLOZ) (Huff and
Adams, 1980). CLOZ, although no longer used clinically,
had relatively few extrapyramidal side effects, yet was
clinically valuable as an antipsychotic medication. The
explanation for its behavior was that it preferentially
acted on the so-called mesolimbic DA system with terminal
fields in the nucleus accumbens, but had little effect on
the nigrostriatal DA system whose nerve endings are primarily in the striatum.

Rats were implanted with an array of four GEC electrodes, two each bilaterally in nucleus accumbens and striatum. These were chronic implants, and 24 hours after recovery from surgery the freely moving rats were ready for
the in vivo electrochemical experiments. All electrodes
were measured until stable baselines were obtained and then
i.p. injections of either CPZ (6 mg/kg) or CLOZ (25 mg/kg)
were given. The signals were usually followed for 1-2 hrs.
As seen in Figure 1, both drugs gave approximately equivalent electrochemical signals in the nucleus accumbens.
However, in the caudate-putamen (striatum), while CPZ showed
an even stronger EChem signal than in accumbens, CLOZ gave
no signal increase--indeed, a slight decrease occurred.
Thus, the electrochemical technique gave results which
agreed with clinical observations. CPZ gave increased EChem
signals in both accumbens and striatum, consistent with its

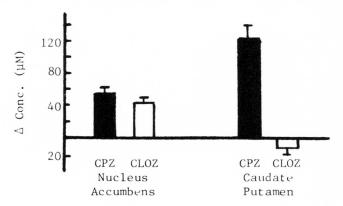

Figure 1

Maximum change in concentration from baseline in the caudate-putamen compared to nucleus accumbens after i.p. injections of chlorpromazine (CPZ), 6 mg/kg (N=4) and clozapine
(CLOZ), 25 mg/kg (N=5).

well-established antipsychotic properties, and moderate-to-strong extrapyramidal side-effects. CLOZ, on the other hand, gave EChem signals in accumbens, in accord with its antipsychotic action, but showed no signal in striatum, consistent with its lack of extrapyramidal disturbances.

Since these electrodes were not pretreated in any way, they undoubtedly responded to the DA metabolite, dihydroxyphenylacetic acid (DOPAC), as well as AA, and some of the recorded signal was certainly due to these components. Despite this, it could be shown that the EChem signals were functionally related to increased activity or turnover at DA nerve terminal regions. Rats were stereotaxically pretreated with 6-hydroxydopamine in the ventral tegmental (A-10) area, which is the source of the cell bodies for DA terminals in the nucleus accumbens. These pretreated animals then showed no signal in accumbens with CLOZ. Hence, it is clear that the electrochemical technique monitored the selective action of CLOZ delivered to two different brain sites (Huff and Adams, 1980).

The above approach can be generalized to other situations involving drug delivery which affects the CNS. If one has EChem electrodes which can monitor some property related to neurotransmitter release implanted in several brain regions, these can serve as detectors for drug delivery. For example, does peripherally injected drug A (assuming it passes blood-brain barrier, of course) affect the frontal cortex and the cerebellum equally--or in the same time frame? The answers to such questions are not automatically known and, in fact, are usually obtained from postmortem assay of the particular tissue regions. Of course, in the electrochemical technique there remains an ambiguity. If one gets EChem response in brain region X and not in Y, the reason for the difference could be that the drug is delivered effectively to X and not to Y--or that the drug is equivalently delivered to both sites, but fails to initiate enhanced transmitter action at site Y. Nevertheless, it would appear that there are numerous instances where EChem signals can be used for such monitoring. This is especially true when one combines the EChem electrodes with ISMs. Here one obtains added information about extracellular ion fluxes which indicate neuronal depolarization (Nagy et al., submitted for publication).

If a given drug is electroactive, its potential inter-

actions with tissue sites can be monitored electrochemically. In this case, the drug is micro-injected close to a
detector electrode so that its local concentration exceeds
that of the endogenous electroactive species (the latter is
not pertinent if the drug oxidizes at considerably higher
potentials than the usual endogenous components). Now one
can essentially monitor the concentration of the drug as a
function of time. If, for example, it reacts quickly with
tissue components, one can observe the rapid decay in concentration; if not, its concentration will decrease more
slowly by mass transport from the site of injection. This
type of experiment was one of the earliest applications of
the in vivo technique and was used to study the rapid interactions of the neurotoxin 6-hydroxydopamine (McCreery et
al., 1974a,b). Here the technique of cyclic voltammetry
enabled one to observe the redox state of the neurotoxin
and its rapid chemical interaction with tissue components.

The in vivo electrochemical study most pertinent to
the present considerations is that concerning the detection
of acetaminophen in the CNS (Morgan and Freed, 1981). This
work was actually designed as an in situ calibration for
EChem electrodes, but if its purpose is turned around, it
is a clear example of drug delivery monitoring. Acetaminophen (ACM) is oxidized at ca. +0.55 V and can be selectively detected by derivative voltammetry techniques. Morgan
and Freed gave i.p. injections of the drug and followed its
EChem signal in the rat caudate as a function of time. Both
blood serum and tissue concentrations were independently
measured by HPLC. The peak blood level was reached in ca.
10 minutes in the rat, whereas the caudate EChem and actual
tissue assay showed a slower rise, reaching a maximum at
ca. 30-60 minutes post-injection. The results are especially satisfying in terms of potential use for monitoring
delivery. Essentially linear dose-response curves measured
electrochemically in the caudate were obtained following
i.p. injections of between 25-100 mg/kg ACM. While this
kind of approach has seldom been used, it deserves further
attention. Naturally, each drug would involve a careful
evaluation. For example, an injected electroactive drug
may be biotransformed into an electroactive metabolite--
indistinguishable from the parent--so that the EChem measurement is really detecting metabolite, rather than parent,
distribution. Alternately, the failure to obtain an EChem
signal may be due to the fact that the original electroactive drug has been converted to a non-oxidizable species

by tissue interaction. Often, these data are known from preliminary metabolic studies and will indicate whether it is possible to employ the electrochemical technique.

Electrochemical on-line monitoring in peripheral tissues, blood vessels, etc. has been practiced for some time. Much of this work has been concerned with pO_2 measurements, but Leland Clark and coworkers have utilized platinum and carbon electrodes for a variety of such measurements in heart and other organs (Clark and Lyons, 1962; Lyons et al., 1963; Clark and Sachs, 1968). A recent monograph surveys a variety of medical applications for electrochemical monitoring devices (Koryta, 1980). These subjects are outside the subject of the present material, but nonetheless illustrate approaches of interest.

In summary, while applications of in vivo electrochemical measurements to specific drug delivery problems are few in number, secondary monitoring through CNS effects appears to be a viable approach. The techniques and instrumentation are actually quite simple, although frequently somewhat unfamiliar to pharmacologists. There are ambiguities in using electrochemical technques--the very nature of the measurement does not afford the specificity of, for example, spectroscopic techniques. There are no "fingerprint" identifications in electrochemistry. On the other hand, there are few techniques which adapt so easily to in situ monitoring, and the sensitivity is extremely good. With the complexity encountered in attempting to monitor the distribution pathways of drugs in living systems, no particular method has general applicability--one must always pick and choose from the wide repertoire of analytical methodology to best fit the individual situation. Hopefully, this brief overview points out some instances in which in vivo electrochemistry can be utilized for certain types of drug delivery problems.

ACKNOWLEDGMENTS

The support of the National Institues of Health via grant NS08740 and the Center for Biomedical Research, University of Kansas, is gratefully acknowledged.

References

Adams, R.N., Applications of modern electroanalytical techniques to pharmaceutical chemistry, J. Pharm. Sci., 58 (1969) 1171-1184.

Adams, R.N. and Marsden, C.A., Electrochemical detection methods for monoamine measurements in vitro and in vivo. In Iversen, L.L., Iversen, S.D. and Snyder, S.H. (Eds.) Handbook of Psychopharmacology, Vol. 15, Plenum, New York, 1982, pp. 1-74.

Blaha, C.D. and Lane, R.L., Chemically modified electrode for in vivo monitoring of brain catecholamines, Brain Res. Bull. 10 (1983) 861-864.

Cespuglio, R., Faradji, H., Hahn, Z. and Jouvet, H., Voltammetric detection of brain 5-hydroxyindolamines by means of electrochemically treated carbon fibre electrodes: chronic recordings for up to one month with movable cerebral electrodes in the sleeping or waking rat. In Marsden, C.A. (Ed.) Measurement of Neurotransmitter Release in vivo, Wiley, New York, 1984, pp. 173-191.

Clark, L.C., Jr. and Lyons, C., Electrode systems for continuous monitoring in cardiovascular surgery, Ann. N.Y. Acad. Sci. 102 (1962) 29-45.

Clark, L.C., Jr. and Sachs, G., Bioelectrodes for tissue metabolism, Ann. N.Y. Acad. Sci. 148 (1968) 133-153.

Ewing, A.G., Wightman, R.M. and Dayton, M.A., In vivo voltammetry with electrodes that discriminate between dopamine and ascorbate, Brain Res. 249 (1982) 361-370.

Falat, L. and Cheng, H.-Y., Voltammetric differentiation of ascorbic acid and dopamine at an electrochemically treated graphite-epoxy electrode, Anal. Chem. 54 (1982) 2108-2111.

Gerhardt, G.A., Oke, A.F., Nagy, G. and Adams, R.N., Nafion-coated electrodes with high selectivity for CNS electrochemistry, Brain Res. 290 (1983) 390-395.

Gonon, F., Buda, M. and Pujol, J.F., Treated carbon fibre electrodes for measuring catechols and ascorbic acid. In Marsden, C.A. (Ed.) Measurement of Neurotransmitter Release in vivo, Wiley, New York, 1984, pp. 153-171.

Huff, R.M. and Adams, R.N., Dopamine release in N. accumbens and striatum by clozapine: simultaneous monitoring by in vivo electrochemistry, Neuropharm. 19 (1980) 587-590.

Koryta, J., Medical and Biological Applications of Electro-
    chemical Devices, Wiley, New York, 1980.
Lyons, C., McArthur, K.T., Clark, L.C., Jr., Edwards, S.
    and Bargeron, L.M., Jr., Functional evaluation of
    surgical procedures for correction of intracardiac
    defects using an autoclavable platinum electrode,
    Surgery 53 (1963) 195-204.
Marsden, C.A., Measurement of Neurotransmitter Release in
    vivo, Wiley, New York, 1984. An excellent comparison
    of electrochemical techniques vs. more traditional in
    vivo techniques such as push-pull perfusion, dialysis
    perfusion, etc.; includes many HPLC approaches.
McCreery, R.L., Dreiling, R. and Adams, R.N., Voltammetry
    in brain tissue: the fate of injected 6-hydroxy-
    dopamine, Brain Res. 73 (1974a) 15-21.
McCreery, R.L., Dreiling, R. and Adams, R.N., Voltammetry
    in brain tissue: quantitative studies of drug inter-
    actions, Brain Res. 73 (1974b) 23-33.
Morgan, M.E. and Freed, C.R., Acetaminophen as an internal
    standard for calibrating in vivo electrochemical elec-
    trodes, J. Pharmacol. Exp. Ther. 219 (1981) 49-53.

THE USE OF SCINTIGRAPHIC METHODS FOR THE EVALUATION OF NOVEL DELIVERY SYSTEMS

S S Davis

Department of Pharmacy
University of Nottingham,
Nottingham, UK.

INTRODUCTION

The advanced delivery systems that are being developed for future clinical use are of increasing complexity and must be evaluated extensively by in vitro and in vivo tests. It is often necessary for research, development and regulatory purposes to have direct information in the following areas:-

i.   The position or distribution of the delivery
     system in the body
ii. The integrity of the delivery system
iii. The in vivo release characteristics

In animal studies it is possible, in theory, to collect such data by sequential sacrifice provided that one has a large enough group and that the rate processes being studied are not too fast. However, with human volunteers, invasive techniques are not applicable, nor can they be used if an important process occurs soon after administration (for example the uptake of colloidal particles by the phagocytic cells of the liver following IV delivery (t50% < 60 seconds).

In our studies on a variety of novel delivery systems we have employed the non-invasive technique of gamma scintigraphy. In this method the drug and/or the delivery system is labelled with a suitable gamma

319

emitting radio-nuclide and the position of the system
and its release characteristics are followed using a
gamma camera. So far to date we have used the method
in studies with animal and human subjects, with
delivery systems administered by a wide variety of
routes (oral, buccal, rectal, pulmonary, nasal,
parenteral). We have borrowed much in the way of
methodology and techniques from the field of nuclear
medicine where aspects of diagnostic imaging have very
similar objectives to drug targeting, namely the
selective delivery of materials to organ or tissue
sites. A book and recent review articles provide for
greater detail than can be given here (Wilson et al,
1982; Davis, 1983; Davis et al, 1984a,b). The reader
is also directed to the pioneering work of Dr George
Digenis and his colleagues at the University of
Kentucky, who were among the first to realise the
applications of scintigraphic methods in the
pharmaceutical sciences (Casey et al, 1976; Digenis,
1982).

RADIONUCLIDE IMAGING

In nuclear medicine techniques are well established for
monitoring the in vivo distribution of gamma emitting
radio-nuclides. A simple device consisting of a small
collimated scintillation detector can be used to follow
changes in activity with time by placing it over an
organ or tissue. This technique has been used with
success to measure circulating levels of activity
(Illum et al, 1982). However, in order to follow and
quantify the distribution of activity on a larger
scale, a gamma camera-computer system is required. A
typical modern camera has a field of view of 40 cm
diameter and consists of a detector made from a large 1
cm thick thallium activated crystal of sodium iodide.
The detector is coupled optically to an array of photomultiplier tubes. A collimator is placed in front of
the detector. This will let through only gamma rays
that fall perpendicular to the camera face. When gamma
irradiation interacts with the crystal, a pulse of
light is produced and the strength and position of the
light is measured by the photomultiplier system. The
detector is linked to a computer system that will
provide display of scintigraphic images. Sophisticated
data recording and handling facilities are normally

available and include colour displays, contour mapping, activity profiles and video tape etc, while various programs allow for data correction, smoothing, subtraction. Tomographic images can be obtained by taking images of the subject from several directions.

PERTURBED ANGULAR CORRELATION

Certain gamma emitting radionuclides can also be used to provide supplementary information about the physical state of a drug delivery system using the method of perturbed angular correlation (PAC) (Digenis, 1982).

Indium-111 decays to cadmium-111 by electron capture and two gamma rays are emitted separated by a small time interval. Coincidence counting techniques can then be used to detect only those emissions having a specific energy and occurring after a specific time interval. Anisotropy in the system will be dependent on the environment of the radionuclide, in particular whether it is in an ordered or disordered state. Drug delivery systems labelled with indium-111 have been used to follow tablet disintegration, the melting of suppositories and the integrity of liposomes (Digenis, 1982; Jay et al, 1983; Mauk et al, 1980).

CHOICE OF RADIONUCLIDE

The radionuclide used in drug delivery studies must be one that emits only minimal amounts of particulate radiation, has the correct energy characteristics for external imaging and an appropriate half-life for the study in question. The optimal energy for gamma rays for detection by the gamma camera are 100–250 keV but lower and higher energies (70–400 keV) can be utilised. If the energy is too low a high proportion of the radiation will be absorbed by the body tissues, while for high energies it is difficult to shield the detector against unwanted radiation (Kelly, 1982). The half-life of the radionuclide should be long enough such that there will be time to prepare the delivery system and perform the study, but (in human studies) short enough to minimize the radiation dose to the subject. Some of the radionuclides used in medical practice that can be utilized in formulation studies are given in Table 1. The available isotopes of

TABLE 1
Radionuclides for use as labels in studies on drug delivery systems

Radio-nuclide	$T_{1/2}$	Energy (keV)	Comments
^{11}C	20.5 m	510	Cyclotron produced positron emitters
^{13}N	10.0 m	510	
^{15}O	2.0 m	510	
^{18}F	110 m	511	
^{75}Se	118.5 d	136 and 265	Good energy characteristics but long half life
^{99m}Tc	6.02 h	140	Ideal character-istics for scintigraphy
^{111}In	2.81 d	171 and 245	
^{113m}In	100 m	393	
^{123}I	13.3 h	159	Good characteristics for imaging but restricted availability
^{125}Sb	2.8 y	408(main intensity)	Poor energy characteristics. Native isotope for Pentostam
^{131}I	8.05 d	360	
^{197}Hg	2.7 d	77 and 69	

carbon, nitrogen and oxygen are all short lived positron emitters that are prepared by a cyclotron method. The positrons combine with electrons with the simultaneous emission of two 511 keV gamma photons in opposite directions. This allows for tomographic imaging using special equipment (PET scanning).

Examples of the utilisation of short lived radionuclides in the study of the tissue distribution of drugs have been given by Digenis (1982). The short half lives and cyclotron preparation necessitate that such systems can only be used in laboratories equipped for production of labelled intermediates and rapid syntheses. The great advantage of such systems is the ability to label a drug compound with a native label and thereby follow pharmacokinetic processes in a non-invasive manner. Native labels are rarely available for studies with drug delivery systems, antimony-125 in sodium stibogluconate (Pentostam) is an exception.

LABELLING OF DRUG DELIVERY SYSTEMS

As discussed above, it is not normally possible to include a native label in a drug molecule and thereby to follow the release, absorption, metabolism and excretion of the compound. Exceptions include those drugs that contain iodine, antimony, mercury, or where it is possible to prepare a labelled compound whose biodistribution mimics those of the unlabelled compound (eg ^{75}Se-labelled bile acids, ^{111}In-labelled bleomycin) (Counsell and Ice, 1975). In studies in drug delivery, model labelled substances can be used to mimic the release behaviour of the drug substance of interest, and/or the carrier system can be labelled. In this way it is possible to follow the distribution and release characteristics of the delivery system. For instance a non-disintegrating controlled release tablet can be labelled with the material ^{99m}Tc-DTPA (diethylenetriaminepentaacetic acid) and the transit and the release behaviour within the gastrointestinal tract can be followed. Alternatively, it is possible to have two labels of different energy levels that can be measured concurrently with the gamma camera. Thus one can follow the fate of the model drug and the delivery system. The release behaviour of the model compound and a real drug can be matched by in vitro tests and the pharmacokinetics of the drug can be measured during the scintigraphic study, using conventional blood or urine level determinations. The quantity of material required to label a delivery system is extremely small in contrast to X-ray methods where the physical nature of the system (especially density) may be modified adversely.

Some examples of the labelled materials used in studies on drug delivery systems are given in Table 2. Chemical modifications of some of these compounds in the form of analogues and prodrugs have been described. As far as labelling the delivery system itself is concerned, the methods depend largely upon the availability of groups within the system to which a label can be attached covalently (eg iodination of double bonds in proteins, phospholipids, oils) or be entrapped. An obvious but essential step in the labelling procedure is the extensive testing in vitro (and in vivo) to ensure that the label remains firmly attached to the material in question (eg model drug, delivery system) or that the release rate is known. In some instances apparently stable labels can be released quite rapidly in vivo (metabolism, transiodination) (Counsell and Ice, 1975). Even the well known sulphur colloid used in radiodiagnosis has poorly defined stability characteristics (Davis et al, 1984b).

In human studies, labelled DTPA is a useful marker since it is not absorbed from the gastrointestinal tract (but is taken up from the nose and lungs). More lipid soluble chelating agents such as oxine and HIDA derivatives of various structures can also be used safely in man. In animal studies ^{131}I labelled rose bengal and iodohippuran are good models for water soluble compounds while ^{75}Se labelled norcholestenol is a good model for lipophilic compounds, particularly steroids.

IMAGING PROCEDURE

Some studies, particularly in the field of gastro-intestinal transit and the evaluation of controlled release systems for oral delivery, are best carried out in human subjects, since animal models are poor predictors of performance in man. Studies on novel drug delivery systems and drug targeting are by

TABLE 2
Radiolabelled compounds used as model drugs in studies
on drug delivery systems

Chemical name	Abbreviation	Label	Application
Diethylenetri-aminepentaacetic acid	DTPA	^{99m}Tc ^{111}In ^{113m}In	Controlled release system GI tract
N-(N'-(2,6-di-methphenyl)) carbonylmethyl iminodiacetic acid	HIDA	^{99m}Tc	Controlled release systems GI transit
4,5,6,7-tetra-chloro-2',4',5', 7'-tetraiodo fluorescein, sodium	Rose bengal	^{131}I	Drug targeting
6 -methyl-(^{75}Se)-selenomethyl 19-norcholest-5(10)-en-3 -ol	Norchol-estenol	^{75}Se	Drug targeting
o-iodohippurate sodium	Iodo-hippuran	^{131}I	Drug targeting
8-hydroxy-quinoline	Oxine	^{111}In	Controlled release systems, GI transit, drug targeting

necessity carried out using animal models. However, in cancer chemotherapy certain delivery (liposomes) and diagnostic systems have been studied in patients. The rabbit is particularly suitable for radio-nuclide imaging studies because of its size and temperament. The dog and monkey are also good candidates but are limited usually by expense. The rat and mouse have been used widely in the liposome field for following drug targeting but they present some difficulties with regard to organ size although these can often be circumvented using focussing (pin hole) collimators. Small rodents have the advantages of low cost and the ease of producing tumour bearing animals.

Imaging is performed with the subject placed next to the collimator and recordings made as dictated by the nature of the study design. Dynamic images of 2 second duration can be made to follow rapid processes while events happening over longer time scales can be followed by static imaging where activity is recorded typically for 60 seconds at intervals over an extended period of time (30 days or longer if the radionuclide has a suitable half-life). Effects due to the attenuation of radioactivity due to depth within the body need to be accounted for, particularly with human subjects. With most modern gamma cameras it is possible to use two radionuclides of different energy spectras concurrently. In this case, corrections have to be made for the "scatterdown effect" from one radionuclide into the photopeak of the lower energy radionuclide (eg ^{111}In and ^{99m}Tc). The choice of dose levels is also important. In a typical study in man the dose levels for ^{99m}Tc and ^{111}In would be 4 MBq and 0.25 MBq respectively, to allow imaging to be undertaken concurrently over a 24 h period.

SELECTED EXAMPLES OF STUDIES ON NOVEL DRUG DELIVERY SYSTEMS

In order to illustrate the manner in which gamma scintigraphy can be used to follow the fate of novel drug delivery systems, some examples will be selected for different types of delivery system, routes of administration and in vivo subjects. To date, in our group at Nottingham we have used the method for a wide variety of systems as an adjunct to biopharmaceutical studies. Since our research camera was purchased more than 100 publicatons have resulted and more detailed accounts are given in the pharmaceutical literature. Other groups elsewhere have been similarly engaged, for example Dr George Digenis in Kentucky, USA, and Dr John Fell, Manchester, UK.

The Gastrointestinal Tract

The transit of novel delivery systems through the gastrointestinal tract can be followed using appropriately labelled formulations. The earlier literature was concerned with aspects of gastric residence and gastric emptying, while more recently intestinal transit times and positioned delivery of drugs have been investigated using normal young or elderly subjects as well as ileostomy subjects. The scintigraphic procedure has been employed to answer one or more of the following questions:-

- does the dosage form get stuck in the oesophagus/stomach/intestine?
- where does the dosage form disintegrate?
- how much spreading occurs with a multiple unit system and how is this controlled?
- what is the release rate from a matrix system in vivo?
- do solutions and suspensions and solid dosage forms have different transit behaviour?
- what is the effect of food/age/position/pathology/drugs on transit?
- how does the pharmacokinetic profile of the drug relate to position of the dosage form in the GIT?
- is it possible to achieve positioned release in the colon or close to an absorption window?
- can transit times be altered by the use of formulation variables, eg density, mucoadhesives, viscosity enhancers?
- how effective is an enteric coating?
- do floating tablets/capsules work?
- is a particular compound absorbed from the colon?

More often than not we have investigated not only pharmaceutical variables, but also physiological and pathological determinants. For example, it is well known that the stomach is able to discriminate between

large particles (> 2 mm) and smaller particles. Large
particles will be retained in the stomach to undergo
digestion, or if non-digestible and non-disintegrating,
to await the end of the digestive phase to then be
cleared from the stomach by the so-called housekeeper
wave (migrating myoelectric complex). Food has an
important effect on the gastric emptying times but very
little effect on transit through the small intestine.
Indeed our recent studies using gamma scintigraphy have
demonstrated that small intestinal transit times are
similar for solutions, pellets and single unit systems
(Davis, 1983). Following emptying from the stomach,
the dosage form will remain in the small intestines for
only 3-4 hours before transit into the colon. Such
figures have implications for the design and evaluation
of controlled release dosage forms intended for once
daily dosing.

The complexity of the study will dictate the type of
radiolabel to be used and the method of incorporation
into the delivery system. For example, a non-released
label firmly entrapped into a matrix or bound to an
ion-exchange resin can be used to follow transit
behaviour. Similarly, simple labelling procedures can
be used to follow all or nothing processes such as
disintegration, the integrity of an enteric coating or
positioned release.

The concurrent use of two radionuclides of different
energies permits a cross-over study to be conducted on
the one occasion. In this way we have compared the
gastrointestinal transit of pellets and osmotic
devices, pellets of different densities and the release
behaviour of matrix tablets formulated using different
excipients. This approach, although more complicated
in terms of data analysis, has the advantage of
providing a direct comparison in the same individual at
the same time, thereby avoiding the considerable
problem of intra-subject variation even when employing
strict controls on diet etc. As illustrations of the
application of the scintigraphic method, Figure 1 shows
the evaluation of a matrix system labelled with
^{111}In-DTPA that breaks up in the lower small
intestine/colon region, while quantitative information
on the transit of an osmotic device (Osmet)
administered concurrently with a labelled pellet system

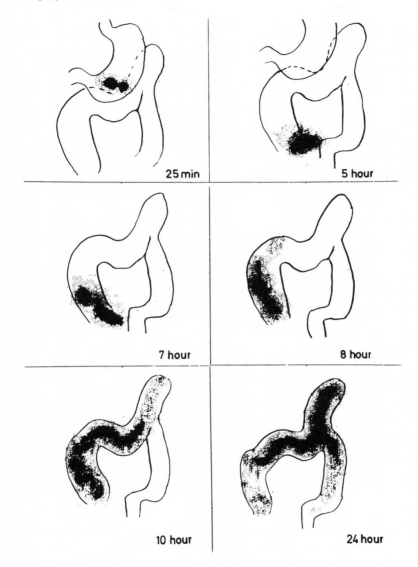

25 min

5 hour

7 hour

8 hour

10 hour

24 hour

FIGURE 1

The gastrointestinal transit and disintegration of a matrix system for positioned release in the colon.

is shown in Figure 2. Not only can the relative
positions of the osmotic device and pellets be
determined but also the quantity of a non-absorbed
marker (^{111}In-DTPA) that has been released from the
osmotic system (Davis et al, 1974c).

Parenteral Administration

Labelled colloidal particles and monoclonal antibodies
are used in diagnostic imaging in order to visualise
tissue sites (eg lung, liver, bone marrow) and
pathological conditions (tumours). Many of the methods
and techniques can be applied directly to drug delivery
and drug targeting. For instance the so-called passive
targeting of drugs to the lungs and liver can be
achieved using microspheres (to include liposomes and
emulsions) of different sizes. Large particles (> 10
um) will be trapped mechanically in the lungs while
small particles (< 5 um) will find their way rapidly to
the cells of the reticuloendothelial system in the
liver and spleen (Illum et al, 1982b). Very small
particles (< 0.2 um) have the possibility to escape to
extravascular sites through small holes or
fenestrations in certain blood vessels (eg liver
sinusoids). Figure 3 shows the different distributions
of activity that can be achieved using colloidal
particles of various sizes. Data describing the
properties of a model system to explore the targeting
of labelled materials to the lung using a microsphere-
ion-exchange system are given in Table 3 (Illum and
Davis, 1982). Subcutaneous and intramuscular
injections can be used to provide sustained release of
pharmacological agents as well as to target of drugs to
the lymphatic system.

Gamma scintigraphy provides an excellent non-invasive
means of following the processes of blood clearance,
organ uptake and redistribution of targeted systems in
the body. As stressed before, attention has to be
taken of the nature of the label, its stability in vivo
and, if studies are conducted on a model drug rather
than the device, the similarities to the final material
to be delivered. Sometimes candidate molecules can be
modified slightly by the incorporation of radionuclides, especially iodine but it should be remembered
that the iodinated compounds may well have different
pharmacokinetic behaviour to the parent compound.

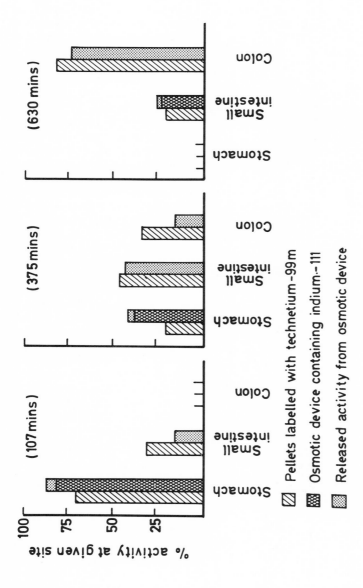

FIGURE 2

Distribution of activity in the gastrointestinal tract from an osmotic device (Osmet)®
and a pellet system.

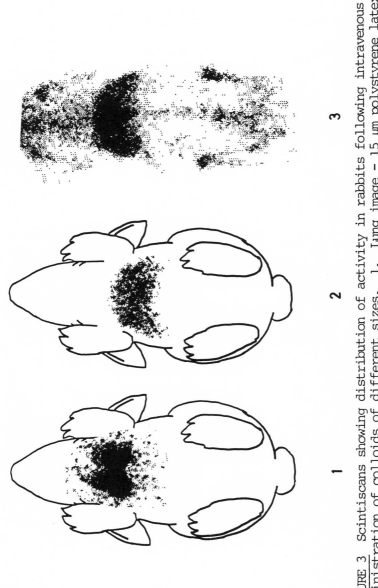

FIGURE 3 Scintiscans showing distribution of activity in rabbits following intravenous administration of colloids of different sizes. 1. Lung image – 15 µm polystyrene latex microspheres labelled with iodine–131. 2. Liver image – 1.27 µm polystyrene latex microspheres labelled with iodine–131. 3. Liver, bone marrow image, technetium–99m–labelled antimony sulphide colloid.

TABLE 3
Delivery of ^{131}I-rose bengal to the lungs using ion-exchange microspheres (DEAE-cellulose)

System	% of initial dose at 3 days	
	Lung	Whole body
Free rose bengal solution	< 1	7
Microsphere delivery system	18	38

Alternatively, model compounds of different physicochemical characteristics can be used to assess the properties of the new delivery system. Thus, scintigraphic methods are usually best employed to explore the properties of the drug delivery system rather than to follow the delivery of one specific pharmacological agent. For example, much has been learnt about the interaction of colloidal particles with the reticuloendothelial system through the use of radiolabelled microspheres, such as polystyrene surface labelled with ^{131}I. The Kupffer cells of the liver are very efficient at removing foreign colloid, and they thereby represent a major obstacle in the targeting of particles to other sites. However, our recent studies indicate that a combination of small particle size and hydrophilic surface coating can result in a significant redistribution (Table 4) (Illum and Davis, 1984a,b).

The kinetics of uptake into tissue sites and the change in tissue levels with time can be followed easily using scintigraphy. Small numbers of animals (n = 3) can be used and large quantities of data can be collected over short and long time scales provided the radionuclide has a suitable half life (eg ^{131}I or ^{75}Se). Figure 4 shows data collected for the intravenous and intramuscular administration of an ethanol/propylene glycol solution containing the labelled steroid ^{75}Se-norcholestenol (Illum and Davis, unpublished results). The initial distribution of the intravenously administered compound to the liver (t50% < 1 min) and the slow clearance from the body (t50% = 1.5d) can be followed in the same small group of animals (n = 3).

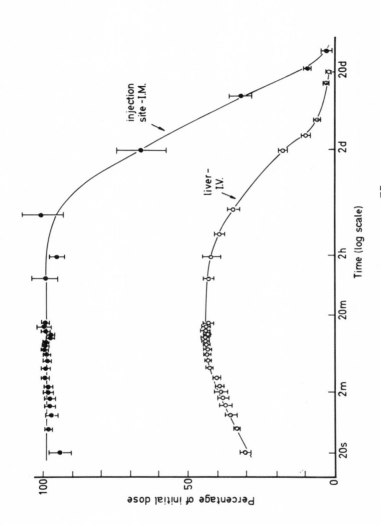

FIGURE 4 The uptake and clearance of a labelled steroid (^{75}Se-labelled norcholestenol) after intramuscular and intravenous administration in an ethanol/propylene glycol solution.

TABLE 4
The effect of particle size and surface coating on the uptake of colloidal polystyrene particles by the body

System	Size μm	Liver/ Spleen	Lung/ Heart	Carcass
Uncoated	1.27	95	5	0
	0.06	90	7	3
Coated with:				
Poloxamer 338	1.27	79	19	2
	0.06	40	30	30
Poloxamer 188	0.06	70	23	7

Pulmonary and Nasal Delivery

The deposition of aerosol formulations in the nose and lungs and their subsequent clearance characteristics can be followed using scintigraphic methods. As for the case of studies on the gastrointestinal tract and parenteral delivery, the study design may well include an investigation of related physiological and pathological factors. Various recent studies have described the use of labelled drugs, eg polymers and albumin microspheres and pertechnetate–drug complexes (Short, 1983; Malton et al, 1982). Our own studies at Nottingham have made use of animal models such as the dog and rabbit. After training both species can be used on a repeated basis to follow aerosol characteristics. The rabbit can be used to study the properties of nebulised systems but is inappropriate for pressurised metered dose systems. The deposition of a test colloid (^{99m}Tc labelled microspheres) in the lungs of the dog is shown in Figure 5. Activity-time profiles through different regions of the lung can be created (Malton, 1984).

Human subjects have been used to determine the deposition and clearance characteristics of novel formulations for nasal delivery (Bond et al, 1984). In healthy volunteers the widespread distribution of the labelled particles (99m-Tc-albumin microspheres) in the

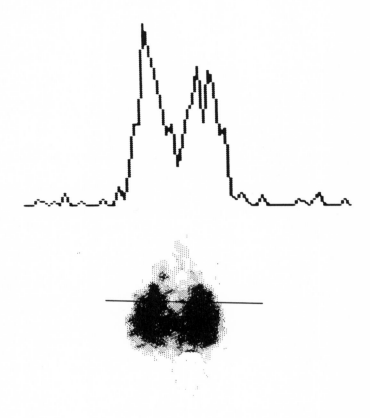

FIGURE 5
Scintiscans showing the deposition of technetium-99m-
labelled albumin microspheres in the lung of the dog and
the horizontal profile of activity through each lung.

nasal cavities was evident. However, in subjects with colds or pathological conditions (nasal polyps) the patterns of distribution and clearance were very different (Lee et al, 1984). Such results have implications for the present attempts to develop novel nasal delivery systems for the delivery of peptides.

CONCLUSIONS

The technique of gamma scintigraphy provides a very useful adjunct to conventional biopharmaceutic and pharmaco-kinetic studies on novel drug delivery systems. In particular it can be used to indicate the fate or position of the delivery system within the body as well as its integrity or release characteristics. Although it is possible to label drug molecules with native labels, such methods are extremely difficult in practice and consequently are restricted to a few specialised centres around the world. Instead radionuclides can be used to label marker molecules or the delivery system itself. The quantities of labelled material are very small, for example less than 1 mg in a matrix tablet, and as a result the physical properties of the system will be unchanged. This is in direct contrast to X-ray methods. X-rays are of course far more suitable than gamma scintigraphy for providing detailed information about anatomical features. However, repeated imaging using normal subjects presents ethical problems. In contrast with scintigraphy the subject is exposed to one decreasing dose that represents normally but a fraction of a conventional abdominal X-ray. Repeated measurements create no further hazard.

An important consideration when using scintigraphic techniques is the stability of the label in vivo and its association with the delivery system. Some studies in the past (particularly the liposome field) have probably followed a label that was rapidly released from the system rather than the system itself. The associated technique of perturbed angular correlation can be used to examine the integrity of a system in vivo.

It should be remembered that gamma scintigraphy is not
the only imaging technique that can be used for studies
on novel drug delivery systems. Ultrasound has a place
in studying subcutaneous implants while future
developments in the field of whole body NMR are awaited
with interest. More powerful magnets and the use of
real time imaging methods (Doyle et al, 1983) could
lead to NMR applications in drug delivery, either by
studying suitable atoms ^{13}C, Na, F etc or by
following drug induced effects.

References

Bond, S.W., Hardy, J.G. and Wilson, C.G., Deposition
and clearance of nasal sprays, Proc. Second European
Congress Biopharmaceutics and Pharmacokinetics, I,
1984, 93-98.

Casey, D.L., Beihn, R.M., Digenis, G.A. and Shambu,
M.B., Method for monitoring hard gelatin capsule
disintegration times in humans using external
scintigraphy, J. Pharm. Sci., 65 (1976) 1412-1413.

Counsell, R.E. and Ice, The design of organ imaging
radiopharmaceuticals, In Ariens, A.J. (Ed.), Drug
Design, Vol. 4, Academic Press, New York, 1975, pp172-
259.

Davis, S.S., The use of scintigraphic methods for the
evaluation of drug dosage forms in the gastrointestinal
tract, In Breimer, D.D. and Speiser, P. (Eds.), Topics
in Pharmaceutical Sciences, 1983, Elsevier, Amsterdam,
1983, pp205-215.

Davis, S.S., Frier, M. and Illum, L., Microparticles as
radiodiagnostic agents, In Guiot, P. and Couvreur, P.
(Eds.), Polymeric Microspheres and Nanoparticles, CRC
Press Inc., Boca Raton, 1984a, in press.

Davis, S.S., Hardy, J.G., Illum, L. and Wilson, C.G.,
Nuclear Medicine Techniques for the Development of
Pharmaceutical Formulations, in Cox, P.H. (Ed.),
Yearbook of Radiopharmacy and Radiopharmacology, Gordon
and Breach, New York, 1984b, in press.

Davis, S.S., Hardy, J.G., Taylor, M.J., Stockwell, A. and Wilson, C.G., The in vivo evaluation of an osmotic device (Osmet) using gamma scintigraphy, J. Pharm. Pharmacol., 1984c, in press.

Digenis, G.A., The utilisation of short-lived radionuclides in the assessment of formulation and in vivo deposition of drugs, In Wilson, C.G., Hardy, J.G., Frier, M. and Davis, S.S. (Eds.), Radionuclide Imaging in Drug Research, Croom Helm, London, 1982, pp103-143.

Doyle, M., Rzedzian, R., Mansfield, P. and Coupland, R.E., Dynamic NMR cardiac imaging in a piglet, Brit. J. Radiol., 56 (1983) 925-930.

Hardy, J.G. and Wilson, C.G., Radionuclide imaging in pharmaceutical, physiological and pharmacological research, Clin. Phys. Physiol. Meas., 2 (1981) 71-121.

Illum, L. and Davis, S.S., Specific intravenous delivery of drugs to the lungs using ion-exchange microspheres, J. Pharm. Pharmac., 34 Suppl. (1982) 89P.

Illum, L. and Davis, S.S., The organ uptake of intravenously administered colloidal particles can be altered using a non-ionic surfactant (Poloxamer 338), FEBS Letters, 167 (1984a) 79-82 (1984).

Illum, L. and Davis, S.S., The kinetics of uptake and organ distribution of colloidal drug carrier particles delivered to rabbits, Proc. Second European Congress on Biopharmaceutics and Pharmacokinetics, II, 1984b, 97.

Illum, L., Hardy, J.G., Wilson, C.G. and Davis, S.S., Gamma ray detection probe for the evaluation of blood activity-time profiles, J. Pharm. Pharmac., 34 Suppl. (1982a) 90P.

Illum, L., Davis, S.S., Wilson, C.G., Frier, M., Hardy, J.G. and Thomas, N.W., Blood clearance and organ deposition of intravenously administered colloidal particles: the effects of particle size, nature and shape, Intern. J. Pharmaceut., 12 (1982b), 135-146.

Jay, M., Beihn, R.M., Syder, G.A., McClanahan, J.S., Digenis, G.A., Caldwell, L. and Mlodozeniec, A., In vitro and in vivo suppository studies with perturbed angular correlation and external scintigraphy, Intern. J. Pharmaceut., 14 (1983) 343-347.

Kelly, J.D., Choice of radionuclides for scintigraphy, In Wilson, C.G., Hardy, J.G., Frier, M. and Davis, S.S. (Eds.), Radionuclide Imaging in Drug Research, Croom Helm, London, 1982, pp39-59.

Lee, S.W., Hardy, J.G., Wilson, C.G. and Smelt, G.J.C., Nasal sprays and polyps, Semin. Nuclear Med., 1984, in press.

Malton, C.A., Biopharmaceutical Studies on Inhalation Aerosols, PhD Thesis, CNAA.

Malton, C.A., Hallworth, G.W., Padfield, J.M., Perkins, A., Wilson, C.G. and Davis, S.S., Deposition and clearance of inhalation aerosols in dogs and rabbits using a gamma camera, J. Pharm. Pharmac., 34 Suppl., 1982, 64P.

Mauk, M.R., Gamble, R.C. and Baldeschweiler, J.D., Targeting of lipid vesicles: specificity of carbohydrate receptor analogues for leukocytes in mice, Proc. Natl. Acad. Sci. USA, 77 (1980) 4430-4434.

Short, M.D., Use of a ^{77}Br-labelled broncho-dilating drug in healthy and asthmatic subjects, Brit. J. Radiol., 56 (1983) 507.

Wilson, C.G., Hardy, J.G., Frier, M. and Davis, S.S. (Eds.), Radionuclide Imaging in Drug Research, Croom Helm, London, 1982, pp330.

APPROACHES TO IMPROVE SPECIFICITY AND SENSITIVITY IN

CHROMATOGRAPHY

Göran Schill

Dept. of Analyt. Pharmaceut. Chem., Uppsala
University Biomedical Center, P.O. Box 574
S-751 23 UPPSALA SWEDEN

The advances in separation and quantification
techniques for organic compounds have been very large
during the last two decades mainly owing to the need for
efficient and mild analytical procedures in biomedical,
biochemical and environmental research. New principles for
liquid-liquid and liquid-solid distribution have been
developed, which have made highly difficult separations
possible.

The problems that meet in the biomedical analysis can
be highly intricate. The analytes (drug, metabolite or
related compound) are often present in concentrations of a
few nanograms or less per ml, and endogenous compounds,
which are often present in much higher concentrations, can
disturb both isolation and quantification. The analytical
approach must be the same as in all kinds of trace
analysis in complex material. Primarily the quantification
method must have sufficient sensitivity. However, the
sensitivity must be combined with selectivity, and this is
often a larger problem since the selectivity depends not
only on the nature of the disturbing sample components but
also on their concentration. This means that the
quantification, as a rule, must be preceeded by an
isolation procedure, and the higher the demand for
sensitivity, the more complete the isolation must be.

341

The nature and concentration of the disturbing (endogenous) compounds are known only to a limited extent and the methodological work cannot be concentrated on the removal of these impurities. It is, instead, necessary to start from the known properties of the analyte with the intention of making the analytical procedures as specific as possible.

Improvement of the selectivity of the method can be achieved along three main lines. 1) Use of phase materials with selective interaction with the sample components to improve the differences in distribution ratios. 2) Use of multicontact procedures, as a rule chromatography, to improve the efficiency of the separations. 3) Use of a selective detection technique as a complement to the improved separation. It is important to have access to a series of different procedures to make combinations possible that will simplify the analysis.

REGULATION OF DISTRIBUTION RATIO AND SELECTIVITY
IN LIQUID SYSTEMS

The separation methods should be constructed so that the distribution ratio and the selectivity can be changed in a systematic way. Organic compounds are by tradition distributed in uncharged form and the distribution ratio can be regulated by the nature of the organic phase, by complexing agents in a liquid organic phase or by pH of the aqueous phase (when the compound is a protolyte). Ionic compounds can only be transferred to an organic phase if they are accompanied by an equivalent amount of an agent of the opposite charge, a counter ion. The distribution can be regulated by the same means as used for uncharged compounds, but the dominating means are the kind and the concentration of the counter ions. This opens unique possibilities for distribution of compounds in charged form which have found wide application in chromatography.

A knowledge of the parameters that govern the distri-

bution equilibria for ionic compounds is a necessary background for the successful application of this technique.
When a charged solute, HA^+, is distributed to an organic
phase of low polarity with the aid of a counter ion, X^-,
ion pairs are usually formed in the organic phase, as
illustrated by the process:

$$HA^+_{aq} + X^-_{aq} = HAX_{org} \qquad \text{Equilibr. const.:} \qquad (1)$$
$$K_{ex(HAX)}$$

If other processes are negligible, the distribution
ratio of HA^+, D_{HA}, is given by the simple relationship:

$$D_{HA} = K_{ex(HAX)} \cdot [X^-]_{aq} \qquad (2)$$

which shows that D_{HA} is governed by the extraction constant, $K_{ex(HAX)}$ and the concentration of the counter ion in
the aqueous phase. Since any kind of counter ion can be
used and the magnitude of $K_{ex(HAX)}$ changes with its
nature, it is obvious that changes of nature and
concentration of the counter ion give almost unlimited
possibilities to regulation of D_{HA} (Schill et al., 1984).

LIQUID CHROMATOGRAPHY

Liquid chromatography, in so called high performance
mode (HPLC), is the dominating isolation technique in the
biomedical analysis. It is characterized by short separation times and high separating efficiency obtained by use
of totally porous micro particles (mean diameter 10 μm
or less) as solid phase.

The techniques for regulation of distribution ratio
and selectivity, mentioned above, are in principle
applicable when the stationary phase is an immobilized
liquid (liquid-liquid chromatography) and when it is a
solid adsorbent (liquid-solid chromatography).

Agents that can bind the analyte to the mobile phase
will decrease its retention while an increase of the bind

ing to the stationary phase by a complexing agent or increase of the adsorbing ability will give a higher retention. An ionic analyte can only be transferred between the
phases if electroneutrality is maintained by a simultaneous transfer of a counter ion or a displacement of an ion
of the same charge as the analyte. The role of the counter
ion as means for regulation of the retention was pointed
out already in the first paper on the technique (Schill et
al., 1965), which has been called ion-pair chromatography
ever since, even if it has not been shown that the process
involves a distribution of ion pairs.

The theoretical relationship between the composition
of the system and the distribution ratio will, in
principle, follow eq. (2) when the stationary phase is a
liquid applied on a solid support, while it is more
complex when the stationary phase is a solid adsorbent
(see Schill et al., 1984 and references therein).

LIQUID–SOLID SYSTEMS

The dominating part of all liquid chromatographic
separations in the biomedical analysis are performed in
the liquid-solid mode with reversed phases, i.e. an
aqueous mobile phase and a hydrophobic adsorbent, usually
surface-modified silica. A solid adsorbing stationary
phase has, contrary to a liquid stationary phase, a
limited binding capacity which opens new, interesting
possibilities for regulation of the selectivity. In a
liquid-solid system, the analyte is retained by adsorption
to the solid phase but mobile phase components might
compete for its limited binding capacity, which will
decrease the retention of the analyte. Both charged and
uncharged mobile phase components can act as competitors
and the effect will increase with the concentration and
the constant for distribution between the phases. The
effect of the charged competitors will also be influenced
by the counter ions. An illustration is given by the
following example.

A series of phenylethyl derivates with substituents in the side chain and in para position in the ring have been chromatographed in a system with a hydrophobic adsorbent (octadecyl phase) and an aqueous, mobile phase containing dimethylcyclohexyl sulfate as counter ion, dimethyloctylammonium as competing cation ("charged modifier") and 1-pentanol as uncharged competing agent (Jansson and Johansson, 1982). The retention can be influenced by all three mobile phase components. Increase of the counter ion concentration (Fig. 1) increases the retention (i.e. the capacity ratio, k') of the amines present in cationic form but to an extent that depends on

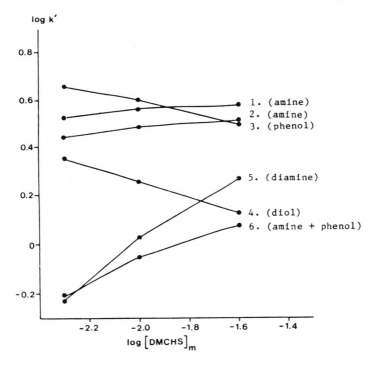

Fig. 1 Influence of counter ion (DMCHS). Mobile phase: DMCHS (dimethylcyclohexyl sulfate) + dimethyloctylamine 0.003 M + 1-pentanol 0.09 M in phosphate buffer pH 2.2. Solid phase: LiChrosorb RP-8. Analytes: phenylethyl derivatives.

the charge and on the nature of the uncharged group in the molecule. Uncharged analytes get a decreased retention owing to competition from adsorbed ion pairs of the mobile phase components. The change in separation selectivity is considerable.

Large changes in the selectivity can also be obtained by increase of the concentration of the charged modifier, dimethyloctylammonium (Fig. 2). All the analytes get decreased retention: largest for the divalent cation and

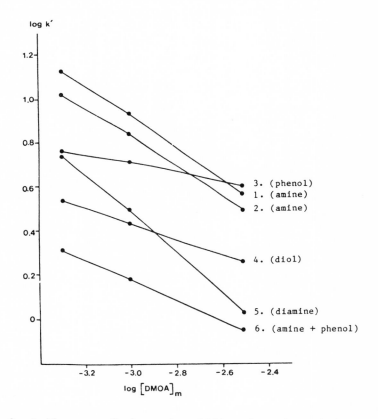

Fig. 2 Influence of charged modifier (DMOA). Mobile phase: DMOA (dimethyloctylamine) + dimethylcyclohexyl sulfate 0.01 M + 1-pentanol 0.09 M in phosphate buffer pH 2.2. Solid phase and Analytes: see Fig. 1.

smallest for the uncharged analyte. A decrease in retention is also obtained on increase of the concentration of
the uncharged competitor, 1-pentanol, but the effects on
the selectivity are much smaller.

APPLICATION OF REVERSED-PHASE LIQUID-SOLID CHROMATOGRAPHY

Reversed-phase systems with a hydrophobic adsorbent
have a widespread use in the biomedical analysis. They are
compatible with aqueous samples which makes them
particularly suitable for hydrophilic analytes. However,
the flexibility of the systems is almost unlimited and
they can be adapted to analytes of widely different
hydrophobicity.

The selectivity of the reversed-phase systems is
often sufficient to allow a direct injection of biological
samples, if the detector has a high selectivity. The
acidic metabolites of acetylsalicylic acid can be determined by direct injection of diluted urine in an ion-pairing system using a mobile phase with pH 7 and tetrabutylammonium as counter ion (Lagerström, 1981). The metabolites (salicylic acid, gentisic acid and salicyluric acid)
are incompletely separated from the endogenous urine components but a satisfying quantification can be obtained by
use of a fluorescence detector that gives response for the
metabolites with a minimum of disturbance from the
endogenous compounds.

The separation between charged and uncharged compounds can be easily improved by use of an ion-pairing
reagent as shown in a method for determination of dopamine
metabolites in rat brain (Magnusson et al., 1980). The
analytes of primary interest are two amines, dopamine and
methoxytyramine, and two carboxylic acid derivatives,
homovanillic acid and 3,4-dihydroxyphenylacetic acid. The
compounds are retained by an hydrophobic adsorbent in
acidic medium, the amines as ion pairs and the acids in
uncharged form. The separation is incomplete in citric
acid buffer, but addition of a hydrophobic anion, hexyl

sulfate, increases the retention of the amines while the
acids are almost unaffected. All the compounds of interest
are phenolic and can be detected amperometrically with
high sensitivity. The only pretreatment of the brain
material is a homogenization in perchloric acid. A clear
chromatogram is obtained which will allow quantification
down to a few picomoles of some of the components.

   Considerable analytical difficulties might appear
when the analyte has about the same polarity as a large
group of endogenous substances, as is the case with one of
the new penicillins, amoxicillin. It is a fairly hydrophilic ampholyte which can be retained in cationic form at
pH < 2.0 and in anionic form at pH > 6.5. The isolation
from urine can be made by a column switching technique in
a system with three separation columns containing the same
hydrophobic adsorbent (octadecyl phase) but different
mobile phases (Schill et al., 1984, p. 153). Amoxycillin
is separated from the impurities in three steps: it is retained in cationic form on the first column, eluted to the
second column in anionic form and finally retained in anionic form on the third column. The selectivity in the analytical process is further improved by a fluorimetric
quantification after post-column coupling to fluorescamine.

LIQUID-LIQUID SYSTEMS

   Liquid-liquid systems for HPLC have for some time
after the introduction of the hydrophobized ("bonded")
solid phases been considered as out of date. Problems with
the instability and quality variations of the bonded
phases have, however, renewed the interest in systems with
a liquid stationary phase.

   Systems with an organic mobile phase and an aqueous
stationary phase applied on silica have been used in the
biomedical analysis for many years. They are suitable for
fairly hydrophobic compounds that can be extracted quantitatively into an organic phase and there are many examples
of the good selectivity that can be obtained with these

systems.

The form for application of the analyte is usually without importance and it will not affect the results if the analyte is injected in uncharged form or as ion pair with any kind of counter ion; the retention is controlled by the properties of the chromatographic system. A method for isolation of apomorphine from a biological sample can give an illustration (Eriksson et al., 1979). Apomorphine is a fairly hydrophilic amine and a highly hydrophobic counter ion (3,5-ditert-butyl-2-hydroxybenzenesulfonate) must be used to get a quantitative ion-pair extraction from the biological fluid. On injection of the extract into the chromatographic system with perchloric acid 1 M as aqueous stationary phase, there is an immediate separation of the components in the ion-pair. Apomorphine migrates with the organic phase as ion pair with perchlorate while the dibutylhydroxybenzenesulfonate migrates (more slowly) with H^+ as counter ion.

Reversed-phase liquid-liquid systems, with a hydrophobic stationary liquid applied on a solid support, have properties that made them an interesting alternative to systems with a solid, hydrophobic adsorbent. With the strongly hydrogen-bonding tributyl phosphate as stationary phase, systems are obtained that are highly suitable for separation of more or less hydrophilic compounds such as catecholamines and related amino acids (Janssen et al., 1980) and carboxylic acids containing several hydrogen-donating groups (Wahlund and Edlén, 1981).

Interesting means for regulation of the separation selectivity exist when the stationary liquid is a solution of a complexing agent in an inert solvent. A method for separation of hydroxy acids and phenols (Stuurman and Wahlund, 1981) uses a solution of the strongly hydrogen-accepting trioctyl phosphineoxide (TOPO) in decane as stationary phase. One molecule of TOPO is coupled to each hydrogen-donating group in the analytes and a change of the TOPO concentration will affect their binding to the stationary phase differently, depending on the

number of binding group. The binding ability of TOPO is
easily regulated by addition of a hydrophobic carboxylic
acid to the aqueous mobile phase.

Further possibilities to change of the separation
selectivity are at hand in systems where the analytes can
migrate both as ion pairs and in uncharged form. Systems
of this kind have been developed for e.g. sulfonamides
(Johansson and Wahlund, 1977) with butyronitrile as
stationary liquid and a buffered solution of tetrabutylammonium as mobile phase. The sulfonamides migrate as
acids at low pH and as ion pairs at high pH. The changes
of the capacity ratio with pH are highly specific for each
analyte and depend on structure-dependent properties such
as pK_a, distribution constant as acid and extraction
constant with tetrabutylammonium.

CONJUGATES

Biological samples are, as a rule, highly complex and
the general goal of the analysis, to give a complete picture of the composition of the sample, can hardly ever be
fulfilled. However, it might even occur that an analytical
method will include an intentional destruction of information. A typical example is the hydrolysis of conjugates
(sulfates, glucuronides) that sometimes precedes the separation and determination procedure. It is, as a rule,
quite needless to destroy this kind of information about
the metabolic changes, since an isolation of such conjugates is easily made in an ion-pair chromatographic
system, c.f. Hoffman et al., 1982.

ENANTIOMERIC COMPOUNDS

Separation and determination of enantiomeric compounds (optical isomers) is a field of highest interest in
the biomedical analysis and important advances have been
made during the last few years. It is well known that
enantiomers of many biologically active compounds often

have widely different effects and there has, for a long
time, been a strong demand for simple methods for determination of the individual isomers of drugs and metabolites in biological material and pharmaceutical formulations. A series of methods based on different principles
have been published lately, c.f. Lindner, 1982.

Our research activities have been concentrated on
liquid chromatographic separations based on interaction
with an optically active (chiral) reagent in the mobile or
the stationary phase. The solid phase has been of a
non-chiral type throughout. Three different principles
have been studied.

Separation of enantiomeric ions as diastereomeric ion
pairs with chiral counter ions has been performed in
systems with a hydrophilic solid phase and the chiral
reagent added to the organic mobile phase. Diastereomeric
ion pairs with different distribution properties can be
obtained if the electrostatic binding between the ions is
supplemented by at least one further attraction and the
work has been concentrated on ions with hydrogen-bonding
substituents. Enantiomeric aminoalcohols, e.g. beta-blocking drugs, have been separated with (+)-camphorsulfonate
as counter ion (Pettersson and Schill, 1982) while chiral
resolution of hydrogen-bonding anions have been made with
counter ions containing an aminoalcohol function
(Pettersson and No, 1983). The fitting between the binding
groups in the interacting ions is of vital importance for
the chiral resolution. Counter ions with the binding
groups in a rigid structure are advantageous: aminoalcohols like quinine, quinidine and cinchonine give considerably better resolution than counter ions with the aminoalcohol function in an aliphatic chain. This indicates
that the topographical conditions on the stationary solid
phase might have influence on the resolution. The separation of the enantiomeric forms of two acids with quinine
as counter ion is demonstrated in Fig. 3. The use of a
UV-absorbing counter ion has the advantage that non-UV-absorbing analytes can be detected with good sensitivity.
The negative peak is due to this indirect detection

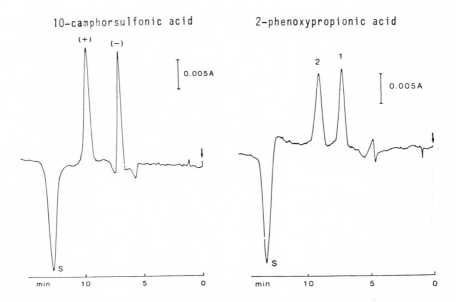

Fig. 3   Separation of enantiomeric acids. Mobile phase:
quinine acetate $3.5 \cdot 10^{-4}$ M in methylene chloride
+ 1-pentanol (99+1). Solid phase: LiChrosorb DIOL.

technique (see below).

    Albumin has a well-known ability to bind enantiomeric
compounds with different strength which can be used in
analytical separation systems. Our studies have been made
with anionic enantiomers in systems with a hydrophobic adsorbent and albumin as a stereoselective coupling reagent
in the aqueous mobile phase (Pettersson et al., 1984). The
chiral selectivity varies strongly with the structure of
the analyte, but separation factors of 5-6 have been
obtained in some cases. The chiral resolution is due to
interaction with albumin in the mobile phase and the analyte is adsorbed to the solid phase in uncomplexed form
only. Good chiral separation can also be made with albumin
or other proteins bound to the solid phase, and it has
lately been reported that cationic enantiomers can be

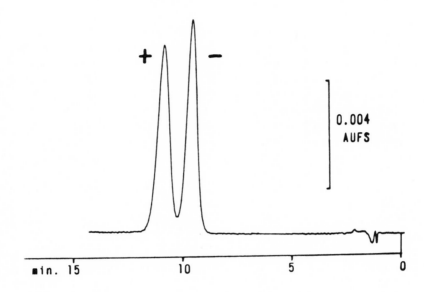

Fig. 4   Separation of norephedrine enantiomers. Mobile phase: potassium hexafluorophosphate 0.09 M in phosphate buffer pH 6. Stationary phase: (+)-di-n-butyltartrate on Phenyl Hypersil.

separated with an α_1-acid glycoprotein-bonded phase (Hermansson, 1984).

   Chiral resolution of aminoalcohols can also be made by ion-pair chromatography in reversed-phase systems with a chiral tartaric acid ester in the stationary phase. The principle has previously been used by liquid-liquid extraction (Prelog et al., 1981) and the studies in our group have been performed with (+)-di-n-butyltartrate applied on a hydrophobic solid phase. Good chiral selectivity has been found for primary and secondary aminoalcohols with moderately hydrophilic character such as ephedrine and pseudoephedrine (Pettersson and Stuurman, 1984) (Fig. 4).

INDIRECT DETECTION

One of the major problems in liquid chromatography is the absence of a simple and general detection technique with high sensitivity. UV, fluorescence and electrochemical detectors will only give high response for analytes with certain specific structures and pre- or postcolumn derivatizations are often necessary to reach a satisfactory sensitivity level. However, the derivatization reactions are also more or less specific and hardly suitable for detection of unknown sample components.

A general and sensitive detection technique, usually called indirect detection, can be based on the ion-pair distribution principle in reversed phase systems (Denkert et al., 1981; Hackzell and Schill, 1982; Rydberg et al., 1983). A UV-absorbing or fluorescent ion is included in the mobile phase and distributed to the hydrophobic adsorbent that is used as stationary phase. The analytes will influence the distribution of the detectable ion by binding or displacement and give rise to a detector response even when they are devoid of inherent detectable properties. The peaks of the analytes can be positive or negative, depending on the retention and charge of the analytes relative to the detectable mobile phase ion (the probe). The latter also gives rise to a peak with constant retention (the system peak), which can be positive or negative depending on the nature of the injected sample (Fig. 5; Crommen, 1984).

The basis for good detection sensitivity is a probe with high detectability owing to molar absorptivity, fluorescence or other properties. In UV-absorbing systems, the probe can be present in such concentration that the base-line absorbance is 0.5 - 0.7, without causing a disturbing increase in noise. The peaks of the analytes correspond to a very limited change in absorbance, usually less than 1%.

The detection sensitivity changes strongly with the retention of the analyte. An illustration is given in Fig.

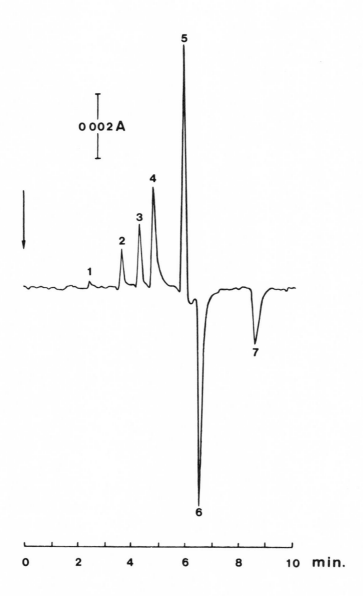

Fig. 5 Separation of amino acids. Mobile phase: DOPA
$2 \cdot 10^{-4}$ M in 0.05 M phosphoric acid. Solid phase:
Ultrasphere ODS. Detection 280 nm.

6 which shows the relationship between the relative retention (k'_{sample}/k'_{system}) and the detection sensitivity obtained with a UV-absorbing cation as probe. The sensitivity is expressed by a conditional molar absorptivity ε^x,
which is the quotient between the peak area expressed in
absorbance units and the amount of analyte injected.

The sensitivity is at a maximum when the relative retention is close to unity. A high response is, however,
obtained in a rather wide range, and a series of

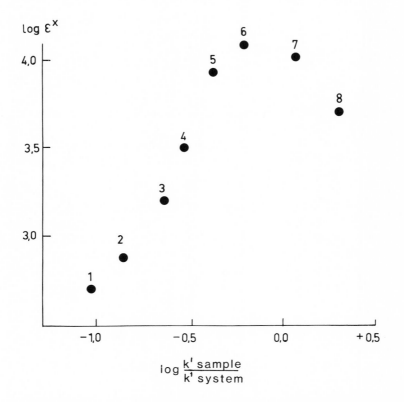

Fig. 6 Detection of hydrophobic, non-UV-absorbing ions.
Mobile phase: N,N-dimethylprotripyline $1.8 \cdot 10^{-5}$ M in
acetic acid 0.01 M. Solid phase: Nucleosil CN. Detection:
292 nm. Analytes: 1 = octylamine, 2 = octanesulfonate, 3 =
octyl sulfate, 4 = decylamine, 5 = tetrabutylammonium, 6 =
undecylamine, 7 = dodecylamine, 8 = tetrapentylammonium.

hydrophobic, non-UV-absorbing analytes with a relative
retention between 0.2 and 2 can be detected in this system
with a sensitivity which corresponds to a molar
absorptivity between 3000 and 12000.

Because the detection sensitivity is so highly dependent on the retention, it is important to adapt the
chromatographic system to the properties of the analyte.
A change in the nature of the probe is the main means for
this adaptation and it is favourable if analyte and probe
have similar retention. The change of probe must often be
supplemented by a change of solid phase and nondetectable
mobile phase components in order to get a suitable retention. Hydrophilic analytes should be detected in systems
with a hydrophilic probe, e.g. sulfanilic acid or methyl-
pyridine but a strongly binding solid phase such as a
rigid polystyrene must then be used as solid phase. Highly
hydrophilic analytes should, on the other hand, be run in
systems with a highly hydrophobic probe, e.g. N,N-di-
methylprotriptyline, using a DIOL phase or similar
adsorbent with low binding ability.

A widespread use of the indirect detection technique
can hardly be expected owing to the fact the theoretical
background is difficult to generalize. The application of
the technique is, however, so simple that it is worthwhile
to develop detection systems of this kind for specific
routine or research purposes.

HIGH DETECTION SENSITIVITY

The research on methods for improved analytical
sensitivity is very intense at present. Concentration
levels of a few ng/ml can today be determined with good
accuracy in many bioanalytical procedures, but all
attempts to reach a considerably lower level, e.g. 10
pg/ml or lower, will face large problems and new analytical procedures must be developed. This will include e.g.
use of microcolumn technique in the chromatographic
systems, c.f. Novotny et al., 1984, in combination with

detection methods with higher sensitivity such as laser
fluorescence and chemiluminescence. The latter technique
has been successfully applied by Imai et al. (1984) who
have determined 2-3 femtomoles of dansylamino acids with
good precision after a chromatographic separation. It
might also be necessary to use new materials in the
analysis equipment to avoid the problem with loss of
analyte by adsorption during the work-up of the sample.

REFERENCES

Crommen, J., Ion-pairing detection technique in
    reversed-phase high-performance liquid chromatography
    of drugs and related compounds. J. Pharm. Biomed.
    Anal. 1 (1983) 549-555.
Denkert, M., Hackzell, L. Schill, G. and Sjögren, E.,
    Reversed-phase ion-pair chromatography with
    UV-absorbing ions in the mobile phase. J. Chromatogr.
    218 (1981) 31-43.
Eriksson, B.-M., Persson, B.-A. and Lindberg, M., Deter-
    mination of apomorphine in plasma and brain tissue by
    ion-pair extraction and liquid chromatography. J.
    Chromatogr. 185 (1979) 575-581.
Hackzell, L. and Schill, G., Detection by ion-pairing
    probes in reversed-phase liquid chromatography.
    Chromatographia 15 (1982) 437-444.
Hackzell, L., Rydberg, T. and Schill, G., Construction of
    systems for detection and quantitation by
    UV-absorbing mobile-phase ions in reversed-phase
    chromatography. J. Chromatogr. 282 (1983) 179-191.
Hermansson, J., Direct liquid chromatographic resolution
    of racemic drugs using α_1-acid glycoprotein as the
    chiral complexing agent in the mobile phase. J.
    Chromatogr. 298 (1984) 67-78.
Hoffman, K.-J., Arfwidsson, A. and Borg, K.O., The
    metabolic disposition of the selective β_1-adrenore-
    ceptor agonist prenalterol in mice, rats, dogs and
    humans. Drug Metabol. Dispos. 10 (1982) 173-179.
Imai, K., Miyaguchi, K. and Honda, K., HPLC-chemilumines-
    cence detection of fluorophores. J. Chromatogr.

(1984) In press.

Janssen, H.L.J., Tjaden, U.R., de Jong, H.J. and Wahlund, K.-G, Reversed-phase ion-pair partition chromatography of biogenic catecholamines and their α-methylhomologues with tributyl phosphate as stationary phase. J. Chromatogr. 202 (1980) 223-232.

Jansson, S.O. and Johansson, S., Regulation of selectivity in the separation of pafenolol and potential impurities by reversed-phase ion-pair chromatography. J. Chromatogr. 242 (1982) 41-50.

Johansson, M.I. and Wahlund, K.-G., Reversed-phase liquid chromatographic separations of sulfonamides and barbituric acids as acids and ion-pairs. Acta Pharm. Suec. 14 (1977) 459-474.

Lagerström, P.-O., Liquid chromatographic determination of drugs in urine by direct injection onto a reversed-phase column. J. Chromatogr. 225 (1981) 476-481.

Lindner, W.F., Resolution of optical isomers by gas and liquid chromatography in Frei, R.W. and Lawrence, J.F. (Eds) Chemical Derivatization in Analytical Chemistry, Vol. 2, Plenum Press, New York, 1982, pp. 145-190.

Magnusson, O., Nilsson, L.B. and Westerlund, D., Simultaneous determination of dopamine, DOPAC and homovanillic acid. Direct injection of supernatants from brain tissue homogenates in a liquid chromatography - electrochemical detection system. J. Chromatogr. 221 (1980) 237-247.

Novotny, M., Karlsson, K.-E., Konishi, M. and Alassandro, M., New biochemical separations using precolumn derivatization and microcolumn liquid chromatography. J. Chromatogr. 292 (1984) 159-167.

Pettersson, C. and Schill, G., Chiral resolution of aminoalcohols by ion-pair chromatography. Chromatographia 16 (1982) 192-197.

Pettersson, C. and No., K., Chiral resolution of carboxylic and sulphonic acids by ion-pair chromatography. J. Chromatogr. 282 (1983) 671-684.

Pettersson, C., Arvidsson, T., Karlsson, A.-L. and Marle, I., Chromatographic resolution of enantiomers by use

of albumin as complexing agent in the mobile phase.
J. Pharm. Biomed. Anal. (1984) In press.

Pettersson, C. and Stuurman, H.W., Direct separation of
enantiomers of ephedrine and some analogues by
reversed-phase LC using (+)-di-n-butyltartrate as the
liquid stationary phase. J. Chromatogr. Sci. (1984)
In press.

Prelog, V., Stojanac, Z. and Kovacevic, K., Über die
Enantiomerentrennung durch Verteilung zwischen
flüssigen Phasen. Helv. Chim. Acta 65 (1982)
377-384.

Schill, G., Modin, R. and Persson, B.-A, Extraction of
amines as complexes with inorganic anions. Acta
Pharm. Suec. 2 (1965) 119-136.

Schill, G., Ehrsson, H., Vessman, J. and Westerlund, D.,
Separation Methods for Drugs and Related Organic
Compounds, Swedish Pharmaceutical Press, Stockholm,
1984.

Stuurman, H.W. and Wahlund, K.-G., Separation of
proton-donating solutes by liquid chromatography with
a strong proton acceptor, tri-n-octylphosphine oxide,
in the liquid stationary phase. J. Chromatogr. 218
(1981) 455-463.

Wahlund, K.-G. and Edlén, B., Tributyl phosphate as
stationary phase in reversed phase liquid
chromatographic separations of hydrophilic carboxylic
acids, amino acids and dipeptides. J. Liq. Chrom.
4(2) (1981) 309-323.

INDEX